Learning from Disease in Pets

CRC One Health One Welfare

Learning from Disease in Pets: A 'One Health' Model for Discovery
Edited by Rebecca A. Krimins

Forthcoming titles:

Animals, Health and Society: Health Promotion, Harm Reduction and Equity in a One Health World
Edited by Craig Stephen

Bond-Centred Veterinary Practice: Applying One Health One Welfare
Edited by Elizabeth Ormerod and Brinda Jegatheesan

For more information about this series, please visit: https://www.routledge.com/CRC-One-Health-One-Welfare/book-series/CRCOHOW

Learning from Disease in Pets

A 'One Health' Model for Discovery

Edited by
Rebecca A. Krimins

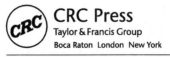

CRC Press
Taylor & Francis Group
Boca Raton London New York

CRC Press is an imprint of the
Taylor & Francis Group, an **informa** business

First edition published 2021
by CRC Press
6000 Broken Sound Parkway NW, Suite 300, Boca Raton, FL 33487-2742

and by CRC Press
2 Park Square, Milton Park, Abingdon, Oxon, OX14 4RN

Library of Congress Cataloging-in-Publication Data
Names: Krimins, Rebecca A., editor.
Title: Learning from disease in pets : a 'one health' model for discovery /
edited by Rebecca A. Krimins.
Description: Boca Raton : Taylor & Francis, 2020. I Series: CRC one health
one welfare I Includes bibliographical references and index. I
Identifiers: LCCN 2020032490 (print) I LCCN 2020032491 (ebook) I ISBN
9780367173166 (hardback) I ISBN 9780367173104 (paperback) I ISBN
9780429056178 (ebook)
Subjects: LCSH: Animals--Diseases.
Classification: LCC SF745 .L48 2020 (print) I LCC SF745 (ebook) I DDC
636.089--dc23
LC record available at https://lccn.loc.gov/2020032490
LC ebook record available at https://lccn.loc.gov/2020032491

ISBN: 978-0-367-17316-6 (hbk)
ISBN: 978-0-367-17310-4 (pbk)
ISBN: 978-0-429-05617-8 (ebk)

Typeset in Times
by Deanta Global Publishing services, Chennai, India

Visit the eResources: www.routledge.com/9780367173166

Contents

Foreword

The inclusion of naturally occurring disease in pet animals is an attractive and increasingly recognized approach to model our understanding of the biology, prevention, and therapy of human disease. Arguably, this comparative and cross-species approach has had the greatest traction in studies of pet dogs with complex medical problems such as cancer, orthopedic, cardiopulmonary, and neuro-inflammatory diseases, and the more recognized study of zoonotic infections. Collectively this traction is based on the existing infrastructure for diagnosis and treatment of pet animals with these spontaneously arising diseases within the veterinary healthcare industry, and the necessary commitment of pet owners who seek out the best care for their pets including their motivation to pursue innovations in care through prospective clinical trials offered from this comparative approach to biomedical medicine. For many reasons the field of Comparative Oncology has been most successful in this win-win, two-species approach to research. Indeed, Comparative Oncology studies have uncovered new understandings of cancer biology, cancer-associated genes, and environmental risk factors common to the dog and the human. A particularly valuable application of Comparative Oncology involves the conduct of clinical trials in pet dogs with naturally occurring cancer to answer human oncology drug or device development questions, which cannot be easily answered in conventional animal cancer models or in human clinical trials. The field has gained support from many groups within the human oncology drug development and cancer research communities. Most notably this includes the launch of the Comparative Oncology Program within the US NIH National Cancer Institute and in both academic and commercial programs around the world. Recent interest in the field included an analysis and meeting on therapeutic translation conducted by the US Institute of Medicine, which included a public comment on the value and perception of the field by the FDA-CDER. It is reasonable that continued adoption of this novel two-species approach will encompass a wide array of disease areas with similar biology between humans and pet animals. In this text, successful examples of this cross-species approach are reviewed in a variety of therapeutic areas, including the notable progress in oncology, alluded to above.

Chand Khanna, DVM, PhD, DACVIM (Onc), DACVP (Hon)
Chief Science Officer, Ethos Veterinary Health
President, Ethos Discovery

Editor

Dr. Rebecca A. Krimins is an Assistant Professor in the Department of Radiology and Radiological Science at Johns Hopkins University, Maryland, with additional appointments in the Department of Anesthesiology and Critical Care Medicine and the Department of Molecular and Comparative Pathobiology. A native of Annapolis, Maryland, Dr. Krimins earned her bachelor's degree in biology from the University of Chicago before entering veterinary school at Ross University School of Veterinary Medicine. After graduating from veterinary school, she completed her veterinary anesthesia and analgesia residency at the Purdue University School of Veterinary Medicine, Indiana. Dr. Krimins has more than 15 years of experience in developing cutting-edge veterinary research trials. As Medical Director of the Veterinary Clinical Trials Network at Johns Hopkins University, Dr. Krimins is able to leverage the expertise and technology available at Johns Hopkins University to transform newly discovered diagnostics and therapeutics into real-life practical approaches that benefit veterinary patients.

Contributors

Karen Gozdan-Aiken
Embark Consulting Group
San Diego, California

Victoria K. Baxter
Department of Pathology &
    Laboratory Medicine
Biocontainment Veterinarian and Head
    of Animal Health Surveillance
Division of Comparative Medicine
University of North Carolina at
    Chapel Hill
Chapel Hill, North Carolina

Philippe Brianceau
Animal Clinical Investigation, LLC
Chevy Chase, Maryland

David Bruyette
Anivive Lifesciences
Long Beach, California

Radford G. Davis
Department of Veterinary Microbiology
    and Preventive Medicine
College of Veterinary Medicine
Iowa State University
Ames, Iowa

Jacob Michael Froehlich
US Food and Drug Administration
Center for Veterinary Medicine
Office of New Animal Drug Evaluation
Rockville, Maryland

Alice Ignaszewski
US Food and Drug Administration
Center for Veterinary Medicine
Office of New Animal Drug Evaluation
Rockville, Maryland

Bryan Jones
Columbus, Ohio

Kristen V. Khanna
Animal Clinical Investigation, LLC
Chevy Chase, Maryland

Timothy Lescun
Large Animal Surgery
and
Preclinical Research Laboratory
College of Veterinary Medicine
Purdue University
West Lafayette, Indiana

Steven M. Niemi
Animal Law & Policy Program
Harvard Law School
Cambridge, Massachusetts

Anna O'Brien
US Food and Drug Administration
Center for Veterinary Medicine,
Office of New Animal Drug Evaluation
Rockville, Maryland

Diane Peters
Department of Pharmacology and
    Molecular Sciences
Johns Hopkins Drug Discovery
Johns Hopkins University School of
    Medicine
Baltimore, Maryland

Alan F. Scott
Genetic Resources Core Facility
McKusick-Nathans Department of
    Genetic Medicine
Johns Hopkins School of Medicine
Baltimore, Maryland

Krista K. Vermillion
Vanderbilt University Medical Center
Nashville, Tennessee

1 The Contribution of Pets to Human and Veterinary Medicine

Rebecca A. Krimins

CONTENTS

INTRODUCTION

Performing veterinary clinical trials is not a novel concept. At veterinary schools, clinical trials benefiting pets have been a focus and a tried-and-true, accepted concept for decades. The American Veterinary Medical Association (AVMA) Animal Health Studies Database provides a platform where veterinarians and pet owners can see if a pet may qualify for a clinical trial; veterinary clinical trials performed in the United States and Canada are listed there (https://ebusiness.av ma.org/aahsd/study_search.aspx). Often these clinical trials enable pets to have access to healthcare not accessible to the main pet population and at little or no cost to the pet owner.

Traditionally, human medical research institutions have used lab animals to translate studies into human therapies. In fact, the US Food and Drug Administration (FDA) *requires* animal testing prior to permitting a drug to be evaluated in a human, with few exceptions (FDA, 2010). The classic model for development of a human therapeutic involves initial chemical/molecular selection or design, *in vitro* testing, and frequently molecular optimization. The FDA preclinical testing for safety for eventual human trials usually requests two animal species to be evaluated (one rodent and one non-rodent). If results at this point still look promising, future steps may be developed for efficacy and safety studies in people. Unfortunately, in practice, this approach has been relatively inefficient

1

and better methods are clearly necessary. For example, an analysis of first-in-man to registration with the FDA or European Medicines Agency from ten large US and European pharmaceutical companies for the period from 1991–2000 demonstrated an ~11% success rate in that roughly nine out of ten compounds developed ultimately failed to gain approval (Kola and Landis 2004). Further, the median capitalized research and development investment to bring a new drug to market (after accounting for the costs of failed trials) was estimated at $985.3 million (Wouters, McKee, and Luyten 2020). A data set published in 2015 analyzed the attrition of drug candidates from four major pharmaceutical companies (AstraZeneca, Eli Lilly and Company, GlaxoSmithKline, and Pfizer) and found a link between the physicochemical properties of compounds and clinical failure due to safety issues (Waring et al. 2015). In 2015, two scientists described the current state of FDA drug approval, where approximately 10,000 compounds were assessed in drug discovery research followed by 250 of these compounds successfully making it to a preclinical research development stage. From those 250 compounds, five compounds would ultimately make it to phase I clinical trials and only one compound would ultimately gain FDA approval (Somerville 2015). A more recent analysis of the probability of success over time in drug development found that there was a decrease in success between 2005 and 2013 and an increase thereafter with an overall success rate in all drug development programs of 13.8% (Wong, Siah, and Lo 2019).

A major reason cited for the inefficiency of drug development is the relatively low power of current rodent models to predict therapeutic efficacy in humans. A review of the scientific literature demonstrates numerous examples in which successful murine studies did not predict success in humans (Bracken 2009, Mak, Evaniew, and Ghert 2014, Masopust, Sivula, and Jameson 2017, Akhtar 2015, Kokolus et al. 2013). For example, in 2017, Bentley and colleagues wrote that although rodent orthotopic xenograft models provide a good basic model for understanding tumor biology, their value in successfully translating preclinical oncology therapeutic triumph into clinical success is "extremely poor" (Bentley et al. 2017). Animal modeling from its origins has always maintained as a goal the tenet to mirror human disease as closely as possible. In accordance with this, a 2019 review focused on optimizing preclinical models for human personalized medicine benefits stated that models that recapitulate as much of the human pathophysiology as possible will be the most predictive of success in man (Tadenev and Burgess 2019).

Development of new therapeutics for veterinary patients faces these and further challenges. Historically, veterinary therapeutics (medical and surgical) have consisted of a subset of those developed and approved for humans (Moulin et al. 2008, Hespel and Cole 2018, Olmstead 1995, Martin 2003, Corradini et al. 2016, DeForge 2019). For pets to gain access to these treatments, one more step is critical, where a successful human therapy is then evaluated and translated for use in veterinary patients (Figure 1.1). Thus, traditionally, pets are the last to benefit from a successful therapy. In the United States, about 60% of the animal health sales are companion animal products and about 40% are food-producing animal

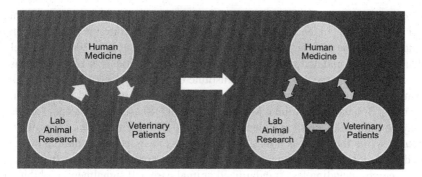

FIGURE 1.1   The traditional method of developing therapies for humans (left half of figure) consists of a unidirectional flow of steps where pets are the last species to receive newly developed treatments. The premise of this book is to demonstrate that in certain disease states, pets with spontaneously occurring disease can be utilized to develop successful diagnostics and treatments (right half of figure). In turn, this will lower the time and costs needed to get successful treatments into humans and pets.

products (AVMA, 2018). As pet owners increase the amount spent per year on maintaining a healthy pet, so has the number of animal health products increased designed specifically for individual species.

The focus of this book is not to change the classic model for how biomedical research is conducted but to demonstrate that an additional, complementary method in certain disease states and for certain problems may be beneficial as well as offer significant value (and in a number of cases as described later in this chapter, has already proven to be beneficial) for both humans and pets. Rather than exclusively evaluating classic lab animal models, pets with spontaneous disease may be a better model for developing therapies that will work in pets and people. In 2015, Kol and colleagues published a list of human diseases and their parallels in companion animals including many cancers, osteoarthritis, cruciate ligament injury, mandibular fracture and reconstruction, intervertebral disk herniation, hemophilia, narcolepsy, cleft palate, lysosomal storage diseases, keratoconjunctivitis sicca, inflammatory bowel disease, dilated cardiomyopathy, hypertrophic cardiomyopathy, and more (Kol et al. 2015). Such models based on animals with spontaneous disease have the potential to be more successful, for example, to find better therapeutics, find undiscovered therapeutics, and build improved diagnostic equipment in a shorter time frame and for less money. In this book, we will demonstrate how pets can be used, in many diseases, to facilitate successful translational research in human and veterinary medicine, in a manner that benefits man and pets, culminating in lower costs to develop treatments and more efficient time frames to get a drug or device from benchtop research to patient bedside. There are numerous examples of the use of a model of naturally occurring disease in an animal to help develop diagnostics and treatments in people. These examples are too abundant to review comprehensively here, but one early example is that of physiologist Augustus Desiré Waller, who recorded the first human electrocardiogram in the late 1800s. Waller used his pet dog "Jimmy" to learn how to use electrodes and measure the recording; this study helped launch the field of electrocardiography (Luderitz 2003). A widely distributed and updated volume of fascicles of Animal Models of Human Disease was published by the Armed Forces Institute of Pathology in 1979. By 1980, the American College of Laboratory Animal Medicine had published a two-volume series on Spontaneous Animal Models of Human Disease. More recent examples may be more relevant to our thesis, and several of these examples are provided below. While the discussion that follows pertains to spontaneous animal models of disease, it is imperative to note that there are numerous limitations to using pets in research, including less standardized animal care and signalment, prohibition of scheduled euthanasia and post-mortem tissue collection, withholding standards of care in negative control groups, and more. Additional information on these limitations is covered in Chapter 7, The Use of Animals in Research. Of note is that although many of the examples provided below are in the field of oncology, this is because the oncologic field is a major source of disease both in veterinary and human medicine. As stated by Cekanova and Rathore in 2014, "The development of *in vivo* animal models that recapitulate the natural history of human cancers and their clinical response to therapy constitute a major prerequisite for rapid bench-to-bedside translation of investigational anticancer therapies and imaging agents that have shown promise in *in vitro* models" (Cekanova and Rathore 2014). Researchers at the University of Vienna, Austria, recently summed up these same concepts stating it would be favorable, especially in academia, if more clinical animal studies would be voluntarily carried out in animal patients with naturally developed disease. This would not only benefit lab animals as well as animal patients, but it is also of translational significance to encourage simultaneous and thus potentially faster development of new drugs (Furdos et al. 2015). And even more recently, Steven Dow of Colorado State University published a paper on cancer types and settings in which the dog model is most likely to impact clinical immuno-oncology research and drug development (Dow 2020). In addition, it is clear that areas of disease besides studies in cancer likewise have benefited from translational research in pets and will continue to do so. Consider the following examples provided below.

CANCER DRUGS

- Toceranib (SU11654) is a receptor tyrosine kinase (RTK) inhibitor that is used to treat canine mast cell tumors. Toceranib phosphate was approved by the FDA for animal use in 2009, under the tradename Palladia™ (Zoetis, Parsippany, NJ). Sunitinib (SU11248) is a receptor tyrosine kinase inhibitor closely related to SU11654 that is used to treat renal cell carcinoma in people as well as specific types of gastrointestinal cancer. Sunitinib was approved by the FDA in 2006 as Sutent®. These two molecules are structural cousins. Pharmaceutical company Sugen conducted the original research on both of these molecules and became interested in targeting KIT receptor tyrosine kinases found in certain human cancers (gastrointestinal stromal tumors, small lung cancers, acute myeloid leukemia) during the late 1990s. At that time, the company became aware of the role of KIT mutations in canine mast cell tumors (a common cancer type found in dogs). A small clinical trial was performed in canine patients with mast cell tumors and results were promising, thereby providing useful proof of concept data to encourage translational research in humans. Furthermore, SU11654 demonstrated pharmacokinetic (PK) properties comparable to SU11248 in dogs. In fact, Sutent does not have a high therapeutic index and the PK properties seen in dogs are much better approximations of human PK properties than that seen in murine models. The fact that some of the same mutations identified in human gastrointestinal stroma tumors were present in canine mast cell tumors made this research especially informative.

London and colleagues concluded in 2003 that orally administered kinase inhibitors exhibit activity against a variety of spontaneous malignancies found in dogs and, based on the similarities between canine and human tumor biology and the presence of analogous RTK dysregulation, that it would be likely that such agents would demonstrate comparable antineoplastic activity in people (London et al. 2003). In 2009, Khanna and Gordon published a commentary on the evaluation of these small molecule tyrosine kinase inhibitors, including parallel opportunities that were discovered and translated between canine and human health (Khanna and Gordon 2009).

Verdinexor and selinexor are examples of compounds where data from canine clinical trials informed the development of similar human therapy (News 2014). In 2018, a research team found the orally bioavailable nuclear export protein Exportin 1 inhibitor, Verdinexor, to be safe and effective in a relevant, spontaneous canine model of cancer. This inhibition prevents the export of tumor suppressor proteins and leads to their accumulation in the nucleus, which reinitiates and amplifies their natural apoptotic function. Nuclear localized tumor suppressor proteins detect cancer-associated DNA damage, leading to the selective apoptosis of cancer cells; normal cells, which do not have significant DNA damage, are spared (Sadowski et al. 2018). The US Food and Drug Administration's Center for Veterinary Medicine has found the effectiveness and safety technical sections for Verdinexor complete to support conditional approval under a New Animal Drug Application (NADA) for the treatment of canine lymphoma. The use of Verdinexor to treat canine lymphoma has been designated a "minor use" in accordance with the Minor Use Minor Species (MUMS) Act. This makes the product eligible for conditional approval similar to orphan drug/accelerated approvals used for submissions of human therapeutics. The utilization of this animal model helped lay the groundwork for evaluation of these same selective inhibitor of nuclear export (SINE) compounds in human cancer (London et al. 2014).

Selinexor (Xpovio®) was approved in July 2019 for use in combination with Dexamethasone for the treatment of adult patients with relapsed or refractory multiple myeloma who have received at least four prior therapies and whose disease is refractory to at least two proteasome inhibitors, at least two immunomodulatory agents, and an anti-CD38 monoclonal antibody.

- Acalabrutinib is a Bruton's tyrosine kinase inhibitor approved by the FDA in 2017 to treat mantle cell lymphoma and in 2019 received supplemental approval for the treatment of chronic lymphocytic leukemia and small lymphocytic leukemia in human patients. Studies performed in dogs with naturally occurring cancer supported research which aided the approval of this drug for human disease. Clinical benefit was observed in 30% (6/20) of dogs. These findings suggested that Acalabrutinib exhibited activity in canine B-cell lymphoma patients, was efficacious and supported the use of canine lymphoma as a relevant model for human non-Hodgkin lymphoma (NHL) (Harrington et al. 2016). Acalabrutinib was developed by Acerta Pharma which was acquired by AstraZeneca in 2016.

CANCER IMMUNOTHERAPY

- Xenogeneic electro-vaccination against CSPG4 has been shown to overcome host unresponsiveness to the "self" antigen and seems to be effective in treating canine melanoma, laying the foundation for its translation to a human clinical setting (Riccardo et al. 2014). Continued work by these same researchers has recently shown identification of CSPG4 as a promising target for translational combinatorial approaches in osteosarcoma (Riccardo et al. 2019). Naturally occurring melanoma in dogs has continued to be studied as a complementary model for human melanoma treatment (Barutello et al. 2018, Piras et al. 2017).
- Research at the University of California, Davis, demonstrated that blocking indolamine-2,3 dioxygenase rebound immune suppression would boost antitumor effects of radio-immunotherapy in both murine models and in dogs with naturally occurring tumors (Monjazeb et al. 2016). Continued research is currently underway further assessing indoleamine dioxygenase inhibitors and their role in cancer treatment (Zhu, Dancsok, and Nielsen 2019).

OTHER ONCOLOGICAL MODALITIES

- Lumicell, Inc. (Newton, MA) is developing a hand-held imaging system that allows human surgeons to assess tumor margins in real time. Studies performed in dogs with soft tissue sarcomas have provided data helpful in getting regulatory approval for initiating phase I and II clinical trials for people (Eward et al. 2013, Bartholf DeWitt et al. 2016, Smith et al. 2018).

- In 2016, researchers at the University of Colorado School of Medicine and Colorado State University College of Veterinary Medicine collaborated on a canine study using photodynamic therapy to treat lung cancer via bronchoscopy (Musani et al. 2018). Like many of the aforementioned studies, dogs with spontaneous disease were used as proof-of-concept in order to aid with translating this work to human patients. Research studies are ongoing in both pets and people as this form of therapy is developed (Chen and Lee 2018).
- Currently, radioactive holmium-166 microspheres injected intratumorally are being evaluated for the treatment of squamous cell carcinoma in both afflicted cats and people (Bakker et al. 2018, van Nimwegen et al. 2018). Quirem Medical BV (Deventer, Netherlands) is developing and commercializing radioactive microspheres based on holmium-166 for selective internal radiation therapy in both human and veterinary medical applications.

INFLAMMATORY BOWEL DISEASE

- Inflammatory bowel disease (IBD) has long been studied in dogs to assess similarities with human disease (Jergens et al. 2009). Recent work compared protein-losing enteropathies in dogs and people to confirm (or investigate) theories for treatment in both species (Craven and Washabau 2019). Bacteria of the genus *Campylobacter* have long been recognized to cause acute diarrhea in humans (Skirrow 1977), and also found in dogs and cats (Skirrow 1977, Blaser et al. 1980). Schneider and colleagues sum up this work in stating that so-called "reverse translational pharmacology", such as that seen with IBD, is an expanding field of research with the promise to improve existing complementary models to characterize the efficacy and safety of candidate drugs and, ultimately, select the most promising therapeutics intended for use in humans. In return, from the perspective of developing veterinary pharmaceuticals for spontaneous diseases in animals, reverse translational pharmacology presents an opportunity to leverage information from pharmacokinetic and pharmacodynamic studies in humans for the benefit of veterinary medicine (Schneider et al. 2018).

OPHTHALMOLOGY

- Eight years prior to the first human approval for topical Cyclosporine A to treat dry eye disease in 2003 (RESTASIS® 0.05%; Allergan pfc, Dublin, Ireland), Intervet Inc. (now part of Merck Animal Health) received FDA approval for OPTIMMUNE® (0.2%) to treat chronic keratoconjunctivitis sicca and chronic keratitis in dogs. Allergan licensed the technology from the University of Georgia and relied on the large amount of data that had been generated in pet dogs to move their product into the market. In 2019, Allergan forecast sales from RESTASIS® to approach $1.2 billion.

CONCLUSION

These are just a few of the latest trends in medicine, in the push to find improved models for developing modernized diagnostics and treatments for both humans and pets. The chapters and discussions that follow in this book are meant to educate and aid researchers in order to demonstrate the detailed facets pertaining to veterinary clinical research. Conventional training and credentialing, advanced skill level, and expert environments are required to perform this work. In summary, this text will help illustrate not only the importance of using spontaneous disease for medical progress but also provide guidance on how to perform clinical trials on veterinary patients. This field is an emerging one and is predicted to grow and mature in the coming decades.

REFERENCES

AVMA. 2018. *AVMA Pet Ownership and Demographics Sourcebook*. AVMA: Schaumburg, IL.

Akhtar, A. 2015. "The flaws and human harms of animal experimentation." *Camb Q Health Eth* 24(4):407–419. doi: 10.1017/S0963180115000079.

Bakker, R. C., R. J. J. van Es, A. J. W. P. Rosenberg, S. A. van Nimwegen, R. Bastiaannet, H. W. A. M. de Jong, J. F. W. Nijsen, and M. G. E. H. Lam. 2018. "Intratumoral injection of radioactive holmium-166 microspheres in recurrent head and neck squamous cell carcinoma: Preliminary results of first use." *Nucl Med Commun* 39(3):213–221. doi: 10.1097/Mnm.0000000000000792.

Bartholf DeWitt, S., W. C. Eward, C. A. Eward, A. L. Lazarides, M. J. Whitley, J. M. Ferrer, B. E. Brigman, D. G. Kirsch, and J. Berg. 2016. "A novel imaging system distinguishes neoplastic from normal tissue during resection of soft tissue sarcomas and mast cell tumors in dogs." *Vet Surg* 45(6):715–722. doi: 10.1111/vsu.12487.

Barutello, G., V. Rolih, M. Arigoni, L. Tarone, L. Conti, E. Quaglino, P. Buracco, F. Cavallo, and F. Riccardo. 2018. "Strengths and weaknesses of pre-clinical models for human melanoma treatment: Dawn of dogs' revolution for immunotherapy." *Int J Mol Sci* 19(3). doi: 10.3390/ijms19030799.

Bentley, R. T., A. U. Ahmed, A. B. Yanke, A. A. Cohen-Gadol, and M. Dey. 2017. "Dogs are man's best friend: In sickness and in health." *Neuro Oncol* 19(3):312–322. doi: 10.1093/neuonc/now109.

Blaser, M. J., F. M. LaForce, N. A. Wilson, and W. L. Wang. 1980. "Reservoirs for human campylobacteriosis." *J Infect Dis* 141(5):665–669. doi: 10.1093/infdis/141.5.665.

Bracken, M. B. 2009. "Why animal studies are often poor predictors of human reactions to exposure." *J R Soc Med* 102(3):120–122. doi: 10.1258/jrsm.2008.08k033.

Cekanova, M., and K. Rathore. 2014. "Animal models and therapeutic molecular targets of cancer: Utility and limitations." *Drug Des Devel Ther* 8:1911–1921. doi: 10.2147/DDDT.S49584.

Chen, K. C., and J. M. Lee. 2018. "Photodynamic therapeutic ablation for peripheral pulmonary malignancy via electromagnetic navigation bronchoscopy localization in a hybrid operating room (OR): A pioneering study." *J Thorac Dis* 10(Suppl 6):S725–S730. doi: 10.21037/jtd.2018.03.139.

Corradini, S., B. Pilosio, F. Dondi, G. Linari, S. Testa, F. Brugnoli, P. Gianella, M. Pietra, and F. Fracassi. 2016. "Accuracy of a flash glucose monitoring system in diabetic dogs." *J Vet Intern Med* 30(4):983–988. doi: 10.1111/jvim.14355.

Craven, M. D., and R. J. Washabau. 2019. "Comparative pathophysiology and management of protein-losing enteropathy." *J Vet Intern Med* 33(2):383–402. doi: 10.1111/jvim.15406.

DeForge, W. F. 2019. "Cardiac pacemakers: A basic review of the history and current technology." *J Vet Cardiol* 22:40–50. doi: 10.1016/j.jvc.2019.01.001.

Dow, S. 2020. "A role for dogs in advancing cancer immunotherapy research." *Front Immunol* 10. doi: 10.3389/fimmu.2019.02935.

Eward, W. C., J. K. Mito, C. A. Eward, J. E. Carter, J. M. Ferrer, D. G. Kirsch, and B. E. Brigman. 2013. "A novel imaging system permits real-time *in vivo* tumor bed assessment after resection of naturally occurring sarcomas in dogs." *Clin Orthop Relat Res* 471(3):834–842. doi: 10.1007/s11999-012-2560-8.

FDA. 2010. "Guidance for industry M3(R2) Nonclinical Safety Studies for the Conduct of Human Clinical Trials and Marketing Authorization for Pharmaceuticals." accessed May 6, 2020 www.fda.gov/media/71542/download.

Furdos, I., J. Fazekas, J. Singer, and E. Jensen-Jarolim. 2015. "Translating clinical trials from human to veterinary oncology and back." *J Transl Med* 13:265. doi: 10.1186/s12967-015-0631-9.

Harrington, B. K., H. L. Gardner, R. Izumi, A. Hamdy, W. Rothbaum, K. R. Coombes, T. Covey, A. Kaptein, M. Gulrajani, B. Van Lith, C. Krejsa, C. C. Coss, D. S. Russell, X. Zhang, B. K. Urie, C. A. London, J. C. Byrd, A. J. Johnson, and W. C. Kisseberth. 2016. "Preclinical evaluation of the novel BTK inhibitor Acalabrutinib in canine models of B-cell non-Hodgkin lymphoma." *PLoS One* 11(7):e0159607. doi: 10.1371/journal.pone.0159607.

Hespel, A. M., and R. C. Cole. 2018. "Advances in high-field MRI." *Vet Clin North Am Small Anim Pract* 48(1):11–29. doi: 10.1016/j.cvsm.2017.08.002.

Jergens, A. E., I. M. Sonea, A. M. O'Connor, L. K. Kauffman, S. D. Grozdanic, M. R. Ackermann, and R. B. Evans. 2009. "Intestinal cytokine mRNA expression in canine inflammatory bowel disease: A meta-analysis with critical appraisal." *Comp Med* 59(2):153–162.

Khanna, C., and I. Gordon. 2009. "Catching cancer by the tail: New perspectives on the use of kinase inhibitors." *Clin Cancer Res* 15(11):3645–3647. doi: 10.1158/1078-0432.Ccr-09-0132.

Kokolus, K. M., M. L. Capitano, C. T. Lee, J. W. Eng, J. D. Waight, B. L. Hylander, S. Sexton, C. C. Hong, C. J. Gordon, S. I. Abrams, and E. A. Repasky. 2013. "Baseline tumor growth and immune control in laboratory mice are significantly influenced by subthermoneutral housing temperature." *Proc Natl Acad Sci U S A* 110(50):20176–20181. doi: 10.1073/pnas.1304291110.

Kol, A., B. Arzi, K. A. Athanasiou, D. L. Farmer, J. A. Nolta, R. B. Rebhun, X. Chen, L. G. Griffiths, F. J. Verstraete, C. J. Murphy, and D. L. Borjesson. 2015. "Companion animals: Translational scientist's new best friends." *Sci Transl Med* 7(308):308ps21. doi: 10.1126/scitranslmed.aaa9116.

Kola, I., and J. Landis. 2004. "Can the pharmaceutical industry reduce attrition rates?." *Nat Rev Drug Discov* 3(8):711–715. doi: 10.1038/nrd1470.

London, C. A., L. F. Bernabe, S. Barnard, W. C. Kisseberth, A. Borgatti, M. Henson, H. Wilson, K. Jensen, D. Ito, J. F. Modiano, M. D. Bear, M. L. Pennell, J. R. Saint-Martin, D. McCauley, M. Kauffman, and S. Shacham. 2014. "Preclinical evaluation of the novel, orally bioavailable Selective Inhibitor of Nuclear Export (SINE) KPT-335 in spontaneous canine cancer: Results of a phase I study." *PLoS One* 9(2):e87585. doi: 10.1371/journal.pone.0087585.

London, C. A., A. L. Hannah, R. Zadovoskaya, M. B. Chien, C. Kollias-Baker, M. Rosenberg, S. Downing, G. Post, J. Boucher, N. Shenoy, D. B. Mendel, G. McMahon, and J. M. Cherrington. 2003. "Phase I dose-escalating study of SU11654, a small molecule receptor tyrosine kinase inhibitor, in dogs with spontaneous malignancies." *Clin Cancer Res* 9(7):2755–2768.

Luderitz, B. 2003. "Augustus Desire Waller (1856–1922) – The first to record the electrical activity of the human heart." *J Interv Card Electrophysiol* 9(1):59–60. doi: 10.1023/a:1025328722646.

Mak, I. W., N. Evaniew, and M. Ghert. 2014. "Lost in translation: Animal models and clinical trials in cancer treatment." *Am J Transl Res* 6(2):114–118.

Martin, M. W. 2003. "Treatment of congestive heart failure a neuroendocrine disorder." *J Small Anim Pract* 44(4):154–160. doi: 10.1111/j.1748-5827.2003.tb00137.x.

Masopust, D., C. P. Sivula, and S. C. Jameson. 2017. "Of mice, dirty mice, and men: Using mice to understand human immunology." *J Immunol* 199(2):383–388. doi: 10.4049/jimmunol.1700453.

Monjazeb, A. M., M. S. Kent, S. K. Grossenbacher, C. Mall, A. E. Zamora, A. Mirsoian, M. Chen, A. Kol, S. L. Shiao, A. Reddy, J. R. Perks, W. T. N. Culp, E. E. Sparger, R. J. Canter, G. D. Sckisel, and W. J. Murphy. 2016. "Blocking Indolamine-2,3-Dioxygenase rebound immune suppression boosts antitumor effects of radio-immunotherapy in murine models and spontaneous canine malignancies." *Clin Cancer Res* 22(17):4328–4340. doi: 10.1158/1078-0432.CCR-15-3026.

Moulin, G., P. Cavalie, I. Pellanne, A. Chevance, A. Laval, Y. Millemann, P. Colin, C. Chauvin, and Agency Antimicrobial Resistance ad hoc Group of the French Food Safety. 2008. "A comparison of antimicrobial usage in human and veterinary medicine in France from 1999 to 2005." *J Antimicrob Chemother* 62(3):617–625. doi: 10.1093/jac/dkn213.

Musani, A. I., J. K. Veir, Z. Huang, T. Lei, S. Groshong, and D. Worley. 2018. "Photodynamic therapy via navigational bronchoscopy for peripheral lung cancer in dogs." *Lasers Surg Med* 50(5):483–490. doi: 10.1002/lsm.22781.

News Science. 2014. "New cancer drug for dogs benefits human research, drug development." *Science Daily.* www.sciencedaily.com/releases/2014/09/140909092119.htm.

Olmstead, M. L. 1995. "The canine cemented modular total hip prosthesis." *J Am Anim Hosp Assoc* 31(2):109–124. doi: 10.5326/15473317-31-2-109.

Piras, L. A., F. Riccardo, S. Iussich, L. Maniscalco, F. Gattino, M. Martano, E. Morello, S. Lorda Mayayo, V. Rolih, F. Garavaglia, R. De Maria, E. Lardone, F. Collivignarelli, D. Mignacca, D. Giacobino, S. Ferrone, F. Cavallo, and P. Buracco. 2017. "Prolongation of survival of dogs with oral malignant melanoma treated by en bloc surgical resection and adjuvant CSPG4-antigen electrovaccination." *Vet Comp Oncol* 15(3):996–1013. doi: 10.1111/vco.12239.

Riccardo, F., S. Iussich, L. Maniscalco, S. Lorda Mayayo, G. La Rosa, M. Arigoni, R. De Maria, F. Gattino, S. Lanzardo, E. Lardone, M. Martano, E. Morello, S. Prestigio, A. Fiore, E. Quaglino, S. Zabarino, S. Ferrone, P. Buracco, and F. Cavallo. 2014. "CSPG-specific immunity and survival prolongation in dogs with oral malignant melanoma immunized with human CSPG4 DNA." *Clin Cancer Res* 20(14):3753–3762. doi: 10.1158/1078-0432.CCR-13-3042.

Riccardo, F., L. Tarone, S. Iussich, D. Giacobino, M. Arigoni, F. Sammartano, E. Morello, M. Martano, F. Gattino, R. De Maria, S. Ferrone, P. Buracco, and F. Cavallo. 2019. "Identification of CSPG4 as a promising target for translational combinatorial approaches in osteosarcoma." *Ther Adv Med Oncol* 11. doi: Unsp 1758835919855491 10.1177/1758835919855491.

Sadowski, A. R., H. L. Gardner, A. Borgatti, H. Wilson, D. M. Vail, J. Lachowicz, C. Manley, A. Turner, M. K. Klein, A. Waite, A. Sahora, and C. A. London. 2018. "Phase II study of the oral selective inhibitor of nuclear export (SINE) KPT-335 (verdinexor) in dogs with lymphoma." *BMC Vet Res* 14(1):250. doi: 10.1186/s12917-018-1587-9.

Schneider, B., V. Balbas-Martinez, A. E. Jergens, I. F. Troconiz, K. Allenspach, and J. P. Mochel. 2018. "Model-based reverse translation Between veterinary and human medicine: The one health initiative." *Cpt Pharmacometr Syst Pharmacol* 7(2):65–68. doi: 10.1002/psp4.12262.

Skirrow, M. B. 1977. "Campylobacter enteritis: a 'new' disease." *Br Med J* 2(6078):9–11. doi: 10.1136/bmj.2.6078.9.

Smith, B. L., M. A. Gadd, C. R. Lanahan, U. Rai, R. Tang, T. Rice-Stitt, A. L. Merrill, D. B. Strasfeld, J. M. Ferrer, E. F. Brachtel, and M. C. Specht. 2018. "Real-time, intraoperative detection of residual breast cancer in lumpectomy cavity walls using a novel cathepsin-activated fluorescent imaging system." *Breast Cancer Res Treat* 171(2):413–420. doi: 10.1007/s10549-018-4845-4.

Somerville, S., and J. H. Kloda 2015. "FDA's expedited review process: The need for speed." [Online Medical Article]. accessed Mar 11, 2015. www.appliedclinicaltrials online.com/fda-s-expedited-review-process-need-speed.

Tadenev, A. L. D., and R. W. Burgess. 2019. "Model validity for preclinical studies in precision medicine: Precisely how precise do we need to be?" *Mamm Genome* 30(5–6):111–122. doi: 10.1007/s00335-019-09798-0.

van Nimwegen, S. A., R. C. Bakker, J. Kirpensteijn, R. J. J. van Es, R. Koole, Mgeh Lam, J. W. Hesselink, and J. F. W. Nijsen. 2018. "Intratumoral injection of radioactive holmium ((166) Ho) microspheres for treatment of oral squamous cell carcinoma in cats." *Vet Comp Oncol* 16(1):114–124. doi: 10.1111/vco.12319.

Waring, M. J., J. Arrowsmith, A. R. Leach, P. D. Leeson, S. Mandrell, R. M. Owen, G. Pairaudeau, W. D. Pennie, S. D. Pickett, J. B. Wang, O. Wallace, and A. Weir. 2015. "An analysis of the attrition of drug candidates from four major pharmaceutical companies." *Nat Rev Drug Discov* 14(7):475–486. doi: 10.1038/nrd4609.

Wong, C. H., K. W. Siah, and A. W. Lo. 2019. "Estimation of clinical trial success rates and related parameters (vol 20, pg 273, 2019)." *Biostatistics* 20(2):366–366. doi: 10.1093/biostatistics/kxy072.

Wouters, O. J., M. McKee, and J. Luyten. 2020. "Estimated Research and Development investment needed to bring a new medicine to market, 2009–2018." *JAMA* 323(9):844–853. doi: 10.1001/jama.2020.1166.

Zhu, M. M. T., A. R. Dancsok, and T. O. Nielsen. 2019. "Indoleamine dioxygenase inhibitors: Clinical rationale and current development." *Curr Oncol Rep* 21(1):2. doi: 10.1007/s11912-019-0750-1.

2 Companion Animals Models of Human Disease

David Bruyette

CONTENTS

INTRODUCTION

The development of *in vivo* animal models that reproduce the natural history of human diseases and their clinical response to therapy constitute a major technique for rapid bench-to-bedside translation of investigational therapies that have shown promise in *in vitro* models [1-10]. This review summarizes spontaneously occurring companion animal disease models of clinical importance to man and pets. Spontaneous disease in companion dogs and cats offers a unique model for human disease biology and translational therapeutics. Companion animals have a relatively high incidence of diseases such as cancers, with biological behavior, response to therapy, and response to cytotoxic agents similar to those occurring in humans. A shorter overall life span and more rapid disease progression are further factors contributing to the advantages of a companion animal model. Following is a discussion with a comparison by organ system of common diseases seen in both man and pets (Table 2.1), as well as leading causes of morbidity and mortality, followed by discussions on nutrition and aging.

A COMPARISON BY ORGAN SYSTEM OF DISEASES SEEN IN BOTH MAN AND PETS

Endocrine Disease/Obesity

Diabetes Mellitus

Much like the historical classification systems used in human diabetics, diabetes in companion animals has been described using phenotypic characteristics, such

TABLE 2.1
Spontaneous Companion Animal Models of Human Disease

Disease or System	Companion Species	Reference #
Endocrine		
Diabetes	Dog, Cat	(140, 141)
Hyperthyroidism	Cat	(142)
Hypothyroidism	Dog	(143)
Cushing's Disease	Dog	(144–150)
Addison's Disease	Dog	(151, 152)
Acromegaly	Cat	(153, 154)
Hyperaldosteronism	Cat	(155–157)
Obesity	Dog, Cat	(158, 159)
Cardiopulmonary		
Heart Failure	Dog	(160)
Dilated Cardiomyopathy	Dog	(161, 162)
Hypertrophic Cardiomyopathy	Cat	(163–166)
Arrhythmogenic	Dog	(167)
Valvular Disease	Dog	(168)
Asthma	Cat	(169)
Pulmonary Fibrosis	Dog	(170, 171)
Patent Ductus Arteriosus	Dog, Cat	(172)
Pulmonic Stenosis	Dog, Cat	(172)
Aortic Stenosis	Dog, Cat	(172)
Ventricular Septal Defect	Dog, Cat	(173, 174)
Atrioventricular Block	Dog	(175, 176)
Endocardiosis, Myocarditis	Dog, Cat	(177, 178)
Tetralogy of Fallot	Dog, Cat	(179)
Portocaval Shunt	Dog	(180)
Sinus Arrhythmia	Dog	(181)
Atrial Fibrillation	Dog	(182)
Wolff-Parkinson-White Syndrome	Dog, Cat	(183, 184)
Sick Sinus Syndrome	Dog	(185)
Renal		
Chronic Renal Disease	Dog, Cat	(186–188)
Glomerulonephritis	Dog, Cat	(189, 190)
Polycystic Renal Disease	Dog, Cat	(191)
Renal Agenesis	Dog, Cat	(192, 193)
Renal Transplant	Dog, Cat	(194, 195)
Renal Amyloidosis	Dog, Cat	(196, 197)
Immunology		
Immunosenescence	Dog	(198, 199)
Allergy, Atopy	Dog, Cat	(200, 201)
Neonatal Isoerythrolysis	Dog, Cat	(202)
Autoimmune Hemolytic Anemia	Dog, Cat	(203)

(Continued)

TABLE 2.1 (CONTINUED)
Spontaneous Companion Animal Models of Human Disease

Disease or System	Companion Species	Reference #
Rheumatoid Arthritis	Dog, Cat	(204, 205)
Anaphylaxis	Dog, Cat	(206)
Thyroiditis	Dog	(207)
Systemic Lupus Erythematosus	Dog, Cat	(208, 209)
Gammopathies	Dog, Cat	(210, 211)
Oncology		
Mast Cell	Dog	(212)
Mammary	Dog, Cat	(213–215)
Melanoma	Dog	(216)
Lymphoma	Dog, Cat	(217, 218)
Osteosarcoma	Dog	(219, 220)
Brain Tumors	Dog, Cat	(221–223)
Gastric and Intestinal Cancer	Dog, Cat	(224)
Leukemia	Dog, Cat	(225)
Hypercalcemia of Malignancy	Dog	(226)
Hepatobiliary/GI/Pancreas		
Copper Storage	Dog	(227–231)
Inflammatory Bowel Disease	Dog, Cat	(232, 233)
Ulcerative Colitis	Dog	(234)
Exocrine Pancreatic Insufficiency	Dog	(235)
Hepatitis	Dog, Cat	(236, 237)
Hepatic Encephalopathy	Dog, Cat	(238)
Megacolon	Cat	(239)
Pancreatitis	Dog, Cat	(240)
Gastroduodenal Ulceration	Dog, Cat	(241, 242)
Megaesophagus	Dog, Cat	(243)
Hepatolenticular Degeneration (Wilson's Disease)	Dog	(244)
Hypertrophic Gastritis (Menetrier's Disease)	Dog	(245)
Granulomatous Enteritis	Dog	(246)
Ophthalmic		
KCS	Dog	(247–249)
Cataract	Dog	(250, 251)
Entropion, Ectropion, Distichiasis	Dog, Cat	(252, 253)
Glaucoma	Dog, Cat	(254, 255)
Retinal Degeneration	Dog, Cat	(256)
Hypertensive Retinopathy	Dog, Cat	(257, 258)
Microphthalmia	Dog, Cat	(259)
Corneal Edema	Dog, Cat	(260)
Persistent Pupillary Membrane	Dog	(261)
Heterochromia Iridis	Dog	(262)
Progressive Retinal Atrophy	Dog	(263)

(Continued)

TABLE 2.1 (CONTINUED)

Spontaneous Companion Animal Models of Human Disease

Disease or System	Companion Species	Reference #
Diabetic Retinopathy	Dog	(264)
Neurologic		
Trauma	Dog	(265, 266)
Spinal Cord	Dog	(267–269)
Alzheimer's-Like Disease	Dog, Cat	(270–273)
Leukoencephalopathy	Dog	(274)
Seizure Disorders	Dog, Cat	(275–278)
Muscular Dystrophies	Dog	(279–282)
Syringomyelia	Dog	(283)
Cerebellar Hypoplasia	Dog, Cat	(284)
Hydrocephalus	Dog	(285)
Chiari Malformation	Dog	(283, 286)
Tremor	Dog	(287)
Brain Atrophy	Dog	(288)
Brachial Plexus Neuropathy	Dog, Cat	(289, 290)
Polyradiculoneuropathy	Dog	(291)
Narcolepsy	Dog, Cat	(292, 293)
Lissencephaly	Dog	(294)
Gangliosidosis	Dog, Cat	(295, 296)
Sphingomyelin Lipidosis	Cat	(297)
Cerebellar Degeneration	Dog, Cat	(298)
Cerebral Ischemia and Infarction (Stroke)	Dog	(299)
Insurance Databases	Dog, Cat	(300–304)
Nutrition		
Diet/Caloric Restriction	Dog	(305–310)
Aging		
Mechanistic	Dog	(311–314)
Reproductive Tract		
Uterine Cancer	Dog	(315)
Pyometra	Dog, Cat	(316)
Ovarian Cancer	Dog, Cat	(317, 318)
Dystocia	Dog, Cat	(319)
Mammary Cancer	Dog, Cat	(320, 321)
Prostate Cancer	Dog	(322)
Testicular Cancer	Dog	(323)
Cryptorchidism	Dog, Cat	(324, 325)
Benign Prostatic Hypertrophy	Dog	(326)
Spontaneous Abortion	Dog, Cat	(327)
Eclampsia, Preeclampsia	Dog, Cat	(328)
Klinefelter's Syndrome and Chimerism	Cat	(329)
Adenomyosis	Dog, Cat	(330, 331)

(Continued)

TABLE 2.1 (CONTINUED)

Spontaneous Companion Animal Models of Human Disease

Disease or System	Companion Species	Reference #
Hematology		
Hereditary spherocytosis	Dog	(332)
Anemia	Dog, Cat	(333–336)
Polycythemia	Dog, Cat	(337)
Hemophilia	Dog, Cat	(338)
Von Willebrand Disease	Dog	(339)
Factor Deficiency	Dog, Cat	(340)
Platelet Function Disorder	Dog, Cat	(341)
Hyperlipidemia	Dog, Cat	(342, 343)
Congenital Porphyria	Cat	(344)
Neutropenic Disorders	Dog, Cat	(345, 346)
Sepsis	Dog, Cat	(347, 348)
Endotoxin	Dog, Cat	(349, 350)
Parasite		
Coccidiosis	Dog	(351)
Ectoparasites	Dog, Cat	(352)
Endoparasites	Dog, Cat	(353)
Histoplasmosis	Dog, Cat	(354)
Leptospirosis	Dog, Cat	(355)
Toxoplasmosis	Cat	(356)
Fungal Disease		
Ringworm	Dog, Cat	(357)
Respiratory		
Pulmonary Hypertension	Dog, Cat	(358, 359)
Asthma	Cat	(360)
Bronchiectasis	Dog, Cat	(361, 362)
Bronchitis	Dog	(363)
Emphysema	Dog, Cat	(364, 365)
Pneumonia	Dog, Cat	(366, 367)
Lung Cancer	Dog, Cat	(368, 369)
Pulmonary Eosinophilia	Dog	(370)
Ear Disease		
Otitis Externa/Media/Interna	Dog, Cat	(371)
Hearing Loss, Deafness	Dog, Cat	(372, 373)
Musculoskeletal Disease		
Atlantoaxial Subluxation	Dog	(374, 375)
Cleft Palate	Dog, Cat	(376)
Degenerative Joint Disease	Dog, Cat	(377)
Developmental Hip Disease	Dog	(378)
Hypertrophic Osteopathy	Dog	(379)
Patellar Luxation	Dog	(380)

(Continued)

TABLE 2.1 (CONTINUED)
Spontaneous Companion Animal Models of Human Disease

Disease or System	Companion Species	Reference #
Myasthenia Gravis	Dog, Cat	(381)
Osteomyelitis	Dog, Cat	(382, 383)
Pectus Excavatum	Dog, Cat	(384, 385)
Polyarthritis	Dog, Cat	(386, 387)
Spina Bifida	Dog, Cat	(388)
Hemivertebra	Dog	(389)
Achondroplasia (Dwarfism)	Dog, Cat	(390, 391)
Spondylitis	Dog, Cat	(392)
Chondrodystrophy	Dog	(393)
Kyphosis	Dog	(394)
Polydactyl	Cat	(395)
Exostosis	Dog, Cat	(396, 397)
Urinary System		
Urolithiasis	Dog	(384)
Cystitis	Dog, Cat	(398, 399)
Urethral, Ureteral Blockage	Dog, Cat	(400, 401)
Ectopic Ureter	Dog	(402)
Incontinence	Dog, Cat	(403, 404)
Cystinuria	Dog	(405)
Diabetes Insipidus	Dog	(406)
Piebald	Dog	(373)
Acne	Dog, Cat	(407, 408)
Alopecia	Dog, Cat	(409)
Dermatitis	Dog, Cat	(410, 411)
Bullous Pemphigoid, Pemphigus	Dog, Cat	(412)
Calcinosis Cutis	Dog, Cat	(413, 414)
Demodicosis	Dog	(415)
Urticaria	Dog	(416)
Acanthosis Nigricans	Dog	(417)
Ehlers-Danlos Syndrome	Dog, Cat	(418, 419)
Panniculitis	Dog	(420)

as insulin dependent or non-insulin dependent diabetes mellitus. In this system, it is clear that dogs are nearly uniformly affected by ß-cell deficiency and are therefore most aligned with human T1DM. Breed predispositions in Samoyeds, Tibetan Terriers, and Cairn Terriers suggested a genetic component that is analogous to ethnic predispositions in human diabetes and subsequent analyses of histocompatibility complex haplotypes (termed Dog Lymphocyte Antigens or DLAs) have demonstrated at least three haplotypes that are associated with increased risk while one other was shown to have a protective effect[11]. The fact that major histocompatibility complex alleles are associated with disease risk in dogs might suggest an immune-mediated etiology and reinforces the similarities with human T1DM. Later studies evaluating single nucleotide polymorphisms in a large population of dogs suggested that several genes associated with human diabetes were found to increase susceptibility in dogs, further confirming the translational value of the canine diabetic model. However, it must be noted that the DLA haplotypes and other candidate genes that are epidemiologically associated with diabetes in dogs can be found in both affected and control dogs within high-risk breeds and may be the result of inbreeding or genetic drift. In addition, despite the fact that canine genetic studies have been supportive of an immune-mediated disease, autoantibodies common islet associated antigens (GAD65 and IA2) are usually not found in the serum of affected dogs at the time of diagnosis. Insulitis (lymphocytic infiltration of islets) is also an inconsistent finding in studies examining pancreatic histology of canine diabetics. Some investigators have theorized that autoimmunity is present in dogs with diabetes mellitus, but that dogs typically present in the late stages of disease, at a time when the complete lack of remaining islet tissue has led to a drop in circulating autoantibodies and to lack of inflammation in the pancreas. An alternative theory is that canine diabetes mellitus may arise secondary to diffuse, non-specific pancreatic injury secondary to pancreatitis, a relatively common condition in dogs. Acute hyperglycemia from this condition may lead to beta cell toxicity, which then progresses to beta cell deficiency and diabetes. In summary, canine diabetes shares many phenotypic and genetic characteristics with human T1DM, although specific disease etiologies are heterogeneous in both populations and careful selection of certain populations of dogs may be required to provide the most valid models for specific human populations[12].

Hyperthyroidism

Since first discovered just 35 years ago, the incidence of spontaneous feline hyperthyroidism has increased dramatically to the extent that it is now one of the most common disorders seen in middle-aged to senior domestic cats[13]. Hyperthyroid cat goiters contain single or multiple autonomously (i.e. TSH-independent) functioning and growing thyroid nodules. Thus, hyperthyroidism in cats is clinically and histologically similar to toxic nodular goiter in humans. The disease in cats is mechanistically different from Graves' disease, because neither the hyperfunction nor growth of these nodules depends on extrathyroidal circulating stimulators. The basic lesion appears to be an excessive intrinsic growth capacity of some thyroid cells, but iodine deficiency, other nutritional goitrogens, or environmental disruptors may play a role in the disease pathogenesis. Clinical features of feline toxic nodular goiter include one or more palpable thyroid nodules, together with signs of hyperthyroidism (e.g. weight loss despite an increased appetite). Diagnosis of feline hyperthyroidism is confirmed by finding the increased serum concentrations of thyroxine (T4) and triiodothyronine (T3), undetectable serum TSH concentrations, or increased thyroid uptake of radioiodine. Thyroid scintigraphy demonstrates a heterogeneous pattern of increased radionuclide uptake, most commonly into both thyroid lobes. Treatment options for toxic nodular goiter in cats are similar to that used in humans and include surgical thyroidectomy, radioiodine, and antithyroid drugs. Most authorities agree that ablative therapy with radioiodine is the treatment of choice for most cats with toxic nodular goiter, because the animals are older, and the disease will never go into remission[13].

Hypothyroidism

Hypothyroidism is a complex clinical condition found in both humans and dogs, thought to be caused by a combination of genetic and environmental factors. A recent study performed a multi-breed analysis of predisposing genetic risk factors for hypothyroidism in dogs using three high-risk breeds—the Gordon Setter, Hovawart, and the Rhodesian Ridgeback[14]. Using a genome-wide association approach and meta-analysis, they identified a major hypothyroidism risk locus shared by these breeds on chromosome 12 ($p = 2.1 \times 10(-11)$). Further characterization of the candidate region revealed a shared ~167 kb risk haplotype (4,915,018–5,081,823 bp), tagged by two SNPs in almost complete linkage disequilibrium. This breed-shared risk haplotype includes three genes (LHFPL5, SRPK1, and SLC26A8) and does not extend to the dog leukocyte antigen (DLA) class II gene cluster located in the vicinity. These three genes have not been identified as candidate genes for hypothyroid disease previously, but have functions that could potentially contribute to the development of the disease. Results implicate the potential involvement of novel genes and pathways for the development of canine hypothyroidism, raising new possibilities for screening, breeding programs, and treatments in dogs. This study may also contribute to the understanding of the genetic etiology of human hypothyroid disease, which is one of the most common endocrine disorders in humans[14].

Cushing's Disease (Hyperadrenocorticism)

Middle-aged to old dogs commonly develop Cushing's disease, through overproduction of glucocorticoids by the adrenal cortex secondary to a functional pituitary adenoma. The associated manifestations are very similar to clinical observations in humans, including changes in the skin, weight gain, abdominal obesity, fatigue, muscle atrophy, hypertension, and renal dysfunction.

In humans, pituitary adenomas (PAs) are common tumors, with an overall prevalence in the general US population estimated at 16.7%[15]. Corticotroph adenomas, comprising functional ACTH-PAs and silent corticotroph adenomas, represent approximately 10% to 15% of all human PAs. Functional ACTH-PAs are the most common cause of Cushing's syndrome (hypercortisolemia from any source), accounting for an estimated 70% of all cases. Prevalence of Cushing's syndrome is estimated to be 1.2 to 2.4 per 1 million people, and it affects approximately 12,000 people in the United States. This number, however, may be much higher, given that Cushing's syndrome is frequently misdiagnosed, and diagnosis is often delayed.

In dogs, functional ACTH-PAs have a reported incidence of 0.2% in all dogs (1–2 cases/1000 dogs/year), with approximately 100,000 dogs affected yearly in the United States. Functional PAs account for approximately 85% to 90% of cases of hyperadrenocorticism, with the remainder of cases resulting from functional adrenal tumors, meal-/food-induced cases, occult, or atypical disease[16–21].

Addison's Disease (Hypoadrenocorticism)

Hypoadrenocorticism is an uncommon disease in dogs and rare in humans, where it is known as Addison's disease (ADD). The disease is characterized by a deficiency in corticosteroid production from the adrenal cortex, requiring lifelong hormone replacement therapy[22,23]. When compared with humans, the pathogenesis of hypoadrenocorticism in dogs is not well established, although the evidence supports a similar autoimmune etiology of adrenocortical pathology. Several immune response genes have been implicated in determining susceptibility to Addison's disease in humans, some of which are shared with other autoimmune syndromes. Indeed, other types of autoimmune disease are common (approximately 50%) in human patients affected with ADD. Several lines of evidence suggest a genetic component to the etiology of canine hypoadrenocorticism. Certain dog breeds are overrepresented in epidemiologic studies, reflecting a likely genetic influence, supported by data from pedigree analysis. Molecular genetic studies have identified similar genes and signaling pathways, involved in ADD in humans, to be also associated with susceptibility to canine hypoadrenocorticism. Immune response genes such as the dog leukocyte antigen (DLA) and cytotoxic T-lymphocyte-associated protein 4 (CTLA4) genes seem to be particularly important. It is clear that there are genetic factors involved in determining susceptibility to canine hypoadrenocorticism, although similar to the situation in humans, this is likely to represent a complex genetic disorder.

Acromegaly

The prevalence of GH (growth hormone)-secreting pituitary tumors in domestic cats (*Felis catus*) is ten-fold greater than in humans. The predominant inhibitory receptors of GH-secreting pituitary tumors are somatostatin receptors (SSTRs) and D_2 dopamine receptors (DRD2). The expression of these receptors is associated with the response to somatostatin analog and dopamine agonist treatment in human patients with acromegaly. A study in cats evaluated pathological features of pituitaries from domestic cats with acromegaly, pituitary receptor expression, and investigated correlates with clinical data, including pituitary volume, time since diagnosis of diabetes, insulin requirement, and serum IGF1 concentration. Loss of reticulin structure was identified in 15 of 21 pituitaries, of which 10 of 15 exhibited acinar hyperplasia. *SSTR1*, *SSTR2*, *SSTR5*, and *DRD2* mRNA were identified in the feline pituitary, whereas *SSTR3* and *SSTR4* were not. Expression of *SSTR1*, *SSTR2*, and *SSTR5* was greater in acromegalic cats compared with controls. A negative correlation was identified between *DRD2* mRNA expression and pituitary volume[24,25].

Primary Hyperaldosteronism

Primary hyperaldosteronism, also referred to as Conn's syndrome, is an adrenocortical disorder characterized by excessive, autonomous secretion of mineralocorticoids, mainly aldosterone, leading to systemic arterial hypertension and/or hypokalemia. After its first description in man in 1955, Conn suggested that as many as 20% of people with arterial hypertension would have primary hyper-aldosteronism. Nevertheless, primary hyperaldosteronism was considered a very rare condition for several decades. With improved screening tests, however, detection has increased, and recent studies have shown that primary hyperaldosteronism is found in about 6% of all human patients with arterial hypertension and up to 11% of those selected for therapy-resistant hypertension. Primary hyperaldosteronism has also been reported in dogs and, much more frequently, in cats. It is probably the most common adrenocortical disorder in cats, and it may be an important cause of arterial hypertension in this species, as it is in man[26–28].

Obesity

There are differences regarding body composition across dog breeds. However, dog obesity is the most common disorder that leads to morbidity, and the range of disorders with which dog obesity has been associated include diabetes mellitus, cardiovascular and musculoskeletal disease, degenerative disorders, decreased immuno-competence, and shortened life span. These are again not related to dog size, but instead promoted by other human factors, like wealth. Thus, restriction of caloric intake might extend the canine life span (see later discussion on caloric restriction)[29,30].

CARDIOPULMONARY DISEASE

The canine heart is a robust physiological model for the human heart[31]. Recently, birth month associations have been reported and replicated in humans using clinical health records[32]. While animals respond readily to their environment in the wild, a systematic investigation of birth season dependencies among pets and specifically canines remains lacking. The Orthopedic Foundation of Animals reported on 129,778 canines representing 253 distinct breeds. Among canines that were not predisposed to cardiovascular disease, a clear birth season relationship is observed with peak risk occurring in June–August. These findings indicate that acquired cardiovascular disease among canines, especially those that are not predisposed to cardiovascular disease, appears birth season dependent. The relative risk of cardiovascular disease for canines not predisposed to cardiovascular disease was as high as 1.47 among July pups. The overall adjusted odds ratio, when mixed breeds were excluded, for the birth season effect was 1.02 (95% CI: 1.002, 1.047, p = 0.032) after adjusting for breed and genetic cardiovascular predisposition effects. Studying birth season effects in model organisms can help to elucidate potential mechanisms behind the reported associations[32]. There are many types of distinct spontaneously occurring cardiac diseases that occur (naturally) in dogs and cats as discussed below.

Heart Failure

The first large animals used to study heart failure were dogs, in which models of myocardial infarction and serial microembolization of the coronary artery were developed. However, the preferred large animal model of heart damage is the pig, because the collateral coronary circulation and arterial anatomy of pigs and humans are very similar and infarct size can be accurately predicted. An additional model of heart failure in large and small animals is pressure overload of the left ventricle, induced by transverse aortic constriction in mice and aortic banding in rats and rabbits. Left ventricle hypertrophy can also be recreated by ventricular pacing in dogs, and renal artery constriction or aortic stenosis.

CARDIOMYOPATHY

Dilated

Large animal models of inherited cardiomyopathies would be extremely useful for the evaluation of novel pharmacological, gene, cell, and device therapies. Several naturally occurring forms of DCM (dilated cardiomyopathy) have been described in dogs, and in fact constitute the most common form of heart disease in large- and giant-breed dogs[33,34]. For example, DCM has been described in Portuguese Water Dogs, Great Danes, Doberman Pinschers, and Boxers. However, the exact genetic basis in each of these breeds remains incompletely understood, with reports showing an association with mutations in genes encoding for sarcomeric, desmosomal, or metabolic proteins. Similarly, an autosomal-dominant form of arrhythmogenic right ventricular cardiomyopathy (ARVC) has been described in Boxers, and while no mutations in desmosomal genes (known to be associated with ARVC in humans) were found in these dogs, there was loss of gap junction plaques resembling the phenotype found in humans. These naturally occurring canine models of cardiomyopathy not only provide a model for testing novel therapies, but (as the gene mutations in these breeds appear different from known gene mutations in humans with DCM and ARVC) also provide an interesting target for genetic screening providing novel genes to be tested, in human forms of DCM and ARVC.

Hypertrophic

Hypertrophic cardiomyopathy (HCM) is the most common cardiac disease in domestic cats, and is characterized by left ventricular hypertrophy (LVH), particularly of the papillary muscles, systolic anterior motion, and myocardial disarray[35-38]. It is a progressive disease that starts in the adolescence (generally after 6 months of age) and can result in heart failure, paralysis of the hind legs due to clot embolization originating in the heart, and sudden cardiac death. HCM is transmitted in an autosomal-dominant trait in the Maine Coon and Ragdoll feline breeds. Two mutations in MYBPC3 have been identified so far. The first one, identified only in the Main Coon breed, is a c.91G>C missense mutation in exon 3, which gives rise to the p.Ala31Pro cardiac myosin-binding protein C (cMyBP-C) mutant in the linker region between the C0 and C1 domains of the protein. Some rare isolated cases of British Longhair, Ragdoll, or Siberian breeds also carry this mutation. The second one, identified only in the Ragdoll breed, is a c.2328C>T transition in exon 26, which results in the p.Arg820Trp cMyBP-C mutant in the C6 domain. Both heterozygous and homozygous cats for MYBPC3 mutations developed LVH (mainly concentric), but some heterozygotes do not exhibit clinical signs of HCM. On the other hand, whereas all homozygotes developed diastolic dysfunction, few heterozygotes developed minor regional myocardial diastolic dysfunction without LVH, suggesting that diastolic dysfunction could be the first feature of the disease, such as observed in heterozygous human patients and mouse model of HCM. Importantly, the c.91G>C mutation results in a lower amount of cMyBP-C protein in the heart in both heterozygous and homozygous Maine Coon cats, such as seen in human HCM. This suggests regulation of mutation expression by protein quality control mechanisms, such as the ubiquitin–protein system, which has been shown to be involved after MYBPC3 gene transfer in cardiac myocytes and *in vivo* in the Mybpc3-targeted knock-in mice. Therefore, cats with HCM represent a good intermediary model between the numerous induced mouse models and human disease states to evaluate different causal therapeutic strategies to prevent the development of heart failure and/ or sudden cardiac death or to rescue the phenotype in both heterozygotes and homozygotes for MYBPC3 mutations. Recent evidence that RNA-based therapies, such as exon skipping or trans-splicing, can repair Mybcp3 mRNA, and more recently, that Mybpc3 gene therapy long term prevents the development of the disease phenotype in Mybpc3-targeted knock-in mice, paved the way to evaluate these strategies in cats.

Arrhythmogenic Right Ventricular Cardiomyopathy

Arrhythmogenic right ventricular cardiomyopathy (ARVC) is associated with a mutation in the striatin gene in Boxer dogs[39]. The disease appeared to be autosomal dominant with incomplete and age-dependent penetrance. A genome wide association study (GWAS) identified a region CFA17 in the Boxer as being highly associated. Evaluation of the underlying gene striatin, calmodulin binding protein (STRN), revealed an 8-bp deletion in the 3' untranslated region. Both homozygotes and heterozygotes were identified, but the dogs that were homozygous for the deletion had a more severe form of the disease. A subsequent study identified the second clinical form of myocardial disease seen in Boxers, dilated cardiomyopathy, as being caused by a deletion in the same gene in at least some families. The encoded protein is believed to serve as a scaffold that functions in a calcium-dependent manner in both signaling and trafficking. The authors made the novel observation that STRN protein colocalizes with the desmosomal proteins plakophilin-2, plakoglobin, and desmoplakin. All are proteins that are involved in the human forms of ventricular cardiomyopathy. STRN now becomes a superb candidate gene for unexplained familial and sporadic forms of the human disease.

Mitral Valve Disease

Age is the greatest risk factor for nearly every major cause of mortality in developed countries. In particular, this is true for heart disease, which is the leading cause of death in the United States. Between the ages of 40 and 60, the risk of dying from heart disease for a typical American adult increases about eightfold, which is greater than the increase in risk associated with having high blood pressure, high cholesterol, and diabetes combined. In addition to cardiovascular disease and cardiomyopathy, degenerative valve disease (DVD) plays an important role in age-related cardiac morbidity in people. It is estimated that more than one out of every eight people over age 75 has moderate to severe DVD and DVD accounts for 10% to 20% of all cardiac surgeries in the United States[40]. Furthermore, its worldwide prevalence is expected to increase dramatically as the aged population increases, raising significant public health concerns.

Animal models play an essential role in the study of heart disease, and species used in this line of research include mice, rats, rabbits, dogs, sheep, and swine, among others. In contrast, DVD induction has not been achieved in rodents to date and their size limits the potential for surgical intervention. Given these limitations, most of the available models of DVD create cardiac pathology in dogs and swine through surgically severing the chordae tendineae, rather than studying DVD in the context of normative aging. While the hemodynamic changes thus created mimic the situation in DVD, the fact that this intervention is performed in young animals in an acute fashion limits its usefulness as a model for changes associated with normative aging, which include gradual age-related alterations to the myocardium in addition to gradual valvular changes. Additionally, all of these models are studied in captive animals maintained in laboratory conditions, which fail to recapitulate important features of the natural environment.

In this context, companion dogs provide a potentially powerful model for understanding how and why DVD is both a cause and consequence of aging. In this species, DVD accounts for roughly 75% of all heart disease, with age also being a significant risk factor[40]. While there have been several studies focusing on individual high-risk breeds such as Cavalier King Charles Spaniels and Dachshunds, and one more recent study that focused on the prevalence of mitral valve disease in dogs diagnosed in a primary care setting, the most recent screening studies of DVD prevalence in the general dog population seem to date from the 1960s. As trivial valvular regurgitation is not uncommon in older dogs and not all dogs with diagnosed valvular regurgitation demonstrate clinical signs of cardiac disease during their lifetimes, it is often assumed that this is a normal part of the aging process, and the extent to which asymptomatic regurgitation and DVD contribute to morbidity and mortality in dogs remains unclear.

It is generally accepted that older, small dogs are more commonly affected by DVD than young, large dogs, and inheritance studies reveal an increased risk of clinical signs among male dogs. A retrospective study of more than 111,967 dogs treated at primary care veterinary practices in the United Kingdom found a prevalence of diagnosed mitral valve disease of 0.4% and a prevalence of heart murmur consistent with DVD but not sufficient to warrant diagnosis of 3.5%. However, the above values are derived from the VetCompass database, which only captures veterinary record data from clinical practice, where screening in the absence of symptoms usually consists of a clinical exam including auscultation. It has been demonstrated that the presence of mild valvular regurgitation in dogs cannot be reliably detected by auscultation and that considerable variation in the ability to detect heart murmurs associated with valvular regurgitation exists among individual veterinarians. In addition, when comparing these clinical data to data obtained by post-mortem examination, the measured prevalence of DVD can increase quite dramatically. For instance, one study demonstrated a prevalence of 391 out of 4,831 dogs (8.1%) seen in private veterinary practice based on clinical diagnosis and/or post-mortem examination. Based on post-mortem examination only, a second study found 139 out of 404 dogs (34.4%) showed valvular disease, and that the prevalence was strongly correlated with age. These observations would seem to indicate that the prevalence of degenerative valve disease in dogs is generally underestimated in clinical practice.

Pulmonary Disease

An extensive body of literature describes the canine pulmonary anatomy and physiology, including the lung mechanics, ventilation, cough reflex, immunobiology, inflammation, pharmacology, and central neuronal control mechanisms. The canine respiratory system shares many similarities with that of humans, and dogs have been used as models for chronic inflammatory diseases, such as induced asthma and chronic obstructive pulmonary disease, which develops from chronic bronchitis and emphysema, again resulting in decreased lifespan.

Asthma

Asthma is a chronic, heterogeneous, and usually recurring inflammatory disease of the lower airways, with exacerbations that feature airway inflammation and bronchial hyperresponsiveness[41]. Asthma has been modeled extensively via disease induction in both wild-type and genetically manipulated laboratory mice (*Mus musculus*). Antigen sensitization and challenge strategies have reproduced numerous important features of airway inflammation characteristic of human asthma, notably the critical roles of type 2 T helper cell cytokines. Recent models of disease induction have advanced to include physiologic aeroallergens with prolonged respiratory challenge without systemic sensitization; others incorporate tobacco, respiratory viruses, or bacteria as exacerbants. Nonetheless, differences in lung size, structure, and physiologic responses limit the degree to which airway dynamics measured in mice can be compared to human subjects. Other rodent allergic airways models, including those featuring the guinea pig (*Cavia porcellus*) might be considered for lung function studies. Finally, domestic cats (*Felis catus*)[42] and horses (*Equus caballus*) develop spontaneous obstructive airway disorders with clinical and pathologic features that parallel human asthma.

Idiopathic Pulmonary Fibrosis

Canine idiopathic pulmonary fibrosis (CIPF) affects middle-aged to older dogs of a single breed, mainly the West Highland White Terrier (WHWT), which is suggestive of a genetic predisposition[43,44]. CIPF causes exercise intolerance, restrictive dyspnea, and coughing. Coarse crackles are heard on thoracic auscultation. Abnormal blood gas parameters and a shortened '6-min walking test' distance are common; secondarily induced pulmonary hypertension and/or airway collapse are frequent. These features of CIPF mimic those of idiopathic pulmonary fibrosis (IPF) in humans and therefore identify CIPF as a possible spontaneously arising model for study of human IPF. However, computed tomographic and histopathological findings of CIPF are not identical to those of human IPF. As in human IPF, the etiology of CIPF is not yet fully elucidated. There are no curative treatments and the prognosis is poor.

RENAL DISEASE

Chronic Renal Disease

Chronic kidney disease (CKD) is defined as the presence of structural or functional abnormalities of one or both kidneys that have been present for an extended period of time[45–47]. CKD is common in cats, with one study reporting that 12% of all cats necropsied over a period of 3 years were suffering from the condition. The prevalence of CKD also increases with age, with reported prevalence rates of 28% in cats over 12 years old and 31% in cats over 15 years old.

The etiology of feline CKD is heterogeneous and includes specific disease processes which initiate renal damage or dysfunction, such as polycystic kidney disease, renal amyloidosis, renal dysplasia, and renal lymphoma. However, in the majority of cats with CKD no inciting cause is identified. One study of a referral population found pathological lesions of a specific renal disease in 50% of cases, another in 33% of cases. A recent study with a large population from first opinion practices identified specific renal lesions in only 16% of cats. The majority of cats with CKD are found to have non-specific renal lesions and the predominant morphological diagnosis in these cases is chronic tubulointerstitial inflammation and fibrosis. The underlying etiology of CKD in the majority of cats, where chronic tubulointerstitial fibrosis is present, is not understood.

Various factors which may contribute to renal damage have been proposed, including diet, vaccination, and ageing. Regardless of the etiology, the progressive nature of renal fibrosis results in deterioration of renal function independent of the initial renal insult. Renal tubulointerstitial fibrosis is recognized as the final common pathway for all kidney diseases in human patients regardless of etiology and is the pathological lesion best correlated with renal function in both humans and cats.

Despite ongoing research there is currently no effective treatment that significantly slows the progression of renal fibrosis in humans or in cats. Therefore, much attention is directed at identifying factors which influence or drive the progression of fibrosis in order to identify potential therapeutic targets.

IMMUNOLOGY

The immune-senescence characteristics of older dogs are shared with elderly people. Old dogs show impairment of cell-mediated immune functions, such as reduced blood CD4+ T-cells, imbalance in Th1 versus Th2 functional activity, elevation of the CD8+ subsets, and reduction in the CD4:CD8 ratio. Furthermore, blood lymphocyte responses to stimulation by mitogens decrease the delayed cutaneous type hypersensitivity response. Conversely, there is relative preservation of the ability to mount humoral immune responses. Serum and salivary immunoglobulin (Ig)A production increases, and IgG concentrations remain unaltered with age. Elderly animals generally have persisting vaccine antibody titers at protective levels, and respond to booster vaccinations with titer elevation. Older dogs show primary humoral responses to novel antigens, but the magnitude of these can be lower relative to the titers of younger animals. There have been few investigations into the phenomenon of 'inflammageing' in dogs, regarding the effects of cumulative antigenic exposure and onset of late life inflammatory disease[48,49].

ONCOLOGIC DISEASE

Dogs spontaneously develop the same types of cancers that humans do, and they are often even treated with the same therapeutic strategies. Several dog breeds are known to have a high incidence and elevated risk of specific cancer subtypes, sometimes even more than one subtype. Additionally, centuries of selective breeding of dogs confers the opportunity to examine polymorphisms that are specific to particular breeds that have exaggerated incidences of particular cancer subtypes. Finally, because dogs cohabitate with their human owners, they are both exposed to the same environmental factors, which might potentiate the development of cancers. Genomic analysis of canine tumors has revealed shared features with humans, which has provided important insight into the genetic basis of tumor development and gives a list of the high-risk breed-specific diseases that have arisen due to the restricted genetic variation produced by consanguinity and inbreeding. This offers an exceptional opportunity to examine the interactions between genetics and environment in the etiologies of various forms of cancer; and the shorter life span of dogs facilitates timely and efficient evaluation of new approaches to cancer diagnosis, treatment, and prevention. A wide variety of cancers are being studied in dogs, which include soft tissue sarcomas, mammary carcinomas, primary and secondary lung carcinomas, malignant melanomas, and cancers of the prostate, bladder, intestine, brain, mouth, and many others. Among all of these, dog lymphomas and canine osteosarcoma are of particular interest in terms of their frequency and pathophysiology, respectively. In dogs (mainly Boxers and Golden Retrievers) and humans, large B-cell non-Hodgkin lymphoma is the most frequent. Canine osteosarcoma affects large breeds such as Great Danes, Wolfhounds, and Rottweilers, where this is generally confined to the long bones, and has similar metastatic rates and destinations as seen for humans. In osteosarcoma, the p53 tumor suppressor pathway, the c-Met proto-oncogene, the chemokineinterleukin-8, and several such mediators are involved in both species. Furthermore, a constitutional 'germline' DNA for cancer predisposition genes in dogs with cancer has been described, which includes BRCA1/BRCA2, which leads to hereditary breast and ovarian cancer syndrome in humans, as well as TP53 germline mutations in dogs, which lead to Li-Fraumeni syndrome in humans, with multiple different cancers. The approach of using single nucleotide poly-morphisms and/or copy number variations and genome-wide association studies has been associated with disease risk in specific dog breeds. Genetic analysis of canine tumors has revealed common features with humans, along with important information about their development. Thus, the consanguinity and inbreeding in the practice of human society for dog breeding has unwittingly created a high-risk model for breed-specific diseases. The limited genetic variation in purebred dogs that is associated with the shorter life span of dogs facilitates timely and efficient evaluation of new approaches to cancer diagnosis, treatment, and prevention[50-74].

Lymphomas

Canine lymphoma (cL) is a common type of neoplasia in dogs with an estimated incidence rate of 20–100 cases per 100,000 dogs and is in many respects com-parable to non-Hodgkin lymphoma in humans[75-77]. Although the exact cause is unknown, environmental factors and genetic susceptibility are thought to play an important role. cL is not a single disease, and a wide variation in clinical pre-sentations and histological subtypes is recognized. Despite this potential varia-tion, most dogs present with generalized lymphadenopathy (multicentric form) and intermediate to high-grade lymphoma, more commonly of B-cell origin. The most common paraneoplastic sign is hypercalcemia that is associated with the T-cell immunophenotype. Chemotherapy is the treatment of choice and a doxo-rubicin-based multidrug protocol is currently the standard of care. A complete remission is obtained for most dogs and lasts for a median period of 7–10 months, resulting in a median survival of 10–14 months. Many prognostic factors have been reported, but stage, immunophenotype, tumor grade, and response to che-motherapy appear of particular importance. Failure to respond to chemotherapy suggests drug resistance, which can be partly attributed to the expression of drug transporters of the ABC-transporter superfamily, including P-gp and BCRP. Ultimately, most lymphomas will become drug resistant and the development of treatments aimed at reversing drug resistance or alternative treatment modalities (e.g. immunotherapy and targeted therapy) are of major importance.

Osteosarcoma

Osteosarcoma (OS) is the most common histological subtype of primary bone cancer both in humans and dogs. It is estimated to occur in over 8,000 dogs each year in the United States.

Although multi-agent chemotherapy has greatly improved the outcome among human patients, mortality is still high. Five-year overall survival rates range from about 15% to 70% for patients with and without visible metastases at the time of diagnosis, respectively. Adding to the severity of this disease, it typically affects children and adolescents, constituting about 5% of pediatric cancers[78,79].

Osteosarcoma accounts for 80% to 90% of canine primary bone tumors. Although rare in the canine population, the rate outnumbers that of the human population, with a lifetime incidence risk about 30 to 50 times higher within the overall canine population. Breed-specific incidence rates of OS differ largely, and estimates within certain breeds even show a lifetime risk exceeding 10%, thereby affecting a substantial number of these dogs. Median survival time for dogs with primary bone cancer of the appendicular skeleton, treated with surgery and chemotherapy, ranges from 5 to 13 months provided there is no visible metastasis at the time of diagnosis, in which case median survival time drops to about 2 months.

Most commonly, OS is diagnosed in middle-aged to older dogs, with a median age of 7 years. A smaller peak in age incidence at 18 to 24 months corresponds with the human peak incidence at late puberty, which has led to the hypothesis of skeletal growth parameters representing some of the possible etiological factors for developing this disease. It is well recognized that giant- and large-breed dogs are at increased risk of developing OS; however, body size alone cannot explain the variation in incidence between different breeds of dogs, as the risk appears to differ extensively among certain breeds of similar body size. Epidemiological studies on human OS have also failed to show a strong correlation between body weight or height and risk of developing OS.

Several studies have demonstrated similarities between canine and human osteosarcoma (OSA) at the molecular level by showing comparable expression of different proteins.

Canine OSA cell lines and tumors frequently contain mutations that inactivate p53 and the phosphatase and tensin homologue (PTEN) family of tumor suppressor genes. Insulin and hepatocyte growth factors influence tumor growth, invasion, and malignant phenotype in canine OSA cell lines. Matrix metalloproteinase 2 (MMP-2) expression has been detected only in high-grade OSAs, while pro-MMP-9 production correlated with the histological grade of OSA, suggesting a potential role of MMPs in the pathogenesis of canine OSA growth and metastasis. STAT3 activation has also been shown to contribute to the survival and proliferation of human and canine OSA cell lines. Recently, the role and expression of the tyrosine kinase receptors (TKRs) have been investigated in veterinary oncology. Overexpression of the erb-B2 gene, encoding for human epidermal growth factor receptor 2 (HER2), was observed in 86% and 40% of canine OSA cell lines and tissue samples, respectively, suggesting an involvement in the pathogenesis of this tumor. Furthermore, as in humans, 79% of canine OSA samples overexpress the MET oncogenes; cell motility and invasiveness appear to be MET-dependent since they can be inhibited by small interfering RNAs (siRNAs) that are specific for MET. Finally, recent evidence demonstrated that PDGF receptors are overexpressed in canine OSA, adding a new potential therapeutic target. Insulin-like growth factor-1 receptor (IGF-1R) is a transmembrane TKR consisting of two extracellular α-subunits responsible for ligand binding, two β-subunits with a transmembrane domain, and an intracellular tyrosine kinase COOH-terminal domain. The specific interaction between IGF-1 and IGF-1R induces the phosphorylation of intracellular tyrosine residue (β-subunit) and results in activation of the receptor. The activated form of IGF-1R is able to activate the PI3K/AKT and mitogen-activated protein kinase (MAPK) signaling pathways.

Brain Tumors

Beyond the advantages of working with a larger animal model, the similarities in tumor biology shared between specific human and canine cancers further contribute to their value as models of human cancer. Intracranial tumors in dogs have an estimated incidence of approximately 14–20 per 100,000[80–82]. Commonly reported primary brain tumors in dogs are meningiomas, gliomas (astrocytomas, oligodendrogliomas), undifferentiated sarcomas, pituitary tumors, and ventricular tumors (choroid plexus tumors and ependymomas). Other primary brain tumors, such as tumors of nerve cells (e.g. gangliocytomas, neuroblastomas), pinealomas, craniopharyngiomas, glioblastoma, and medulloblastomas, are less commonly described. Middle-aged to older dogs have the highest incidence of brain tumors among domestic animals and of these, meningiomas may be the most frequent and occur at a significantly older age than other tumor types.

Brain tumors in dogs share striking similarities to human brain tumors in neuro-imaging characteristics, gross and histological appearance, expression of growth factors and receptors, as well as their initial cytogenetic expressions.

HEPATIC/BILIARY DISEASE

Copper Storage Disease

Copper is an essential trace nutrient metal involved in a multitude of cellular processes.

Hereditary defects in copper metabolism result in disorders with a severe clinical course such as Wilson disease and Menkes disease. In Wilson disease, copper accumulation leads to liver cirrhosis and neurological impairments. A lack in genotype-phenotype correlation in Wilson disease points toward the influence of environmental factors or modifying genes. In a number of Non-Wilsonian forms of copper metabolism, the underlying genetic defects remain elusive. Several purebred dog populations are affected with copper-associated hepatitis showing similarities to human copper metabolism disorders. Gene-mapping studies in these populations offer the opportunity to discover new genes involved in copper metabolism. Furthermore, due to the relatively large body size and long life span of dogs, they are excellent models for development of new treatment strategies. One example is the recent use of canine organoids for disease modeling and gene therapy of copper storage disease. Further, possibilities for the use of dogs in development of new treatment modalities for copper storage disorders, including gene repair in patient-derived hepatic organoids, are possible.

The deleterious effects of a disrupted copper metabolism are illustrated by hereditary diseases caused by mutations in the genes coding for the copper transporters ATP7A and ATP7B. Menkes disease, involving ATP7A, is a fatal neurodegenerative disorder of copper deficiency. Mutations in ATP7B lead to Wilson disease, which is characterized by a predominantly hepatic copper accumulation. The low incidence and the phenotypic variability of human copper toxicosis hamper identification of causal genes or modifier genes involved in the disease pathogenesis. The Labrador Retriever was recently characterized as a new canine model for copper toxicosis. Purebred dogs have reduced genetic variability, which facilitates identification of genes involved in complex heritable traits that might influence phenotype in both humans and dogs. A genome-wide association study in 235 Labrador Retrievers identified two chromosome regions containing ATP7A and ATP7B that were associated with variation in hepatic copper levels. DNA sequence analysis identified missense mutations in each gene. The amino acid substitution ATP7B:p.Arg1453Gln was associated with copper accumulation, whereas the amino acid substitution ATP7A:p.Thr327Ile partly protected against copper accumulation. Confocal microscopy indicated that aberrant copper metabolism upon expression of the ATP7B variant occurred because of mis-localization of the protein in the endoplasmic reticulum. Dermal fibroblasts derived from ATP7A:p.Thr327Ile dogs showed copper accumulation and delayed excretion. Attenuation of copper accumulation by the ATP7A mutation sheds an interesting light on the interplay of copper transporters in body copper homeostasis and warrants a thorough investigation of ATP7A as a modifier gene in copper-metabolism disorders. The identification of two new functional variants in ATP7A and ATP7B contributes to the biological understanding of protein function, with relevance for future development of therapy[83–88].

GASTROINTESTINAL DISEASE

Inflammatory Bowel Disease

Inflammatory bowel disease (IBD) is a multifactorial disorder with many different putative influences mediating disease onset, severity, progression, and diminution. Spontaneous natural IBD is classically expressed as Crohn's disease (CD) and ulcerative colitis (UC) commonly found in primates; lymphoplasmacytic enteritis, eosinophilic gastritis and colitis, and ulcerative colitis with neuronal hyperplasia in dogs; and colitis in horses. Spontaneous inflammatory bowel disease has been noted in a number of rodent models which differ in genetic strain background, induced mutation, microbiota influences, and immunopathogenic pathways. Histological lesions in Crohn's disease feature non-caseating granulomatous inflammation, while UC lesions typically exhibit ulceration, lamina propria inflammatory infiltrates, and lack of granuloma development. Intestinal inflammation caused by CD and UC is also associated with increased incidence of intestinal neoplasia[89–91].

Protein-losing enteropathy, or PLE, is not a disease but a syndrome that develops in numerous disease states of differing etiologies, often involving the lymphatic system, such as lymphangiectasia and lymphangitis in dogs. The pathophysiology of lymphatic disease is incompletely understood, and the disease is challenging to manage. Understanding of PLE mechanisms requires knowledge of lymphatic system structure and function, which are reviewed here. The mechanisms of enteric protein loss in PLE are identical in dogs and people, irrespective of the underlying cause. In people, PLE is usually associated with primary intestinal lymphangiectasia, suspected to arise from genetic susceptibility, or 'idiopathic' lymphatic vascular obstruction. In dogs, PLE is most often a feature of inflammatory bowel disease (IBD), and less frequently intestinal lymphangiectasia, although it is not proven which process is the true driving defect. In cats, PLE is relatively rare. Review of the veterinary literature (1977–2018) reveals that PLE was life-ending in 54.2% of dogs compared to published disease-associated deaths in IBD of <20%, implying that PLE is not merely a continuum of IBD spectrum pathophysiology. In people, diet is the cornerstone of management, whereas dogs are often treated with immunosuppression for causes of PLE including lymphangiectasia, lymphangitis, and crypt disease. Currently, however, there is no scientific, extrapolated, or evidence-based support for an autoimmune or immune-mediated mechanism. Moreover, people with PLE have disease-associated loss of immune function, including lymphopenia, severe CD4+ T-cell depletion, and negative vaccinal titers.

Pancreatic Insufficiency

Exocrine pancreatic insufficiency (EPI) is a disorder wherein the pancreas fails to secrete adequate amounts of digestive enzymes. In dogs, EPI is usually the consequence of an autoimmune disease known as pancreatic acinar atrophy. Originally believed to be a simple autosomal recessive disorder, a test-breeding recently revealed that EPI has a more complex mode of inheritance[92]. The contributions of multiple genes, combined with environmental factors, may explain observed variability in clinical presentation and progression of this disease. Research efforts aim to identify genetic variations underlying EPI to assist breeders in their efforts to eliminate this disease from their breed and provide clinicians with new targets for therapeutic intervention and/or disease prevention. Genome-wide linkage, global gene expression, and candidate gene analyses have failed to identify a major locus or genetic variations in German Shepherd dogs with EPI. Recently, genome-wide association studies revealed numerous genomic regions associated with EPI. Current studies are focused on alleles of the canine major histocompatibility complex[92].

OPHTHALMIC DISEASE

Keratoconjunctivitis Sicca (KCS)

Spontaneous keratoconjunctivitis sicca seen in pet dogs has the advantage of being similar in pathogenesis to human dry eye. The condition occurs through autoimmune destruction of the lacrimal gland similar to that occurring in Sjogren's syndrome in the human patient and is particularly valuable in that it exists in an animal larger than the laboratory rodents and rabbits otherwise used. It does have the disadvantage of being less readily controlled in its time and severity of onset than a rodent model and the fact that it occurs on a more varied genetic background could be seen as a disadvantage in that it complicates matters by bringing into play a number of uncontrollable variables. On the other hand, this outbred genetic background could be seen as advantageous given that it more closely models the real world of human patients where disease occurs against different genetic and environmental backgrounds. The ocular disease in canine keratoconjunctivitis sicca is similar to human dry eye, although in many cases more severe often with complete absence of tear production to warrant consideration as an example of translational medicine in a 'one health' scenario[93–95].

Dry eye occurs very commonly in dogs kept as companion animals. The first survey of canine keratoconjunctivitis sicca was undertaken by Professor Lloyd Helper, a key player at the beginning of modern veterinary ophthalmology, who noted only 0.4% of the canine population to be affected with a deficiency in tear production in 1976. After 20 years, Dr. Renee Kaswan, a leader in canine dry eye research, reported a prevalence of up to 35% in the patients she surveyed. The truth is that the number of animals affected is probably somewhere in between these two figures. Research undertaken in Cambridge to measure the Schirmer tear test (STT) in 1,000 dogs demonstrated levels of tear production lower than 15 mm of tear strip wetting in 1 min in 131 dogs giving a prevalence of 13%. In a recent survey of cases seen in the clinic of the Queen's Veterinary School Hospital, University of Cambridge, United Kingdom, 181 of the last thousand cases seen were affected by keratoconjunctivitis sicca. This high prevalence of the condition means that a population for evaluation of new products to be used in canine dry eye can readily be accessed.

Cataracts

Cataracts are one of the most significant ophthalmologic diseases in veterinary medicine. Dogs are more prone to develop cataracts than other domestic animals. Cataracts are a leading cause of blindness in dogs with approximately 100 breeds affected by primary hereditary forms. Some canine breeds such as the Australian Shepherd exhibit a pronounced tendency toward inherited cataracts, and some diseases such as diabetes are also known to cause cataracts owing to a change in the crystalline lens metabolic pathway.

Most cases of cataracts are inherited; for instance, Miniature Poodles, American Cocker Spaniels, Miniature Schnauzers, Golden Retrievers, Boston Terriers, and Siberian Huskies are all predisposed to cataracts. The results of a published study suggest that the majority of dogs with diabetes will develop cataracts within 5–6 months from the time of diagnosis of the disease (diabetes), and that approximately 80% of dogs will develop cataracts within 16 months of diagnosis[96].

Despite the large number of breeds affected with hereditary cataracts (HC), little is known about the genetics of the condition, and to date only a single gene, HSF4, has been implicated in the development of the disease in dogs. Using DNA samples from almost 400 privately owned Australian Shepherds, researchers have investigated the association between the deletion mutation in HSF4 and cataracts in this breed. The authors have revealed that the mutation is significantly associated with cataracts and that a dog carrying the mutation is approximately 17 times more likely to develop binocular cataracts than dogs that are clear of the mutation.

The data also indicate that additional mutations associated with the development of cataracts are likely to be co-segregating in the Australian Shepherd population.

Clinical data from 72 dog breeds of varying size and life expectancy were grouped according to breed body mass and tested for prevalence at ages 4 to 5, ages 7 to 10, and lifetime incidence of non-hereditary, age-related cataract. The incidence of age-related cataract was found to be directly related to the relative life expectancies in the breed groups: the smallest dog breeds had a lower age-related cataract prevalence between ages 4 and 5 than mid-size breeds and these, in turn, had a lower prevalence than the giant breeds. A similar sequence was evident for ages 7 to 10 and for overall lifetime incidence of age-related cataract. These differences became more significant when comparing small and giant breeds only. The results have shown that body size, life expectancy, and age-related cataract incidence are interrelated in dogs. Oxidative stress on lens components has been recognized as an important mechanism in the development of cataracts. Given that age-related cataract has been shown to be at least partially caused by oxidative damage to lens epithelial cells and the internal lens, it has been suggested that it can be considered not only as a general biomarker for life expectancy in the canine and possibly other species, but also for the systemic damages produced by reactive oxygen species (ROS).

The prevalence of cataract is also influenced by age in most purebred dogs and affects 16.80% of the mixed-breed/hybrid dog population between the ages of 7 and 15+. For the most part cataract is the disruption of the normal arrangement of the lens fibers in the eye, which causes the loss in the transparency of the lens, causing vision loss. A retrospective study of all dogs that presented with cataracts to veterinary medical teaching hospitals in North America between 1964 and 2003 was conducted to determine cataract prevalence. The different decades, breeds, gender, and age at time of presentation with cataract were compared. The prevalence of dogs presented with cataract varied by decade and ranged from 0.95% (1964–1973), 1.88% (1974–1983), 2.42% (1994–2003), to 3.5% (1984–1993). The total number of dogs presented with cataracts over the 40-year period was 39,229. From 1964 to 2003 the prevalence of cataract formation in this patient population increased by about 255%. Fifty-nine breeds of dogs were affected with cataracts above the baseline prevalence of 1.61% seen in mixed breed/hybrid dogs. The breeds with the highest cataract prevalence included: Smooth Fox Terrier (11.70%), Havanese (11.57%), Bichon Frise (11.45%), Boston Terrier (11.11%), Miniature Poodle (10.79%), Silky Terrier (10.29%), and Toy Poodle (10.21%). The breeds with the highest incidence of cataracts in dogs during the entire four decades were the Boston Terrier (11.11%), Miniature Poodle (10.79%), American Cocker Spaniel (8.77%), Standard Poodle (7.00%), and Miniature Schnauzer (4.98%)[96,97].

NEUROLOGIC AND NEUROMUSCULAR DISEASE

Trauma

Dogs with clinical spinal cord injury (SCI) can address an important translational gap in the field of SCI research. The clinical dog model of SCI parallels the human condition with respect to patient and lesion heterogeneity, clinical management, available outcome assessment tools, and spinal cord histopathology[98,99]. Compared with most laboratory animals, the dog spinal cord is of more comparable size to that of humans, allowing for the study of interventions at a relevant scale and with outcome assessments similar to those used in human trials. Moreover, there is a large group of chronically paralyzed pet dogs available for study of chronic injury. Despite being considered a research priority by the human SCI community, experimental studies specifically aimed at the chronic injury state are costly and logistically challenging. The canine clinical model of SCI presents a unique opportunity to study chronic injury in a group of pet dogs living with SCI, and treatment effects in this model may be more predictive of outcome in human trials than laboratory studies.

A multicenter international consortium, CANSORT-SCI, manages a high volume of both acute and chronic clinical SCI in dogs. This offers the opportunity to efficiently conduct rigorous clinical trials in the veterinary setting before taking an intervention into humans. The significant body of published work indicates that the strength of the model lies in its utilization for translational studies to provide important assessments of promising laboratory interventions. Further, CANSORT-SCI is an example of the One Health Initiative, a worldwide strategy for expanding interdisciplinary collaborations and communications in all aspects of health care for humans, animals, and the environment. The studies support continued and expanded use of dogs with clinical SCI to enhance translation from benchtop to the human bedside with the overall goal being to improve functional outcome for persons and animals affected by SCI.

DEGENERATIVE

Spinal Cord

Canine degenerative myelopathy (CDM) represents a unique naturally occurring animal model for human amyotrophic lateral sclerosis (ALS) because of similar clinical signs, neuropathologic findings, and involvement of the superoxide dismutase 1 (SOD1) mutation[100–102]. A definitive diagnosis can only be made postmortem through microscopic detection of axonal degeneration, demyelination, and astroglial proliferation, which is more severe in the dorsal columns of the thoracic spinal cord and in the dorsal portion of the lateral funiculus. Interestingly, the muscle acetylcholine receptor complexes are intact in CDM prior to functional impairment, thus suggesting that muscle atrophy in CDM does not result from physical denervation. Moreover, since sensory involvement seems to play an important role in CDM progression, a more careful investigation of the sensory pathology in ALS is also warranted. The importance of SOD1 expression remains unclear, while oxidative stress and denatured ubiquinated proteins appear to play a crucial role in the pathogenesis of CDM. A better understanding of the factors that determine the disease progression in CDM may be beneficial for the development of effective treatments for ALS.

Brain

Alzheimer's-Like Disease

Domesticated species, such as dogs and cats, represent interesting model systems for aging. Even though the average canine life span of 10–12 years discourages longevity studies, dogs spontaneously develop many age-related phenotypes, such as muscular and neurological decline, as well as cardiovascular disease. Rodents, however, do not develop significant neurodegeneration with age unless severely genetically manipulated. Dogs may therefore be particularly interesting in the study of cognitive deterioration and age-associated neurodegenerative disorders. In addition, the physiology and pathology of dogs have been extremely well characterized. Similarly, cats represent another physiologically well-characterized domesticated animal that has been used in aging studies. As in dogs, several pathological age-associated processes occur in felines, including kidney disease, arthritis, sarcopenia, and neurological decline. Cats live an average of 12–14 years, and life span studies in this species are therefore also problematic; however, their aging phenotype may make them attractive models.

In recent years cats and dogs have been considered as a useful animal model for Alzheimer's disease (AD) due to the close proximity of canine and human brain aging[103–106]. Behavioral changes can be divided into four general categories, which are: loss of cognition and recognition, loss of house training, disorientation, and changes in their sleep-wake cycle. There is a scale termed CCDR (canine cognitive dysfunction rating), which allows assessment of the severity of the cognitive dysfunction scale. Affected dogs exhibit a change in behavior and daily routines, e.g. they do not recognize family members, forget former housetraining, get lost in their houses, get stuck in the corners, and act peculiarly by whining, scratching the floor without reason, and barking a lot.

Geriatric dogs develop cognitive impairment and central nervous system pathologies that mimic the changes that occur in human neurodegenerative diseases, such as Alzheimer's disease. Canine cognitive dysfunction, or 'canine dementia', is a neurobehavioral syndrome in aged dogs that is characterized by deficits in learning, memory, and spatial awareness, and changes in social interactions and sleeping patterns. Like humans, aged dogs suffer from cognitive impairment that appears to resemble Alzheimer's disease, where this is apparently characterized by deposition of significant amounts of amyloid protein (Aß) and development of diffuse plaques that correlate with cognitive decline. Unlike humans, however, dogs with cognitive impairment do not appear to develop neurofibrillary tangles. This appears to be because the amino-acid sequence of the Aß peptide is identical in dogs and humans, while this is not the case for the tau amino acid sequence. Therapeutic strategies that include antioxidant medications, diets, and behavioral enrichment have been shown to improve Alzheimer's disease pathology in dogs, and at the same time, anti-inflammatory drugs, statins, and immunization against Aß peptide have also been pursued in aged dogs.

Domestic cats display several behavioral changes in their elderly years. The most common is spatial disorientation or confusion, for example getting trapped in the corners or forgetting the location of the litter box. It is also frequently observed that social relationships with their owners or other animals in the house are altered, e.g. cats become more aggressive or passive. Geriatric cats change their daily schedule, including their sleep-wake pattern and their interest in food and they decrease grooming. They sometimes exhibit inappropriate vocalization, like crying loudly during the night.

Several studies have identified senile plaques in the cats' brains but only in those aged 10 and more. Aβ can also aggregate as oligomers in younger cats, aged 8. Curiously, there were cases found with Aβ deposits that were not associated with tau immunoreactivity, but no cases were found with neurofibrillary tangle (NFT) in the absence of Aβ deposits. Additionally, in cats, Aβ aggregates differently in the cerebral cortex and hippocampus, which may be due to different neuronal cell types in both regions, and/or environments surrounding neurons in these regions.

The association between Aβ depositions in the brain and cognitive dysfunction in cats remains clarified, as it was proven multiple times, that the brains from aged cats, who exhibited altered behavior, were found to contain diffuse senile plaques. Interestingly, SPs of cats seem to be more diffuse than those that can be found in dogs with ALD.

Since domestic cats can spontaneously develop Aβ deposition, neurofibrillary tangles formation, neuronal loss, and neuronal degeneration (in contrast to other animals) during their short life span, they could serve as a valuable natural model of human Alzheimer's disease.

Leukoencephalopathies

Canine leukoencephalomyelopathy (LEMP) is a juvenile-onset neurodegenerative disorder of the CNS white matter currently described in Rottweiler and Leonberger dogs[107]. Genome-wide association study (GWAS) allowed LEMP mapping in a Leonberger cohort to dog chromosome 18. Subsequent whole genome re-sequencing of a Leonberger case enabled the identification of a single private homozygous non-synonymous missense variant located in the highly conserved metallo-beta-lactamase domain of the N-acyl phosphatidylethanolamine phospholipase D (NAPEPLD) gene, encoding an enzyme of the endocannabinoid system. Sequencing this gene in LEMP-affected Rottweilers identified a different frameshift variant, which is predicted to replace the C-terminal metallo-beta-lactamase domain of the wild type protein. Haplotype analysis of SNP array genotypes revealed that the frameshift variant was present in diverse haplotypes in Rottweilers, and also in Great Danes, indicating an old origin of this second NAPEPLD variant. The identification of different NAPEPLD variants in dog breeds affected by leukoencephalopathies with heterogeneous pathological features, implicates the NAPEPLD enzyme as important in myelin homeostasis, and suggests a novel candidate gene for myelination disorders in people.

Seizure Disorders

Epilepsy is one of the most pervasive neurological disorders affecting mammals, with a prevalence in domestic dogs of ~0.6–1%, and an estimated 1–3%

prevalence in the human population. Spontaneous seizures in companion animals demonstrate good construct validity, with the etiologies of canine epilepsies being broad and representative of what is observed in humans. Brain tumors, encephalitides, neurodegenerative diseases, stroke, and traumatic brain injury are common causes of structural/metabolic epilepsies, and confirmed and suspected gene mutations have been observed in cases of idiopathic/genetic epilepsies. A robust body of literature has documented the etiologic, epidemiologic, pharmacologic, and electrophysiologic similarities that exist between human and canine epilepsies. These studies indicate that canine epilepsies demonstrate considerable seizure phenotypic and electroencephalographic (EEG) face validity with humans, encompassing numerous focal and generalized epileptic syndromes. Emerging evidence also indicates that epileptic humans and dogs are afflicted by similar cognitive and behavioral symptoms. Although much less is known about the neuropathology of the majority of companion animal epilepsies, hallmark features of neuronal death, impaired neurogenesis, microglial activation, and blood-brain barrier compromise have been described.

In humans and companion animals, the health burden of epilepsy is significant in terms of its association with chronic disability, premature death, and negative socioeconomic impact.

Nearly 60% of epileptic dogs will experience one or more episodes of status epilepticus (SE) during their lives. SE remains one of the most immediately life-threatening neurological conditions for humans and dogs, with associated mortality rates approaching 25% for both species[108–111].

Treatment for refractory seizures, which are reported in 33% and 25% of epileptic humans and dogs, respectively, is also a significant challenge. Thus, epileptic dog populations offer a unique avenue to investigate the predictive validity of novel anticonvulsant drug, diet, or device candidates using safety, pharmacokinetic, or efficacy end-points in both acute emergent and chronic clinical settings.

Muscular Dystrophies

In Duchenne muscular dystrophy (DMD) patients, one-third of cases are due to de novo mutations in the DMD gene which is composed of 79 exons made up of 2.2 million base pairs. Similarly, DMD mutations within dystrophin-deficient dogs occur spontaneously. Dystrophin-deficient muscular dystrophy in dogs has been reported in several breeds: Alaskan Malamute, Bergamasco, Belgian Groenendael Shepherd, Cavalier King Charles Spaniel, Cocker Spaniel, German Short-Haired Pointer, Golden Retriever, Grand Basset Griffon Vendéen, Irish Terrier, Japanese Spitz, Labrador Retriever, Lurcher siblings, Norfolk Terrier, Old English Sheepdog, Pembroke Welsh Corgi, Rat Terrier, Rottweiler, Tibetan Terrier, Unknown Mix, and Weimaraner. While correlation between incidence of the disease and the particular breed of dog has yet to be determined, it seems that the occurrence of dystrophin deficiency in dogs is unrelated to its genetic background. Additionally, the mutation spectrum is unknown in dystrophin-deficient dogs due to limited numbers of cases and unidentified mutations in most of the affected dogs. A mutation of the canine DMD gene in the Golden Retriever muscular dystrophy (GRMD) has become the most extensively examined and characterized canine model in several institutes. Since then at least nine patterns of spontaneous dystrophin mutations have been reported in different breeds: a large deletion mutation of whole exons in the dystrophin gene of German Short-Haired Pointers, an acceptor splice site mutation of intron 6 in the Golden Retriever, a deletion mutation of exons 8–29 in Tibetan Terriers, long interspersed repetitive element-1 insertion in intron 13 of Pembroke Welsh Corgis, an inversion mutation with a break point in intron 19 of the Japanese Spitz, an insertion of repetitive element in intron 19 of Labrador Retrievers, a point mutation at donor splice site in intron 50 of Cavalier King Charles Spaniels, a nonsense mutation in exon 58 of the Rottweiler and lastly a small deletion mutation of four nucleotides in exon 65 of Cocker Spaniels.

Over the years, several dystrophin-deficient canine models have been established. The GRMD dogs were backcrossed with the Beagle breed by Shimatsu et al. at the National Center of Neurology and Psychiatry (NCNP), Japan, to produce the Canine X-linked muscular dystrophy in Japan (CXMDJ). Although a colony has not been established for DMD-like Cavalier King Charles Spaniel muscular dystrophy (CKCS-MD), another canine model candidate, it has been reported and tested for exon skipping therapy *in vitro*. At Auburn University (United States), a colony of dystrophin-deficient Pembroke Welsh Corgi was established by outbreeding with Beagles. Of the various canine models, GRMD and CXMDJ are currently maintained as active colonies for analysis of muscular dystrophy pathogenesis and new drug development. The biggest advantage of these canine models compared to mouse models is that they show phenotypes closer to human DMD in skeletal muscle and cardiac muscles at a young age. While cardiac symptoms are one of the main causes of death for human patients, mouse models do not show severe cardiac symptoms. On the other hand, GRMD and CXMDJ models show severe clinical symptoms such as body wide muscle weakness and cardiac symptoms. They also show various human DMD-like phenotypes such as joint contracture and kyphosis. The early onset of disease phenotypes in GRMD and CXMDJ enables more detailed analysis such as clinical grading, magnetic resonance imaging, electrocardiogram (ECG), and echocardiography. The models also have larger body weights and longer life spans compared to mouse models making them more reflective of human disease for use in toxicological studies. Overall the canine models display more accurate representations of human DMD symptoms compared to the widely used mouse models[112–115].

INFECTIOUS DISEASE

A complex biological system is often required to study the myriad of host-pathogen interactions associated with infectious diseases, especially since the current basis of biology has reached the molecular level. The use of animal models is important for understanding the very complex temporal relationships that occur in infectious disease involving the body, its neuroendocrine and immune systems, and the infectious organism. Because of these complex interactions, the choice of animal model must be a thoughtful and clearly defined process in order to provide relevant, translatable scientific data and to ensure the most beneficial use of the animals. While many animals respond similarly to humans from physiological, pathological, and therapeutic perspectives, there are also significant species-by-species differences. A well-designed animal model requires a thorough understanding of similarities and differences in the responses between humans and animals and incorporates that knowledge into the goals of the study. Determining the intrinsic and extrinsic factors associated with the disease and creating a biological information matrix to compare the animal model and human disease courses is a useful tool to help choose the appropriate animal model. Confidence in the correlation of results from a model to the human disease can be achieved only if the relationship of the model to the human disease is well understood[116,117].

As an example, canine oral papillomavirus (COPV) causes florid warty lesions in the mucosa of the oral cavity within 4–8 weeks post exposure in experimental settings. The mucosatrophic nature of these viruses and the resulting oropharyngeal papillomas that are morphologically similar to human vaginal papillomas caused by HPV-6 and HPV-11 make this a useful model. These lesions typically spontaneously regress 4–8 weeks after appearing; this model is therefore useful in understanding the interplay between the host immune defense and viral pathogenesis. Male and female Beagles, aged 10 weeks to 2 years, with no history of COPV, are typically used for these studies. Infection is achieved by the application of a 10 ml droplet of virus extract to multiple 0.5 cm^2 scarified areas within the mucosa of the upper lip of anesthetized beagles.

Pain

Chronic pain is common in companion animals such as dogs and cats, and associated with the same diseases as in people, for example OA, osteosarcoma, intervertebral disk disease. Carefully studying novel interventions in these companion animals, using validated outcome measures, has the potential to lead to important pain treatment breakthroughs for both species. Most drugs fail in the transition from safety-focused studies to efficacy-focused studies, suggesting that proof-of-efficacy studies could be performed in companion animals at the same time as safety studies in humans, or even earlier, following basic preclinical safety profiling. Information gained could help in determining the go/no-go decision prior to expensive human clinical trials. However, if spontaneous disease models in companion animals are to be successfully used in translational research, outcome measures of the many dimensions of pain, reflecting the complexity of the disease in humans, need to be well developed, and their use needs to be feasible. Outcome measures related to pain in companion animal OA have been particularly well developed, and these spontaneous models can be used to gain translational advantages in the field of OA pain research[118–121].

Biomechanically, structurally, histologically, genomically, and molecularly human and canine OA are similar. OA in cats also appears to be very similar to the human condition. Estimates of the number of dogs with clinical signs associated with OA are 20% of the population, translating to at least 15 million dogs in the United States alone. Recent studies have indicated that up to 93% of all cats have radiographic signs of OA, and it is estimated that about half of these have clinical signs associated with the condition. OA in companion animals is often initiated early in life, with pets generally presenting at a more advanced age for clinical signs, for example in a recent clinical study involving dogs with OA, the mean ages were 7 to 9 years old. Overall, outcome measures for OA pain are very well developed in the dog although less so in the cat. The effects of joint pain can be measured in both species by measuring changes in limb use (kinetic variables) using force plates or pressure-sensitive walkways. Kinetic evaluation of parameters such as peak vertical force and vertical impulse have been able to detect the analgesic effects of non-steroidal anti-inflammatories in dogs.

ORAL HEALTH/DENTISTRY

In the dental research fields, such as in the field of periodontics, dogs, especially captive Beagle dogs, have been extensively utilized to elucidate mechanisms of periodontal disease due to their similarity to human periodontal tissues and tooth sizes[122,123]. Although differences exist, such as not having occlusal contacts in the premolar teeth or open contacts between the teeth, the prevalence of gingivitis and periodontitis increases in severity with age in dogs even faster than in humans with similar etiologic factors. Studies in Beagle dogs have shown using a plaque-induced model, Beagle dogs develop calculus, have loss of attachment or periodontal tissue breakdown, and bone loss. Experimental periodontitis induced by ligatures in Beagle dogs has revealed osteoclasts appearing during later stages of inflammation and that IL-11 is capable of slowing the progression of attachment and bone loss.

Although these studies have provided useful information to the field of periodontics, considering the life span of Beagle dogs to be 11–12 years, with 10% survival age about 16 years, the majority of these studies suffer from the same limitations of those performed in mice, in that they have been performed on young animals.

LEADING CAUSES OF MORBIDITY AND MORTALITY OF COMPANION ANIMALS

From 1995 to the present, Agria Insurance, Sweden, has provided data on both health care and life insurance claims for descriptive and analytical research[124–129]. Over the periods studied most extensively, 1995–2002 for dogs, 1997–2004 for horses, and 1999–2006 for cats, Agria has insured approximately 200,000 dogs, 100,000 horses, and up to 200,000 cats per year. Estimates based on formal research or market surveys suggest that Agria insures approximately 40% of both the Swedish dog and horse populations and 50% of the purebred cat population. Where animal insurance is so widely embraced, the Agria-insured populations are likely to be representative of the national population.

An increase in survival over the years for dogs and cats is undoubtedly affected by owner, societal, and veterinary factors relative to the availability of, and willingness and ability to, access, and continue, veterinary care. In addition, marked differences in survival across breeds suggest that comparisons between people and companion animals in terms of health, disease, and longevity must consider these complexities.

For many disease conditions the risk of death increases with age. This can be seen in the overall pattern of death with age for males and females. An important consideration when considering age effects in dogs is the extreme differences between breeds. The average yearly mortality among life-insured dogs (10 years of age and younger) was approximately 4% yearly. However, among the 100 most common breeds of dogs (those with at least 250 dogs at risk yearly) the risk ranged from 0.6% per year to over 18%.

One way of looking at the age pattern is to examine survival analysis of the proportion of animals surviving to various ages. Overall in the insured population, they found a small but statistically significant increase from 64% to 68% of dogs surviving to 10 years of age in the period 1999–2002 compared with 1995–1998. This rather unexpected result coincided with an increase in the risk of dogs having at least one veterinary care event (a veterinary visit that exceeded the deductible). Similar differences were seen in many, but not all, breeds.

One could hypothesize that as more dogs receive veterinary care, the longer they live. It is likely that the statistics reflect a societal shift to accessing more care and/or instituting or continuing treatment for older dogs. Interestingly, pain management pharmaceuticals (e.g. non-steroidal anti-inflammatory drugs; NSAIDS) specifically for dogs became available in Sweden in 1998–1999. It is possible that improved quality of life in ageing animals had an influence on the survival statistics.

Another way of examining survival is to look at conditional survival. For example, in these data, a Bernese Mountain Dog that was alive at 8 years of age had a 50% chance of being dead by 10 years of age, whereas for Border Collies the risk was less than 10%. It is clear that, regardless of calendar age, the biological age across breeds is very different and health control programs with age-based recommendations that target all dogs without reference to specific breeds are likely unsupportable.

There has been an overall decrease in deaths before 10 years of age, with an increase in the percentage of dogs with at least one veterinary care event in 1999–2002 compared with 1995–1998. How much this reflects owner/societal attitudes about accessing care can only be hypothesized. Deaths due to traumatic causes decrease with age. Inflammatory problems are high in the very young, lower in dogs 2–4 years of age, and then increase with age. In the Swedish dog population, pyometra is the most common cause of disease in female dogs and accounts for some of this pattern. However, diseases such as outer ear infection and pyoderma have rather similar patterns. The decrease at the highest ages is likely due, at least partly, to owner decisions about care. Patterns of disease also vary by body system. Dogs display a similar U-shaped pattern for respiratory disease as is seen in man and other species with younger and older animals at an increased risk of infectious respiratory disease as the result of immunoincompetency.

In a study from North American teaching hospitals, young dogs died more commonly of gastrointestinal and infectious causes, whereas older dogs died of neurologic and neoplastic causes. Increasing age was associated with an increasing risk of death because of cardiovascular, endocrine, and urogenital causes, but not because of hematopoietic or musculoskeletal causes. Dogs of larger breeds died more commonly of musculoskeletal and gastrointestinal causes, whereas dogs of smaller breeds died more commonly of endocrine causes. Cats insured at Agria are relatively representative of the purebred cat population in Sweden, with the limitation that cats over 13 years of age are not included, and the median age of death is >12.5 years. The life-insured domestic cats are likely not representative of the total population of owned domestic cats in Sweden. The overall mortality varied with age and breed but not with sex. Cause-specific mortality varied with age and breed. Urinary problems, trauma, neoplasia, infections, and cardiovascular problems were the five most common categories of causes of death. The fact that the overall survival rate increased with time period likely reflects both a willingness to keep pet cats longer and the increased level of veterinary care.

THE ROLE OF NUTRITION

Dogs and cats are outbred animals that are willing to consume a consistent diet for long periods, so are ideal candidates for prospective studies of naturally occurring disease[130–135]. In some studies, the effect of diet on survival has been substantial. Food restriction, for example, slows the development of osteoarthritis and increases the life span of Labrador Retrievers by 2 years, protein (P) and P restriction more than doubles the median survival time of dogs and cats with chronic kidney disease, and adding n-3 fats and arginine to the diet of dogs with stage 3 lymphoma improves median survival time by one quarter. Obesity is also very common in both dogs and cats and is also associated with disease as in human subjects. When interpreting these results, however, it is essential to take into account pathophysiological differences among species. Dogs and cats do not display all the characteristics of metabolic disease seen in human subjects; dogs and cats metabolize fat well and atherosclerosis and cardiac infarction are uncommon. Such differences should not, however, preclude further study because differences among species often clarify knowledge. Monitoring of disease in companion animals may also provide a surveillance system for the safety of the food supply, as illustrated by recent outbreaks of acute renal failure and liver failure in cats and dogs in the United States caused respectively by melamine and mycotoxin contamination of pet foods.

AGING

Dogs have been used in the recent past as subjects for intervention studies in two main contexts that are highly relevant for aging and aging-associated diseases[136–139]. The first of these is calorie restriction. Given the pattern of parallel evolution of the digestive physiology in man and dogs, the results of dietary manipulations in dogs have a particularly high translational value. Reduction of calorie intake without malnutrition is a well-established protocol to prolong the life span of laboratory rodents, and to delay the onset of a large number of age-associated conditions. Later studies showed, however, that responses to calorie restriction depend on the genetic background, which introduces a confounding effect in rodent studies. Whether calorie restrictions would elicit the same effects in larger mammals, and ultimately humans, has remained unanswered for a long time, and is partially still a matter of speculation. In the mid-1980s, a calorie restriction experiment in dogs was launched roughly in coincidence with the launch of primate calorie restriction trials that are partially still ongoing. This study demonstrated that a 25% food restriction induced a significant life span extension, coupled with improvements in glucose homeostasis. This study showed for the first time that calorie restriction can prolong the life span of a mammalian species, the size and diet of which is more comparable to humans, and also showed the potential of longitudinal observations in dogs. A major drawback for the study was that it was based on Labrador Retrievers, which is a breed known to be highly prone to obesity, as of all the dog breeds for which data have been reported, Labrador Retrievers have the greatest documented prevalence of obesity. This is partially because they carry a loss-of-function mutation in the proopiomelanocortin (POMC) gene, which codes for an anorexigenic peptide that is a key component of the core appetite control pathway. It is therefore of great importance to repeat similar experiments in other breeds or in mongrels. However, the link between weight and mortality is not linear; in particular, the relationship between all-cause mortality and body mass index defines a U-shaped curve, which indicates that extreme leanness as well as obesity tends to be associated with increased mortality. Furthermore, a number of other dietary manipulations that are more feasible in a translational context have recently emerged, such as alternate fasting (e.g. two non-consecutive fasting days per week), periodic fasting (e.g. a few consecutive days of fasting every few months), and the use of fasting-mimicking diets.

REFERENCES

1. van der Worp HB, Howells DW, Sena ES, Porritt MJ, Rewell S, O'Collins V, Macleod MR. Can animal models of disease reliably inform human studies? *PLoS Med* 2010 Mar 30;7(3):e1000245.
2. McGonigle P, Ruggeri B. Animal models of human disease: Challenges in enabling translation. *Biochem Pharmacol* 2014 Jan 1;87(1):162–171.
3. Schoenebeck JJ, Ostrander EA. Insights into morphology and disease from the dog genome project. *Annu Rev Cell Dev Biol* 2014;30:535–560.
4. Olson PN, Ganzert RR. A new medical research model: Ethically and responsibly advancing health for humans and animals. *Annu Rev Anim Biosci* 2015;3:265–282.
5. Bon C, Toutain PL, Concordet D, Gehring R, Martin-Jimenez T, Smith J, Pelligand L, Martinez M, Whittem T, Riviere JE, Mochel JP. Mathematical modeling and simulation in animal health. Part III: Using nonlinear mixed-effects to characterize and quantify variability in drug pharmacokinetics. *J Vet Pharmacol Ther* 2018 Apr;41(2):171–183.

6. Kol A, Arzi B, Athanasiou KA, Farmer DL, Nolta JA, Rebhun RB, Chen X, Griffiths LG, Verstraete FJ, Murphy CJ, Borjesson DL. Companion animals: Translational scientist's new best friends. *Sci Transl Med* 2015 Oct 7;7(308):308ps2.
7. Dickinson PA, Kesisoglou F, Flanagan T, Martinez MN, Mistry HB, Crison JR, Polli JE, Cruañes MT, Serajuddin ATM, Müllertz A, Cook JA, Selen A. Optimizing clinical drug product performance: Applying biopharmaceutics risk assessment roadmap (BioRAM) and the BioRAM scoring grid. *J Pharm Sci* 2016 Nov;105(11):3243–3255.
8. Wendler A, Wehling M. Translatability score revisited: Differentiation for distinct disease areas. *J Transl Med* 2017 Nov 3;15(1):226.
9. van Steenbeek FG, Hytönen MK, Leegwater PA, Lohi H. The canine era: The rise of a biomedical model. *Anim Genet* 2016 Oct;47(5):519–527.
10. Bentley RT, Ahmed AU, Yanke AB, Cohen-Gadol AA, Dey M. Dogs are man's best friend: In sickness and in health. *Neuro Oncol* 2017 Mar 1;19(3):312–322.
11. Adin CA, Gilor C. The diabetic dog as a translational model for human islet transplantation. *Yale J Biol Med* 2017 Sep 25;90(3):509–515.
12. Vrabelova D, Adin C, Gilor C, Rajab A. Pancreatic islet transplantation: From dogs to humans and back again. *Vet Surg* 2014 Aug;43(6):631–641.
13. Peterson ME. Animal models of disease: Feline hyperthyroidism: An animal model for toxic nodular goiter. *J Endocrinol* 2014 Nov;223(2):T97–114.
14. Bianchi M, Dahlgren S, Massey J, Dietschi E, Kierczak M, Lund-Ziener M, Sundberg K, Thoresen SI, Kämpe O, Andersson G, Ollier WE. A multi-breed genome-wide association analysis for canine hypothyroidism identifies a shared major risk locus on CFA12. *PLoS One* 2015;10(8): e0134720.
15. Castillo VA, Gallelli MF. Corticotroph adenoma in the dog: Pathogenesis and new therapeutic possibilities. *Res Vet Sci* 2010 Feb;88(1):26–32.
16. Galac S, Korpershoek E. Pheochromocytomas and paragangliomas in humans and dogs. *Vet Comp Oncol* 2017 Dec;15(4):1158–1170.
17. Galac S. Cortisol-secreting adrenocortical tumours in dogs and their relevance for human medicine. *Mol Cell Endocrinol* 2016 Feb 5;421:34–39.
18. Galac S, Wilson DB. Animal models of adrenocortical tumorigenesis. *Endocrinol Metab Clin North Am* 2015 Jun;44(2):297–310.
19. Miller MA, Bruyette DS, Scott-Moncrieff JC, Owen TJ, Ramos-Vara JA, Weng HY, Vanderpool AL, Chen AV, Martin LG, DuSold DM, Jahan S. Histopathologic findings in canine pituitary glands. *Vet Pathol* 2018 Nov;55(6):871–879.
20. Miller MA, Owen TJ, Bruyette DS, Scott-Moncrieff JC, Ramos-Vara JA, Weng HY, Chen AV, Martin LG, DuSold DM. Immunohistochemical evaluation of canine pituitary adenomas obtained by transsphenoidal hypophysectomy. *Vet Pathol* 2018 Nov;55(6):889–895.
21. Sanders K, Kooistra HS, Galac S. Treating canine Cushing's syndrome: Current options and future prospects. *Vet J* 2018 Nov;241:42–51.
22. Klein SC, Peterson ME. Canine hypoadrenocorticism: Part I. *Can Vet J* 2010 Jan;51(1):63–69.
23. Klein SC, Peterson ME. Canine hypoadrenocorticism: Part II. *Can Vet J* 2010 Feb;51(2):179–184.
24. Scudder CJ, Mirczuk SM, Richardson KM, Crossley VJ, Regan JTC, Gostelow R, Forcada Y, Hazuchova K, Harrington N, McGonnell IM, Church DB, Kenny PJ, Korbonits M, Fowkes RC, Niessen SJM. Pituitary pathology and gene expression in acromegalic cats. *J Endocr Soc* 2018 Oct 16;3(1):181–200.
25. Borgeat K, Niessen SJM, Wilkie L, Harrington N, Church DB, Luis Fuentes V, Connolly DJ. Time spent with cats is never wasted: Lessons learned from feline

acromegalic cardiomyopathy, a naturally occurring animal model of the human disease. *PLoS One* 2018 Mar 29;13(3):e0194342.

26. Schulman RL. Feline primary hyperaldosteronism. *Vet Clin North Am Small Anim Pract* 2010 Mar;40(2):353–359.

27. Djajadiningrat-Laanen S, Galac S, Kooistra H. Primary hyperaldosteronism: Expanding the diagnostic net. *J Feline Med Surg* 2011 Sep;13(9):641–650.

28. Javadi S, Djajadiningrat-Laanen SC, Kooistra HS, van Dongen AM, Voorhout G, van Sluijs FJ, van den Ingh TS, Boer WH, Rijnberk A. Primary hyperaldosteronism, a mediator of progressive renal disease in cats. *Domest Anim Endocrinol* 2005 Jan;28(1):85–104.

29. Bartges J, Kushner RF, Michel KE, Sallis R, Day MJ. One health solutions to obesity in people and their pets. *J Comp Pathol* 2017 May;156(4):326–333.

30. Raubenheimer D, Machovsky-Capuska GE, Gosby AK, Simpson S. Nutritional ecology of obesity: From humans to companion animals. *Br J Nutr* 2015 Jan;113(Suppl):S26–39.

31. Zaragoza C, Gomez-Guerrero C, Martin-Ventura JL, Blanco-Colio L, Lavin B, Mallavia B, Tarin C, Mas S, Ortiz A, Egido J. Animal models of cardiovascular diseases. *J Biomed Biotechnol* 2011;2011:497841.

32. Boland MR, Kraus MS, Dziuk E, Gelzer AR. Cardiovascular disease risk varies by birth month in canines. *Sci Rep* 2018 May 17;8(1):7130.

33. England J, Loughna S, Rutland CS. Multiple species comparison of cardiac troponin T and dystrophin: Unravelling the DNA behind dilated cardiomyopathy. *J Cardiovasc Dev Dis* 2017 Jul 7;4(3):8.

34. Simpson S, Edwards J, Ferguson-Mignan TF, Cobb M, Mongan NP, Rutland CS. Genetics of human and canine dilated cardiomyopathy. *Int J Genomics* 2015;2015:204823.

35. Kittleson MD, Meurs KM, Harris SP. The genetic basis of hypertrophic cardiomyopathy in cats and humans. *J Vet Cardiol* 2015 Dec;17(Suppl 1):S53–73.

36. Freeman LM, Rush JE, Stern JA, Huggins GS, Maron MS. Feline hypertrophic cardiomyopathy: A spontaneous large animal model of human HCM. *Cardiol Res* 2017 Aug;8(4):139–142.

37. Duncker DJ, Bakkers J, Brundel BJ, Robbins J, Tardiff JC, Carrier L. Animal and in silico models for the study of sarcomeric cardiomyopathies. *Cardiovasc Res* 2015 Apr 1;105(4):439–448.

38. Prat V, Rozec B, Gauthier C, Lauzier B. Human heart failure with preserved ejection versus feline cardiomyopathy: What can we learn from both veterinary and human medicine? *Heart Fail Rev* 2017 Nov;22(6):783–794.

39. Vischer AS, Connolly DJ, Coats CJ, Fuentes VL, McKenna WJ, Castelletti S, Pantazis AA. Arrhythmogenic right ventricular cardiomyopathy in Boxer dogs: The diagnosis as a link to the human disease. *Acta Myol* 2017 Sep 1;36(3):135–150.

40. Urfer SR, Kaeberlein TL, Mailheau S, Bergman PJ, Creevy KE, Promislow DE, Kaeberlein M. Asymptomatic heart valve dysfunction in healthy middle-aged companion dogs and its implications for cardiac aging. *GeroScience* 2017 Feb;39(1):43–50.

41. Ver Heul A, Planer J, Kau AL. The human microbiota and asthma. *Clin Rev Allergy Immunol* 2019 Dec;57(3):350–363.

42. Reinero CR, DeClue AE, Rabinowitz P. Asthma in humans and cats: Is there a common sensitivity to aeroallegens in shared environments? *Environ Res* 2009 Jul;109(5):634–640.

43. Clercx C, Fastrès A, Roels E. Idiopathic pulmonary fibrosis in West Highland white terriers: An update. *Vet J* 2018 Dec;242:53–58.

44. Tashiro J, Rubio GA, Limper AH, Williams K, Elliot SJ, Ninou I, Aidinis V, Tzouvelekis A, Glassberg MK. Exploring animal models that resemble idiopathic pulmonary fibrosis. *Front Med (Lausanne)* 2017 Jul 28;4:118.

45. Geddes RF, Finch NC, Syme HM, Elliott J. The role of phosphorus in the pathophysiology of chronic kidney disease. *J Vet Emerg Crit Care (San Antonio)* 2013 Mar–Apr;23(2):122–133.

46. Klosterman ES, Pressler BM. Nephrotic syndrome in dogs: Clinical features and evidence-based treatment considerations. *Top Companion Anim Med* 2011 Aug;26(3):135–142.

47. Lawson J, Elliott J, Wheeler-Jones C, Syme H, Jepson R. Renal fibrosis in feline chronic kidney disease: Known mediators and mechanisms of injury. *Vet J* 2015 Jan;203(1):18–26.

48. Garden OA, Pinheiro D, Cunningham F. All creatures great and small: Regulatory T cells in mice, humans, dogs and other domestic animal species. *Int Immunopharmacol* 2011 May;11(5):576–588.

49. Day MJ. Ageing, immunosenescence and inflammageing in the dog and cat. *J Comp Pathol* 2010 Jan;142(Suppl 1):S60–69.

50. Axiak-Bechtel SM, Maitz CA, Selting KA, Bryan JN. Preclinical imaging and treatment of cancer: The use of animal models beyond rodents. *Q J Nucl Med Mol Imaging* 2015 Sep;59(3):303–316.

51. National Cancer Policy Forum; Board on Health Care Services; Institute of Medicine; National Academies of Sciences, Engineering, and Medicine. *The Role of Clinical Studies for Pets with Naturally Occurring Tumors in Translational Cancer Research: Workshop Summary*. Washington (DC): National Academies Press (US); 2015.

52. National Cancer Policy Forum; Board on Health Care Services; Institute of Medicine; National Academies of Sciences, Engineering, and Medicine. *The Role of Clinical Studies for Pets with Naturally Occurring Tumors in Translational Cancer Research: Workshop Summary*. Washington (DC): National Academies Press (US). PMID: 26803853.

53. Garden OA, Volk SW, Mason NJ, Perry JA. Companion animals in comparative oncology: One Medicine in action. *Vet J* 2018 Oct;240:6–13.

54. Gardner HL, Fenger JM, London CA. Dogs as a model for cancer. *Annu Rev Anim Biosci* 2016;4:199–222.

55. Willmann M, Hadzijusufovic E, Hermine O, Dacasto M, Marconato L, Bauer K, Peter B, Gamperl S, Eisenwort G, Jensen-Jarolim E, Müller M, Arock M, Vail DM, Valent P. Comparative oncology: The paradigmatic example of canine and human mast cell neoplasms. *Vet Comp Oncol* 2019 Mar;17(1):1–10.

56. Kieslinger M, Swoboda A, Kramer N, Pratscher B, Wolfesberger B, Burgener IA. Companion animals as models for inhibition of STAT3 and STAT5. *Cancers (Basel)* 2019 Dec 17;11(12):E2035.

57. Nolan MW, Kent MS, Boss MK. Emerging translational opportunities in comparative oncology with companion canine cancers: Radiation oncology. *Front Oncol* 2019 Nov 22;9:1291.

58. Gingrich AA, Modiano JF, Canter RJ. Characterization and potential applications of dog natural killer cells in cancer immunotherapy. *J Clin Med* 2019 Oct 27;8(11):1802.

59. Tarone L, Barutello G, Iussich S, Giacobino D, Quaglino E, Buracco P, Cavallo F, Riccardo F. Naturally occurring cancers in pet dogs as pre-clinical models for cancer immunotherapy. *Cancer Immunol Immunother* 2019 Nov;68(11): 1839–1853.

60. Børresen B, Hansen AE, Kjaer A, Andresen TL, Kristensen AT. Liposome- encapsulated chemotherapy: Current evidence for its use in companion animals. *Vet Comp Oncol* 2018 Mar;16(1):E1–15.

61. Goebel K, Merner ND. A monograph proposing the use of canine mammary tumours as a model for the study of hereditary breast cancer susceptibility genes in humans. Version 2. *Vet Med Sci* 2017 Mar 21;3(2):51–62.

62. Adega F, Borges A, Chaves R. Cat mammary tumors: Genetic models for the human counterpart. *Vet Sci* 2016 Aug 16;3(3):17.

63. Harman RM, Curtis TM, Argyle DJ, Coonrod SA, Van de Walle GR. A comparative study on the *in vitro* effects of the DNA methyltransferase Inhibitor 5-azacytidine (5-AzaC) in breast/mammary cancer of different mammalian species. *J Mammary Gland Biol Neoplasia* 2016 Jun;21(1–2):51–66.

64. Paterson YZ, Kafarnik C, Guest DJ. Characterization of companion animal pluripotent stem cells. *Cytom A* 2018 Jan;93(1):137–148.

65. Park JS, Withers SS, Modiano JF, Kent MS, Chen M, Luna JI, Culp WTN, Sparger EE, Rebhun RB, Monjazeb AM, Murphy WJ, Canter RJ. Canine cancer immunotherapy studies: Linking mouse and human. *J Immunother Cancer* 2016 Dec 20;4:97.

66. Spugnini EP, Fais S, Azzarito T, Baldi A. Novel instruments for the implementation of electrochemotherapy protocols: From bench side to Veterinary Clinic. *J Cell Physiol* 2017 Mar;232(3):490–495.

67. Hare JI, Lammers T, Ashford MB, Puri S, Storm G, Barry ST. Challenges and strategies in anti-cancer nanomedicine development: An industry perspective. *Adv Drug Deliv Rev* 2017 Jan 1;108:25–38.

68. Nishiya AT, Massoco CO, Felizzola CR, Perlmann E, Batschinski K, Tedardi MV, Garcia JS, Mendonça PP, Teixeira TF, Zaidan Dagli ML. Comparative aspects of canine melanoma. *Vet Sci* 2016 Feb 19;3(1):7.

69. Riccardo F, Aurisicchio L, Impellizeri JA, Cavallo F. The importance of comparative oncology in translational medicine. *Cancer Immunol Immunother* 2015 Feb;64(2):137–148.

70. Cekanova M, Rathore K. Animal models and therapeutic molecular targets of cancer: Utility and limitations. *Drug Des Devel Ther* 2014 Oct 14;8:1911–1921.

71. Alvarez CE. Naturally occurring cancers in dogs: Insights for translational genetics and medicine. *ILAR J* 2014;55(1):16–45.

72. Davis BW, Ostrander EA. Domestic dogs and cancer research: A breed-based genomics approach. *ILAR J* 2014;55(1):59–68.

73. Di Cerbo A, Palmieri B, De Vico G, Iannitti T. Onco-epidemiology of domestic animals and targeted therapeutic attempts: Perspectives on human oncology. *J Cancer Res Clin Oncol* 2014 Nov;140(11):1807–1814.

74. Pinho SS, Carvalho S, Cabral J, Reis CA, Gärtner F. Canine tumors: A spontaneous animal model of human carcinogenesis. *Transl Res* 2012 Mar;159(3):165–172.

75. O'Connor CM, Wilson-Robles H. Developing T cell cancer immunotherapy in the dog with lymphoma. *ILAR J* 2014;55(1):169–181.

76. Zandvliet M. Canine lymphoma: A review. *Vet Q* 2016 Jun;36(2):76–104.

77. Marconato L, Gelain ME, Comazzi S. The dog as a possible animal model for human non-Hodgkin lymphoma: A review. *Hematol Oncol* 2013 Mar;31(1):1–9.

78. Simpson S, Dunning MD, de Brot S, Grau-Roma L, Mongan NP, Rutland CS. Comparative review of human and canine osteosarcoma: Morphology, epidemiology, prognosis, treatment and genetics. *Acta Vet Scand* 2017 Oct 24;59(1):71.

79. Makielski KM, Mills LJ, Sarver AL, Henson MS, Spector LG, Naik S, Modiano JF. Risk factors for development of canine and human osteosarcoma: A comparative review. *Vet Sci* 2019 May 25;6(2):48.

80. Jue TR, McDonald KL. The challenges associated with molecular targeted therapies for glioblastoma. *J Neurooncol* 2016 May;127(3):427–434.

81. Hicks J, Platt S, Kent M, Haley A. Canine brain tumours: A model for the human disease? *Vet Comp Oncol* 2017 Mar;15(1):252–272.

82. MacDiarmid JA, Langova V, Bailey D, Pattison ST, Pattison SL, Christensen N, Armstrong LR, Brahmbhatt VN, Smolarczyk K, Harrison MT, Costa M, Mugridge NB, Sedliarou I, Grimes NA, Kiss DL, Stillman B, Hann CL, Gallia GL, Graham RM, Brahmbhatt H. Targeted doxorubicin delivery to brain tumors via minicells: Proof of principle using dogs with spontaneously occurring tumors as a model. *PLoS One* 2016 Apr 6;11(4):e0151832.

83. Kruitwagen HS, Fieten H, Penning LC. Towards bioengineered liver stem cell transplantation studies in a preclinical dog model for inherited copper toxicosis. *Bioengineering (Basel)* 2019 Sep 25;6(4):88.

84. Wu X, Leegwater PA, Fieten H. Canine models for copper homeostasis disorders. *Int J Mol Sci* 2016 Feb 4;17(2):196.

85. Fieten H, Leegwater PA, Watson AL, Rothuizen J. Canine models of copper toxicosis for understanding mammalian copper metabolism. *Mamm Genome* 2012 Feb;23(1–2):62–75.

86. Favier RP, Spee B, Penning LC, Rothuizen J. Copper-induced hepatitis: The COMMD1 deficient dog as a translational animal model for human chronic hepatitis. *Vet Q* 2011 Mar;31(1):49–60.

87. Nantasanti S, de Bruin A, Rothuizen J, Penning LC, Schotanus BA. Concise review: Organoids are a powerful tool for the study of liver disease and personalized treatment design in humans and animals. *Stem Cells Transl Med* 2016 Mar;5(3):325–330.

88. Gonçalves NN, Ambrósio CE, Piedrahita JA. Stem cells and regenerative medicine in domestic and companion animals: A multispecies perspective. *Reprod Domest Anim* 2014 Oct;49(Suppl 4):2–10.

89. Meneses AMC, Schneeberger K, Kruitwagen HS, Penning LC, van Steenbeek FG, Burgener IA, Spee B. Intestinal organoids-current and future applications. *Vet Sci* 2016 Oct 21;3(4):31.

90. Gootenberg DB, Turnbaugh PJ. Companion animals symposium: Humanized animal models of the microbiome. *J Anim Sci* 2011 May;89(5):1531–1537.

91. Prattis S, Jurjus A. Spontaneous and transgenic rodent models of inflammatory bowel disease. *Lab Anim Res* 2015 Jun;31(2):47–68.

92. Clark LA, Cox ML. Current status of genetic studies of exocrine pancreatic insufficiency in dogs. *Top Companion Anim Med* 2012 Aug;27(3):109–112.

93. Dodi PL. Immune-mediated keratoconjunctivitis sicca in dogs: Current perspectives on management. *Vet Med (Auckl)* 2015 Oct 30;6:341–347.

94. Williams DL. Optimising tear replacement rheology in canine keratoconjunctivitis sicca. *Eye (Lond)* 2018 Feb;32(2):195–199.

95. Williams DL. Immunopathogenesis of keratoconjunctivitis sicca in the dog. *Vet Clin North Am Small Anim Pract* 2008 Mar;38(2):251–268.

96. Park YW, Kim JY, Jeong MB, Kim SH, Yoon J, Seo K. A Retrospective study on the association between vitreous degeneration and cataract in dogs. *Vet Ophthalmol* 2015 Jul;18(4):304–308.

97. Donzel E, Arti L, Chahory S. Epidemiology and clinical presentation of canine cataracts in France: A retrospective study of 404 cases. *Vet Ophthalmol* 2017 Mar;20(2):131–139.

98. Partridge B, Rossmeisl JH Jr. Companion animal models of neurological disease. *J Neurosci Methods* 2020 Feb 1;331:108484.

99. Moore SA, Granger N, Olby NJ, Spitzbarth I, Jeffery ND, Tipold A, Nout-Lomas YS, da Costa RC, Stein VM, Noble-Haeusslein LJ, Blight AR, Grossman RG, Basso DM, Levine JM. Targeting translational successes through CANSORT-SCI: Using pet dogs to identify effective treatments for spinal cord injury. *J Neurotrauma* 2017 Jun 15;34(12):2007–2018.

100. Ohl K, Tenbrock K, Kipp M. Oxidative stress in multiple sclerosis: Central and peripheral mode of action. *Exp Neurol* 2016 Mar;277:58–67.

101. Coates JR, Wininger FA. Canine degenerative myelopathy. *Vet Clin North Am Small Anim Pract* 2010 Sep;40(5):929–950.

102. Nardone R, Höller Y, Taylor AC, Lochner P, Tezzon F, Golaszewski S, Brigo F, Trinka E. Canine degenerative myelopathy: A model of human amyotrophic lateral sclerosis. *Zoology (Jena)* 2016 Feb;119(1):64–73.

103. Gołaszewska A, Bik W, Motyl T, Orzechowski A. Bridging the gap between Alzheimer's disease and Alzheimer's-like diseases in animals. *Int J Mol Sci* 2019 Apr 3;20(7):1664.

104. Rajendran L, Paolicelli RC. Microglia-mediated synapse loss in Alzheimer's disease. *J Neurosci* 2018 Mar 21;38(12):2911–2919.

105. Vanderheyden WM, Lim MM, Musiek ES, Gerstner JR. Alzheimer's disease and sleep-wake disturbances: Amyloid, astrocytes, and animal models. *J Neurosci* 2018 Mar 21;38(12):2901–2910.

106. Laurijssens B, Aujard F, Rahman A. Animal models of Alzheimer's disease and drug development. *Drug Discov Today Technol* 2013 Sep;10(3):e319–327.

107. Minor KM, Letko A, Becker D, Drögemüller M, Mandigers PJJ, Bellekom SR, Leegwater PAJ, Stassen QEM, Putschbach K, Fischer A, Flegel T, Matiasek K, Ekenstedt KJ, Furrow E, Patterson EE, Platt SR, Kelly PA, Cassidy JP, Shelton GD, Lucot K, Bannasch DL, Martineau H, Muir CF, Priestnall SL, Henke D, Oevermann A, Jagannathan V, Mickelson JR, Drögemüller C. Canine NAPEPL associated models of human myelin disorders. *Sci Rep* 2018 Apr 11;8(1):5818.

108. Kitz S, Thalhammer JG, Glantschnigg U, Wrzosek M, Klang A, Halasz P, Shouse MN, Pakozdy A. Feline temporal lobe epilepsy: Review of the experimental literature. *J Vet Intern Med* 2017 May;31(3):633–640.

109. Podell M, Volk HA, Berendt M, Löscher W, Muñana K, Patterson EE, Platt SR. 2015 ACVIM small animal consensus statement on seizure management in dogs. *J Vet Intern Med* 2016 Mar–Apr;30(2):477–490.

110. Charalambous M, Brodbelt D, Volk HA. Treatment in canine epilepsy—A systematic review. *BMC Vet Res* 2014 Oct 22;10:257.

111. De Risio L, Bhatti S, Muñana K, Penderis J, Stein V, Tipold A, Berendt M, Farqhuar R, Fischer A, Long S, Mandigers PJ, Matiasek K, Packer RM, Pakozdy A, Patterson N, Platt S, Podell M, Potschka H, Batlle MP, Rusbridge C, Volk HA. International veterinary epilepsy task force consensus proposal: Diagnostic approach to epilepsy in dogs. *BMC Vet Res* 2015 Aug 28;11:148.

112. Amoasii L, Hildyard JCW, Li H, Sanchez-Ortiz E, Mireault A, Caballero D, Harron R, Stathopoulou TR, Massey C, Shelton JM, Bassel-Duby R, Piercy RJ, Olson EN. Gene editing restores dystrophin expression in a canine model of Duchenne muscular dystrophy. *Science* 2018 Oct 5;362(6410):86–91.

113. Chamberlain JR, Chamberlain JS. Progress toward gene therapy for Duchenne muscular dystrophy. *Mol Ther* 2017 May 3;25(5):1125–1131.

114. Kornegay JN. The golden retriever model of Duchenne muscular dystrophy. *Skelet Muscle* 2017 May 19;7(1):9.

115. Yu X, Bao B, Echigoya Y, Yokota T. Dystrophin-deficient large animal models: Translational research and exon skipping. *Am J Transl Res* 2015 Aug 15;7(8):1314–1331.
116. Day MJ. One health: The importance of companion animal vector-borne diseases. *Parasit Vectors* 2011 Apr 13;4:49.
117. Jacob J, Lorber B. Diseases transmitted by man's best friend: The dog. *Microbiol Spectr* 2015 Aug;3(4). doi:10.1128/microbiolspec.IOL5-0002-2015.
118. Perry JA, Douglas H. Immunomodulatory effects of surgery, pain, and opioids in cancer patients. *Vet Clin North Am Small Anim Pract* 2019 Nov;49(6):981–991.
119. Lascelles BDX, Brown DC, Maixner W, Mogil JS. Spontaneous painful disease in companion animals can facilitate the development of chronic pain therapies for humans. *Osteoarthr Cartil* 2018 Feb;26(2):175–183.
120. Cimino Brown D. What can we learn from osteoarthritis pain in companion animals? *Clin Exp Rheumatol* 2017 Sep–Oct;35(Suppl 107(5)):53–58.
121. Littlewood KE, Mellor DJ. Changes in the welfare of an injured working farm dog assessed using the five domains model. *Animals (Basel)* 2016 Sep 21;6(9):58.
122. Bonner M, Fresno M, Gironès N, Guillén N, Santi-Rocca J. Reassessing the role of Entamoeba gingivalis in periodontitis. *Front Cell Infect Microbiol* 2018 Oct 29;8:379.
123. An JY, Darveau R, Kaeberlein M. Oral Health in geroscience: Animal models and the aging oral cavity. *GeroScience* 2018 Feb;40(1):1–10.
124. Egenvall A, Nødtvedt A, Häggström J, Ström Holst B, Möller L, Bonnett BN. Mortality of life-insured Swedish cats during 1999–2006: Age, breed, sex, and diagnosis. *J Vet Intern Med* 2009 Nov–Dec;23(6):1175–1183.
125. Bonnett BN, Egenvall A. Age patterns of disease and death in insured Swedish dogs, cats and horses. *J Comp Pathol* 2010 Jan;142(Suppl 1):S33–38.
126. Egenvall A, Bonnett BN, Häggström J, Ström Holst B, Möller L, Nødtvedt A. Morbidity of insured Swedish cats during 1999–2006 by age, breed, sex, and diagnosis. *J Feline Med Surg* 2010 Dec;12(12):948–959.
127. Bonnett BN, Egenvall A, Hedhammar A, Olson P. Mortality in over 350,000 insured Swedish dogs from 1995–2000: I. Breed-, gender-, age- and cause-specific rates. *Acta Vet Scand* 2005;46(3):105–120.
128. Egenvall A, Nødtvedt A, Häggström J, Ström Holst B, Möller L, Bonnett BN. Mortality of life-insured Swedish cats during 1999–2006: Age, breed, sex, and diagnosis. *J Vet Intern Med* 2009 Nov–Dec;23(6):1175–1183.
129. Egenvall A, Bonnett BN, Hedhammar A, Olson P. Mortality in over 350,000 insured Swedish dogs from 1995–2000: II. Breed-specific age and survival patterns and relative risk for causes of death. *Acta Vet Scand* 2005;46(3):121–136.
130. Carlos G, Dos Santos FP, Fröehlich PE. Canine metabolomics advances. *Metabolomics* 2020 Jan 18;16(2):16.
131. Román GC, Jackson RE, Gadhia R, Román AN, Reis J. Mediterranean diet: The role of long-chain ω-3 fatty acids in fish; polyphenols in fruits, vegetables, cereals, coffee, tea, cacao and wine; probiotics and vitamins in prevention of stroke, age-related cognitive decline, and Alzheimer disease. *Rev Neurol (Paris)* 2019 Dec;175(10):724–741.
132. Hill TL. Gastrointestinal tract dysfunction with critical illness: Clinical assessment and management. *Top Companion Anim Med* 2019 Jun;35:47–52.
133. Buddington RK, Sangild PT. Companion animals symposium: Development of the mammalian gastrointestinal tract, the resident microbiota, and the role of diet in early life. *J Anim Sci* 2011 May;89(5):1506–1519.

134. Hill RC. Conference on "Multidisciplinary approaches to nutritional problems". Symposium on "Nutrition and health". Nutritional therapies to improve health: Lessons from companion animals. *Proc Nutr Soc* 2009 Feb;68(1):98–102.

135. Lawler DF, Larson BT, Ballam JM, Smith GK, Biery DN, Evans RH, Greeley EH, Segre M, Stowe HD, Kealy RD. Diet restriction and ageing in the dog: Major observations over two decades. *Br J Nutr* 2008 Apr;99(4):793–805.

136. Mazzatenta A, Carluccio A, Robbe D, Giulio CD, Cellerino A. The companion dog as a unique translational model for aging. *Semin Cell Dev Biol* 2017 Oct;70:141–153.

137. Kaeberlein M, Creevy KE, Promislow DE. The dog aging project: Translational geroscience in companion animals. *Mamm Genome* 2016 Aug;27(7–8):279–288.

138. Creevy KE, Austad SN, Hoffman JM, O'Neill DG, Promislow DE. The companion dog as a model for the longevity dividend. *Cold Spring Harb Perspect Med* 2016 Jan 4;6(1):a026633.

139. Kaeberlein M. The biology of aging: Citizen scientists and their pets as a bridge Between research on model organisms and human subjects. *Vet Pathol* 2016 Mar;53(2):291–298.

140. Engelhardt, A., K. F. Stock, H. Hamann, R. Brahm, H. Grussendorf, C. U. Rosenhagen, and O. Distl. 2007. "Analysis of systematic and genetic effects on the prevalence of primary cataract, persistent pupillary membrane and distichiasis in the two color variants of English Cocker Spaniels in Germany." *Berl Munch Tierarztl Wochenschr* 120(11–12):490–498.

141. De Risio, L., S. Bhatti, K. Munana, J. Penderis, V. Stein, A. Tipold, M. Berendt, R. Farqhuar, A. Fischer, S. Long, P. J. J. Mandigers, K. Matiasek, R. M. A. Packer, A. Pakozdy, N. Patterson, S. Platt, M. Podell, H. Potschka, M. P. Batlle, C. Rusbridge, and H. A. Volk. 2015. "International veterinary epilepsy task force consensus proposal: Diagnostic approach to epilepsy in dogs." *BMC Vet Res* 11(1). doi:ARTN 148.10.1186/s12917-015-0462-1.

142. Adin, C. A. 2006. "Canine renal transplantation: The next steps." *Vet Surg* 35(2):103–104. doi:10.1111/j.1532-950X.2006.00120.x.

143. Hill, T. L. 2019. "Gastrointestinal tract dysfunction with critical illness: Clinical assessment and management." *Top Companion Anim Med* 35:47–52. doi:10.1053/j.tcam.2019.04.002.

144. Dodi, P. L. 2015. "Immune-mediated keratoconjunctivitis sicca in dogs: Current perspectives on management." *Vet Med (Auckl)* 6:341–347. doi:10.2147/VMRR. S66705.

145. Khan, F. A., C. J. Gartley, and A. Khanam. 2018. "Canine cryptorchidism: An update." *Reprod Domest Anim* 53(6):1263–1270. doi:10.1111/rda.13231.

146. Szczerbal, I., P. Krzeminska, S. Dzimira, T. M. Tamminen, S. Saari, W. Nizanski, M. Gogulski, J. Nowacka-Woszuk, and M. Switonski. 2018. "Disorders of sex development in cats with different complements of sex chromosomes." *Reprod Domest Anim* 53(6):1317–1322. doi:10.1111/rda.13263.

147. Little, S. 2011. "Feline reproduction: Problems and clinical challenges." *J Feline Med Surg* 13(7):508–515. doi:10.1016/j.jfms.2011.05.008.

148. Parry, B. W. 1989. "Laboratory evaluation of hemorrhagic coagulopathies in small animal practice." *Vet Clin North Am Small Anim Pract* 19(4):729–742. doi:10.1016/s0195-5616(89)50081-0.

149. Biezus, G., P. E. Ferian, L. H. H. D. Pereira, J. A. Withoeft, M. M. Antunes, M. G. N. Xavier, J. Volpato, T. G. de Cristo, J. H. Fonteque, and R. A. Casagrande. 2019. "Clinical and haematological disorders in cats with natural and progressive infection by feline leukemia virus (FeLV)." *Acta Sci Vet* 47(1). doi:A RTN1629.10.22456/1679-9216.90027.

150. Orima, H., M. Fujita, S. Aoki, M. Washizu, T. Yamagami, M. Umeda, and M. Sugiyama. 1992. "A case of lobar emphysema in a dog." *J Vet Med Sci* 54(4):797–798. doi:10.1292/jvms.54.797.

151. Freeman, L. M., J. E. Rush, J. A. Stern, G. S. Huggins, and M. S. Maron. 2017. "Feline hypertrophic cardiomyopathy: A spontaneous large animal model of human HCM." *Cardiol Res* 8(4):139–142. doi:10.14740/cr578w.

152. Adega, F., A. Borges, and R. Chaves. 2016. "Cat mammary tumors: Genetic models for the human counterpart." *Vet Sci* 3(3). doi:10.3390/vetsci3030017.

153. Fujita, A., M. Tsuboi, K. Uchida, and R. Nishimura. 2016. "Complex malformations of the urogenital tract in a female dog: Gartner duct cyst, ipsilateral renal agenesis, and ipsilateral hydrometra." *Jpn J Vet Res* 64(2):147–152.

154. Clercx, C., and D. Peeters. 2007. "Canine eosinophilic bronchopneumopathy." *Vet Clin North Am Small Anim Pract* 37(5):917–935, vi. doi:10.1016/j.cvsm.2007.05.007.

155. Gootenberg, D. B., and P. J. Turnbaugh. 2011. "Companion animals symposium: Humanized animal models of the microbiome." *J Animal Sci* 89(5):1531–1537. doi:10.2527/jas.2010-3371.

156. Aguirre, G. 1973. "Hereditary retinal diseases in small animals." *Vet Clin North Am* 3(3):515–528. doi:10.1016/s0091-0279(73)50065-0.

157. Naor, A. W., M. J. Wilkerson, M. Meindel, M. Morton, and L. M. Pohlman. 2017. "Pathology in practice. Systemic lupus erythematosus (SLE) in a dog." *J Am Vet Med Assoc* 250(6):627–629. doi:10.2460/javma.250.6.627.

158. Prattis, S., and A. Jurjus. 2015. "Spontaneous and transgenic rodent models of inflammatory bowel disease." *Lab Anim Res* 31(2):47–68. doi:10.5625/lar.2015.31.2.47.

159. Segev, G., L. D. Cowgill, S. Jessen, A. Berkowitz, C. F. Mohr, and I. Aroch. 2012. "Renal amyloidosis in dogs: A retrospective study of 91 cases with comparison of the disease between Shar-Pei and non-Shar-Pei dogs." *J Vet Intern Med* 26(2):259–268. doi:10.1111/j.1939-1676.2011.00878.x.

160. Schrope, D. P., and W. J. Kelch. 2006. "Signalment, clinical signs, and prognostic indicators associated with high-grade second- or third-degree atrioventricular block in dogs: 124 cases (January 1, 1997–December 31, 1997)." *J Am Vet Med Assoc* 228(11):1710–1717. doi:10.2460/javma.228.11.1710.

161. Smith, E. J., D. J. Marcellin-Little, O. L. Harrysson, and E. H. Griffith. 2016. "Influence of chondrodystrophy and brachycephaly on geometry of the humerus in dogs." *Vet Comp Orthop Traumatol* 29(3):220–226. doi:10.3415/VCOT-15-11-0181.

162. Lusson, D., B. Billiemaz, and J. L. Chabanne. 1999. "Circulating lupus anticoagulant and probable systemic lupus erythematosus in a cat." *J Feline Med Surg* 1(3):193–196. doi:10.1016/S1098-612X(99)90208-5.

163. Mai, W., and C. Weisse. 2011. "Contrast-enhanced portal magnetic resonance angiography in dogs with suspected congenital portal vascular anomalies." *Vet Rad Ultrasound* 52(3):284–288. doi:10.1111/j.1740-8261.2010.01771.x.

164. Berry, C. R., and C. W. Lombard. 1986. "ECG of the month. Wolff-Parkinson-White syndrome in a cat." *J Am Vet Med Assoc* 189(12):1542–1543.

165. Ward, J. L., T. C. DeFrancesco, S. P. Tou, C. E. Atkins, E. H. Griffith, and B. W. Keene. 2016. "Outcome and survival in canine sick sinus syndrome and sinus node dysfunction: 93 cases (2002–2014)." *J Vet Cardiol* 18(3):199–212. doi:10.1016/j.jvc.2016.04.004.

166. Degl'Innocenti, S., N. Asiag, O. Zeira, C. Falzone, and C. Cantile. 2017. "Neuroaxonal dystrophy and cavitating leukoencephalopathy of Chihuahua dogs." *Vet Pathol* 54(5):832–837. doi:10.1177/0300985817712557.

167. Lawler, D. F., B. T. Larson, J. M. Ballam, G. K. Smith, D. N. Biery, R. H. Evans, E. H. Greeley, M. Segre, H. D. Stowe, and R. D. Kealy. 2008. "Diet restriction and ageing in the dog: Major observations over two decades." *Br J Nutr* 99(4):793–805. doi:10.1017/S0007114507871686.

168. Mazzatenta, A., A. Carluccio, D. Robbe, C. Di Giulio, and A. Cellerino. 2017. "The companion dog as a unique translational model for aging." *Semin Cell Dev Biol* 70:141–153. doi:10.1016/j.semcdb.2017.08.024.

169. Norris, C. R., and V. F. Samii. 2000. "Clinical, radiographic, and pathologic features of bronchiectasis in cats: 12 cases (1987–1999)." *J Am Vet Med Assoc* 216(4):530–534. doi:10.2460/javma.2000.216.530.

170. Hosoya, K., S. Takagi, and M. Okumura. 2013. "Iatrogenic tumor seeding after ureteral stenting in a dog with urothelial carcinoma." *J Am Anim Hosp Assoc* 49(4):262–266. doi:10.5326/JAAHA-MS-5865.

171. Smith, K. F., R. L. Quinn, and L. J. Rahilly. 2015. "Biomarkers for differentiation of causes of respiratory distress in dogs and cats: Part 1--Cardiac diseases and pulmonary hypertension." *J Vet Emerg Crit Care (San Antonio)* 25(3):311–329. doi:10.1111/vec.12318.

172. Marconato, L., M. E. Gelain, and S. Comazzi. 2013. "The dog as a possible animal model for human non-Hodgkin lymphoma: A review." *Hematol Oncol* 31(1):1–9. doi:10.1002/hon.2017.

173. Aitken, M. M. 2019. "Treating rheumatoid arthritis in dogs." *Vet Rec* 185(3):86–87. doi:10.1136/vr.14704.

174. Kittleson, M. D., K. M. Meurs, and S. P. Harris. 2015. "The genetic basis of hypertrophic cardiomyopathy in cats and humans." *J Vet Cardiol* 17:S53–73. doi:10.1016/j.jvc.2015.03.001.

175. Kaszak, I., A. Ruszczak, S. Kanafa, K. Kacprzak, M. Krol, and P. Jurka. 2018. "Current biomarkers of canine mammary tumors." *Acta Vet Scand* 60(1):66. doi:10.1186/s13028-018-0417-1.

176. Dewey, C. W., E. Davies, and J. L. Bouma. 2016. "Kyphosis and kyphoscoliosis associated with congenital malformations of the thoracic vertebral bodies in dogs." *Vet Clin North Am Small Anim Pract* 46(2):295–306. doi:10.1016/j.cvsm.2015.10.009.

177. Churcher, R. K., and A. D. Watson. 1997. "Canine histiocytic ulcerative colitis." *Aust Vet J* 75(10):710–713. doi:10.1111/j.1751-0813.1997.tb12250.x.

178. O'Neill, D. G., A. Riddell, D. B. Church, L. Owen, D. C. Brodbelt, and J. L. Hall. 2017. "Urinary incontinence in bitches under primary veterinary care in England: Prevalence and risk factors." *J Small Anim Pract* 58(12):685–693. doi:10.1111/jsap.12731.

179. Gelberg, H. B., and K. McEntee. 1985. "Feline ovarian neoplasms." *Vet Pathol* 22(6):572–576. doi:10.1177/030098588502200610.

180. Chamberlain, J. R., and J. S. Chamberlain. 2017. "Progress toward gene therapy for Duchenne muscular dystrophy." *Mol Ther* 25(5):1125–1131. doi:10.1016/j.ymthe.2017.02.019.

181. Gershwin, L. J. 2018. "Current and newly emerging autoimmune diseases." *Vet Clin North Am Small Anim Pract* 48(2):323–338. doi:10.1016/j.cvsm.2017.10.010.

182. Pool, R. R., and C. B. Carrig. 1972. "Multiple cartilaginous exostoses in a cat." *Vet Pathol* 9(5):350–359. doi:10.1177/030098587200900505.

183. Bunel, M., G. Chaudieu, C. Hamel, L. Lagoutte, G. Manes, N. Botherel, P. Brabet, P. Pilorge, C. Andre, and P. Quignon. 2019. "Natural models for retinitis pigmentosa: Progressive retinal atrophy in dog breeds." *Hum Genet* 138(5):441–453. doi:10.1007/s00439-019-01999-6.

184. Shelton, G. D. 2016. "Myasthenia gravis and congenital myasthenic syndromes in dogs and cats: A history and mini-review." *Neuromuscul Disord* 26(6):331–334. doi:10.1016/j.nmd.2016.03.002.

185. Jaffey, J. A., G. Bullock, E. Teplin, J. Guo, N. A. Villani, T. Mhlanga-Mutangadura, R. D. Schnabel, L. A. Cohn, and G. S. Johnson. 2019. "A homozygous ADAMTS2 nonsense mutation in a Doberman Pinscher dog with Ehlers Danlos syndrome and extreme skin fragility." *Anim Genet* 50(5):543–545. doi:10.1111/age.12825.

186. Miller, M. A., D. S. Bruyette, J. C. Scott-Moncrieff, T. J. Owen, J. A. Ramos-Vara, H. Y. Weng, A. L. Vanderpool, A. V. Chen, L. G. Martin, D. M. DuSold, and S. Jahan. 2018. "Histopathologic findings in canine pituitary glands." *Vet Pathol* 55(6):871–879. doi:10.1177/0300985818766211.

187. Meekins, J. M. 2015. "Acute blindness." *Top Companion Anim Med* 30(3):118–125. doi:10.1053/j.tcam.2015.07.005.

188. Mueller, R. S., and S. Unterer. 2018. "Adverse food reactions: Pathogenesis, clinical signs, diagnosis and alternatives to elimination diets." *Vet J* 236:89–95. doi:10.1016/j.tvjl.2018.04.014.

189. Gotthelf, L. N. 2004. "Diagnosis and treatment of otitis media in dogs and cats." *Vet Clin North Am Small Anim Pract* 34(2):469–487. doi:10.1016/j.cvsm.2003.10.007.

190. Gow, A. G. 2017. "Hepatic encephalopathy." *Vet Clin North Am Small Anim Pract* 47(3):585–599. doi:10.1016/j.cvsm.2016.11.008.

191. Vanderheyden, W. M., M. M. Lim, E. S. Musiek, and J. R. Gerstner. 2018. "Alzheimer's disease and sleep-wake disturbances: Amyloid, astrocytes, and animal models." *J Neurosci* 38(12):2901–2910. doi:10.1523/Jneurosci.1135-17.2017.

192. Rosenkrantz, W. S. 2004. "Pemphigus: Current therapy." *Vet Dermatol* 15(2):90–98. doi:10.1111/j.1365-3164.2004.00360.x.

193. Devine, L., P. J. Armstrong, J. C. Whittemore, L. Sharkey, N. Bailiff, A. Huang, and M. Rishniw. 2017. "Presumed primary immune-mediated neutropenia in 35 dogs: A retrospective study." *J Small Anim Pract* 58(6):307–313. doi:10.1111/jsap.12636.

194. Kellihan, H. B., and R. L. Stepien. 2010. "Pulmonary hypertension in dogs: Diagnosis and therapy." *Vet Clin North Am Small Anim Pract* 40(4):623–641. doi:10.1016/j.cvsm.2010.03.011.

195. Schulman, R. L. 2010. "Feline primary hyperaldosteronism." *Vet Clin North Am Small Anim Pract* 40(2):353–359. doi:10.1016/j.cvsm.2009.10.006.

196. Rajendran, L., and R. C. Paolicelli. 2018. "Microglia-mediated synapse loss in Alzheimer's disease." *J Neurosci* 38(12):2911–2919. doi:10.1523/Jneurosci.1136-17.2017.

197. Loj, M., M. Garncarz, and M. Jank. 2012. "Genomic and genetic aspects of heart failure in dogs - A review." *Acta Vet Hung* 60(1):17–26. doi:10.1556/AVet.2012.002.

198. Soderstrom, M. J., S. D. Gilson, and N. Gulbas. 1995. "Fatal reexpansion pulmonary edema in a kitten following surgical correction of pectus excavatum." *J Am Anim Hosp Assoc* 31(2):133–136. doi:10.5326/15473317-31-2-133.

199. Prat, V., B. Rozec, C. Gauthier, and B. Lauzier. 2017. "Human heart failure with preserved ejection versus feline cardiomyopathy: What can we learn from both veterinary and human medicine?" *Heart Fail Rev* 22(6):783–794. doi:10.1007/s10741-017-9645-0.

200. Terragni, R., M. Vignoli, H. J. van Bree, L. Gaschen, and J. H. Saunders. 2014. "Diagnostic imaging and endoscopic finding in dogs and cats with gastric tumors: A review." *Schweiz Arch Tierheilkd* 156(12):569–576. doi:10.1024/0036-7281/a000652.

201. Sparkes, A. 2018. "Understanding feline idiopathic cystitis." *Vet Rec* 182(17):486. doi:10.1136/vr.k1848.

202. Kruitwagen, H. S., H. Fieten, and L. C. Penning. 2019. "Towards bioengineered liver stem cell transplantation studies in a preclinical dog model for inherited copper toxicosis." *Bioengineering (Basel)* 6(4). doi:10.3390/bioengineering6040088.
203. Bianchi, M., S. Dahlgren, J. Massey, E. Dietschi, M. Kierczak, M. Lund-Ziener, K. Sundberg, S. I. Thoresen, O. Kampe, G. Andersson, W. E. R. Ollier, A. Hedhammar, T. Leeb, K. Lindblad-Toh, L. J. Kennedy, F. Lingaas, and G. R. Pielberg. 2015. "A multi-breed genome-wide association analysis for canine hypothyroidism identifies a shared major risk locus on CFA12." *PLoS One* 10(8). doi:ARTN, e.0134720.10.1371/Journal.Pone.0134720.
204. Hagman, R. 2018. "Pyometra in small animals." *Vet Clin North Am Small Anim Pract* 48(4):639–661. doi:10.1016/j.cvsm.2018.03.001.
205. Xenoulis, P. G. 2015. "Diagnosis of pancreatitis in dogs and cats." *J Small Anim Pract* 56(1):13–26. doi:10.1111/jsap.12274.
206. Hart, T. M., and C. D. Stauthammer. 2010. "ECG of the month." *JAVMA J Am Vet Med Assoc* 237(6):641–643. doi:10.2460/javma.237.6.641.
207. Raubenheimer, D., G. E. Machovsky-Capuska, A. K. Gosby, and S. Simpson. 2015. "Nutritional ecology of obesity: From humans to companion animals." *Br J Nutr* 113(Suppl):S26–39. doi:10.1017/S0007114514002323.
208. Laurijssens, B., F. Aujard, and A. Rahman. 2013. "Animal models of Alzheimer's disease and drug development." *Drug Discov Today Technol* 10(3):e319–327. doi:10.1016/j.ddtec.2012.04.001.
209. Borns-Weil, S. 2019. "Inappropriate urination." *Vet Clin North Am Small Anim Pract* 49(2):141–155. doi:10.1016/j.cvsm.2018.10.003.
210. MacDiarmid, J. A., V. Langova, D. Bailey, S. T. Pattison, S. L. Pattison, N. Christensen, L. R. Armstrong, V. N. Brahmbhatt, K. Smolarczyk, M. T. Harrison, M. Costa, N. B. Mugridge, I. Sedliarou, N. A. Grimes, D. L. Kiss, B. Stillman, C. L. Hann, G. L. Gallia, R. M. Graham, and H. Brahmbhatt. 2016. "Targeted doxorubicin delivery to brain tumors via minicells: Proof of principle using dogs with spontaneously occurring tumors as a model." *PLoS One* 11(4):e0151832. doi:10.1371/journal.pone.0151832.
211. Makielski, K. M., L. J. Mills, A. L. Sarver, M. S. Henson, L. G. Spector, S. Naik, and J. F. Modiano. 2019. "Risk factors for development of canine and human osteosarcoma: A comparative review." *Vet Sci* 6(2). doi:10.3390/vetsci6020048.
212. Lowrie, M., and L. Garosi. 2016. "Classification of involuntary movements in dogs: Tremors and twitches." *Vet J* 214:109–116. doi:10.1016/j.tvjl.2016.05.011.
213. Leonard, C. A., and M. Tillson. 2001. "Feline lameness." *Vet Clin North Am Small Anim Pract* 31(1):143–163, vii. doi:10.1016/s0195-5616(01)50042-x.
214. Hoffman, A. M., and S. W. Dow. 2016. "Concise review: Stem cell trials using companion animal disease models." *Stem Cells* 34(7):1709–1729. doi:10.1002/stem.2377.
215. Bogers, S. H. 2018. "Cell-based therapies for joint disease in veterinary medicine: What we have learned and what we need to know." *Front Vet Science* 5. doi:ARTN70.10.3389/fvets.2018.00070.
216. Klosterman, E. S., and B. M. Pressler. 2011. "Nephrotic syndrome in dogs: Clinical features and evidence-based treatment considerations." *Top Companion Anim Med* 26(3):135–142. doi:10.1053/j.tcam.2011.04.004.
217. O'Brien, C. R., and J. S. Wilkie. 2001. "Calcinosis circumscripta following an injection of proligestone in a Burmese cat." *Aust Vet J* 79(3):187–189. doi:10.1111/j.1751-0813.2001.tb14575.x.
218. Garden, O. A., L. Kidd, A. M. Mexas, Y. M. Chang, U. Jeffery, S. L. Blois, J. E. Fogle, A. L. MacNeill, G. Lubas, A. Birkenheuer, S. Buoncompagni, J. R. S. Dandrieux, A. Di Loria, C. L. Fellman, B. Glanemann, R. Goggs, J. L. Granick,

D. N. LeVine, C. R. Sharp, S. Smith-Carr, J. W. Swann, and B. Szladovits. 2019. "ACVIM consensus statement on the diagnosis of immune-mediated hemolytic anemia in dogs and cats." *J Vet Intern Med* 33(2):313–334. doi:10.1111/jvim.15441.

219. Slanina, M. C. 2016. "Atlantoaxial instability." *Vet Clin North Am Small Anim Pract* 46(2):265–275. doi:10.1016/j.cvsm.2015.10.005.

220. Greenbarg, E. H., D. A. Jimenez, L. A. Nell, and C. W. Schmiedt. 2018. "Pilot study: Use of contrast-enhanced ultrasonography in feline renal transplant recipients." *J Feline Med Surg* 20(4):393–398. doi:10.1177/1098612x17713855.

221. Galac, S., and D. B. Wilson. 2015. "Animal models of adrenocortical tumorigenesis." *Endocrinol Metab Clin North Am* 44(2):297. doi:10.1016/j.ecl.2015.02.003.

222. Wilkie, D. A. 1990. "Control of ocular inflammation." *Vet Clin North Am Small Anim Pract* 20(3):693–713. doi:10.1016/s0195-5616(90)50058-3.

223. Steinberg, H. S. 1988. "Brachial plexus injuries and dysfunctions." *Vet Clin North Am Small Anim Pract* 18(3):565–580. doi:10.1016/s0195-5616(88)50055-4.

224. Lawson, J., J. Elliott, C. Wheeler-Jones, H. Syme, and R. Jepson. 2015. "Renal fibrosis in feline chronic kidney disease: Known mediators and mechanisms of injury." *Vet J* 203(1):18–26. doi:10.1016/j.tvjl.2014.10.009.

225. Borgeat, K., S. J. M. Niessen, L. Wilkie, N. Harrington, D. B. Church, V. L. Fuentes, and D. J. Connolly. 2018. "Time spent with cats is never wasted: Lessons learned from feline acromegalic cardiomyopathy, a naturally occurring animal model of the human disease." *PLoS One* 13(3). doi:ARTN, e.0194342.10.1371/journal.pone.0194342.

226. Davidson, M. G. 2000. "Toxoplasmosis." *Vet Clin North Am Small Anim Pract* 30(5):1051–1062. doi:10.1016/s0195-5616(00)05006-3.

227. Bailey, C. S., and J. P. Morgan. 1992. "Congenital spinal malformations." *Vet Clin North Am Small Anim Pract* 22(4):985–1015. doi:10.1016/s0195-5616(92)50089-4.

228. Amoasii, L., J. C. W. Hildyard, H. Li, E. Sanchez-Ortiz, A. Mireault, D. Caballero, R. Harron, T. R. Stathopoulou, C. Massey, J. M. Shelton, R. Bassel-Duby, R. J. Piercy, and E. N. Olson. 2018. "Gene editing restores dystrophin expression in a canine model of Duchenne muscular dystrophy." *Science* 362(6410):86–90. doi:10.1126/science.aau1549.

229. Baker, H. J., P. A. Wood, D. A. Wenger, S. U. Walkley, K. Inui, T. Kudoh, M. C. Rattazzi, and B. L. Riddle. 1987. "Sphingomyelin lipidosis in a cat." *Vet Pathol* 24(5):386–391. doi:10.1177/030098588702400504.

230. Djajadiningrat-Laanen, S., S. Galac, and H. Kooistra. 2011. "Primary hyperaldosteronism expanding the diagnostic net." *J Feline Med Surg* 13(9):641–650. doi:10.1016/j.jfms.2011.07.017.

231. Demko, J., and R. McLaughlin. 2005. "Developmental orthopedic disease." *Vet Clin North Am Small Anim Pract* 35(5):1111–1135, v. doi:10.1016/j.cvsm.2005.05.002.

232. Cotchin, E. 1964. "Spontaneous uterine cancer in animals." *Br J Cancer* 18:209–227. doi:10.1038/bjc.1964.23.

233. Di Dona, F., G. Della Valle, and G. Fatone. 2018. "Patellar luxation in dogs." *Vet Med (Auckl)* 9:23–32. doi:10.2147/VMRR.S142545.

234. Minor, K. M., A. Letko, D. Becker, M. Drogemuller, P. J. J. Mandigers, S. R. Bellekom, P. A. J. Leegwater, Q. E. M. Stassen, K. Putschbach, A. Fischer, T. Flegel, K. Matiasek, K. J. Ekenstedt, E. Furrow, E. E. Patterson, S. R. Platt, P. A. Kelly, J. P. Cassidy, G. D. Shelton, K. Lucot, D. L. Bannasch, H. Martineau, C. F. Muir, S. L. Priestnall, D. Henke, A. Oevermann, V. Jagannathan, J. R. Mickelson, and C. Drogemuller. 2018. "Canine NAPEPLD-associated models of human myelin disorders." *Sci Rep* 8(1). doi:ARTN 5818.10.1038/s41598-018-23938-7.

235. Peterson, M. E. 2014. "Animal models of disease: Feline hyperthyroidism: An animal model for toxic nodular goiter." *J Endocrinol* 223(2):T97–114. doi:10.1530/JOE-14-0461.

236. Ellinwood, N. M., P. Wang, T. Skeen, N. J. Sharp, M. Cesta, S. Decker, N. J. Edwards, I. Bublot, J. N. Thompson, W. Bush, E. Hardam, M. E. Haskins, and U. Giger. 2003. "A model of mucopolysaccharidosis IIIB (Sanfilippo syndrome type IIIB): N-acetyl-alpha-D-glucosaminidase deficiency in Schipperke dogs." *J Inherit Metab Dis* 26(5):489–504. doi:10.1023/a:1025177411938.

237. Preiswerk, G., and K. Breitenfeld. 1984. "Examination of the fundus of the eye of renal hypertensive dogs." *Experientia* 40(5):458–459. doi:10.1007/bf01952384.

238. Johnson, G. S., M. A. Turrentine, and K. H. Kraus. 1988. "Canine von Willebrand's disease. A heterogeneous group of bleeding disorders." *Vet Clin North Am Small Anim Pract* 18(1):195–229. doi:10.1016/s0195-5616(88)50017-7.

239. Geddes, R. F., N. C. Finch, H. M. Syme, and J. Elliott. 2013. "The role of phosphorus in the pathophysiology of chronic kidney disease." *J Vet Emerg Crit Care* 23(2):122–133. doi:10.1111/vec.12032.

240. Dubey, J. P., and D. S. Lindsay. 2019. "Coccidiosis in dogs-100 years of progress." *Vet Parasitol* 266:34–55. doi:10.1016/j.vetpar.2018.12.004.

241. Shively, J. N., and R. D. Phemister. 1968. "Fine structure of the iris of dogs manifesting heterochromia iridis." *Am J Ophthalmol* 66(6):1152–1162. doi:10.1016/0002-9394(68)90826-x.

242. Golaszewska, A., W. Bik, T. Motyl, and A. Orzechowski. 2019. "Bridging the gap between Alzheimer's disease and Alzheimer's-like diseases in animals." *Int J Mol Sci* 20(7). doi:ARTN 1664.10.3390/ijms20071664.

243. Davidson, A. P., and J. L. Westropp. 2014. "Diagnosis and management of urinary ectopia." *Vet Clin North Am Small Anim Pract* 44(2):343–353. doi:10.1016/j.cvsm.2013.11.007.

244. Dear, J. D. 2014. "Bacterial pneumonia in dogs and cats." *Vet Clin North Am Small Anim Pract* 44(1):143. doi:10.1016/j.cvsm.2013.09.003.

245. Greco, D. S. 2001. "Congenital and inherited renal disease of small animals." *Vet Clin North Am Small Anim Pract* 31(2):393–399, viii. doi:10.1016/s0195-5616(01)50211-9.

246. Werner, A. H., and H. T. Power. 1994. "Retinoids in veterinary dermatology." *Clin Dermatol* 12(4):579–586. doi:10.1016/0738-081x(94)90226-7.

247. Miller, M. A., T. J. Owen, D. S. Bruyette, J. C. Scott-Moncrieff, J. A. Ramos-Vara, H. Y. Weng, A. V. Chen, L. G. Martin, and D. M. DuSold. 2018. "Immunohistochemical evaluation of canine pituitary adenomas obtained by transsphenoidal hypophysectomy." *Vet Pathol* 55(6):889–895. doi:10.1177/0300985818784160.

248. Thomas, W. B. 1999. "Nonneoplastic disorders of the brain." *Clin Tech Small Anim Pract* 14(3):125–147. doi:10.1016/S1096-2867(99)80030-9.

249. Willmann, M., E. Hadzijusufovic, O. Hermine, M. Dacasto, L. Marconato, K. Bauer, B. Peter, S. Gamperl, G. Eisenwort, E. Jensen-Jarolim, M. Muller, M. Arock, D. M. Vail, and P. Valent. 2019. "Comparative oncology: The paradigmatic example of canine and human mast cell neoplasms." *Vet Comp Oncol* 17(1). doi:10.1111/vco.12440.

250. England, J., S. Loughna, and C. S. Rutland. 2017. "Multiple species comparison of cardiac troponin T and dystrophin: Unravelling the DNA behind dilated cardiomyopathy." *J Cardiovasc Dev Dis* 4(3). doi:ARTN 8.10.3390/jcdd4030008.

251. Clercx, C., A. Fastres, and E. Roels. 2018. "Idiopathic pulmonary fibrosis in West Highland white terriers: An update." *Vet J* 242:53–58. doi:10.1016/j.tvjl.2018.10.007.

252. Moore, M. P. 1992b. "Discospondylitis." *Vet Clin North Am Small Anim Pract* 22(4):1027–1034. doi:10.1016/s0195-5616(92)50091-2.

253. Stormont, C. 1975. "Neonatal isoerythrolysis in domestic animals: A comparative review." *Adv Vet Sci Comp Med* 19:23–45.

254. Klein, S. C., and M. E. Peterson. 2010a. "Canine hypoadrenocorticism: Part I." *Can Vet J Rev Vet Canadienne* 51(1):63–69.

255. Lee, K. I., C. Y. Lim, B. T. Kang, and H. M. Park. 2011. "Clinical and MRI findings of lissencephaly in a mixed breed dog." *J Vet Med Sci* 73(10):1385–1388. doi:10.1292/jvms.11-0117.

256. Williams, D. L. 2018. "Optimising tear replacement rheology in canine keratoconjunctivitis sicca." *Eye (Lond)* 32(2):195–199. doi:10.1038/eye.2017.272.

257. Foil, C. S. 1995. "Facial, pedal, and other regional dermatoses." *Vet Clin North Am Small Anim Pract* 25(4):923–944. doi:10.1016/s0195-5616(95)50135-4.

258. McDonald, J. E., and A. M. Knollinger. 2019. "The use of hyaluronic acid subdermal filler for entropion in canines and felines: 40 cases." *Vet Ophthalmol* 22(2):105–115. doi:10.1111/vop.12566.

259. Martinez, S., J. Valdes, and R. A. Alonso. 2000. "Achondroplastic dog breeds have no mutations in the transmembrane domain of the FGFR-3 gene." *Can J Vet Res Rev Canadienne Rech Vet* 64(4):243–245.

260. Reinero, C. R., A. E. DeClue, and P. Rabinowitz. 2009. "Asthma in humans and cats: Is there a common sensitivity to aeroallegens in shared environments?" *Environ Res* 109(5):634–640. doi:10.1016/j.envres.2009.02.001.

261. Guillaumin, J., and S. P. DiBartola. 2017. "Disorders of sodium and water homeostasis." *Vet Clin North Am Small Anim Pract* 47(2):293–312. doi:10.1016/j.cvsm.2016.10.015.

262. Webster, C. R. L., S. A. Center, J. M. Cullen, D. G. Penninck, K. P. Richter, D. C. Twedt, and P. J. Watson. 2019. "ACVIM consensus statement on the diagnosis and treatment of chronic hepatitis in dogs." *J Vet Intern Med* 33(3):1173–1200. doi:10.1111/jvim.15467.

263. Vaden, S. L. 2011. "Glomerular disease." *Top Companion Anim Med* 26(3):128–134. doi:10.1053/j.tcam.2011.04.003.

264. Pariaut, R. 2017. "Atrial fibrillation current therapies." *Vet Clin North Am Small Anim Pract* 47(5):977–988. doi:10.1016/j.cvsm.2017.04.002.

265. Chesney, C. 2011. "Canine atopy - Inside out, or outside in?" *Vet Rec* 168(20):533–534. doi:10.1136/vr.d3005.

266. Thomsen, B. B., H. Gredal, M. Wirenfeldt, B. W. Kristensen, B. H. Clausen, A. E. Larsen, B. Finsen, M. Berendt, and K. L. Lambertsen. 2017. "Spontaneous ischaemic stroke lesions in a dog brain: Neuropathological characterisation and comparison to human ischaemic stroke." *Acta Vet Scand* 59(1):7. doi:10.1186/s13028-016-0275-7.

267. Ragni, R. A., and D. Fews. 2008. "Ureteral obstruction and hydronephrosis in a cat associated with retroperitoneal infarction." *J Feline Med Surg* 10(3):259–263. doi:10.1016/j.jfms.2007.10.009.

268. Zandvliet, M. 2016. "Canine lymphoma: A review." *Vet Q* 36(2):76–104. doi:10.1080/01652176.2016.1152633.

269. Biddle, D., and D. K. Macintire. 2000. "Obstetrical emergencies." *Clin Tech Small Anim Pract* 15(2):88–93. doi:10.1053/svms.2000.6803.

270. Partridge, B., and J. H. Rossmeisl. 2020. "Companion animal models of neurological disease." *J Neurosci Methods* 331. doi:ARTN108484.10.1016/j.jneumeth.2019.108484.

271. Strain, G. M. 2012. "Canine deafness." *Vet Clin North Am Small Anim Pract* 42(6):1209–1224. doi:10.1016/j.cvsm.2012.08.010.

272. Scansen, B. A. 2018. "Cardiac interventions in small animals: Areas of uncertainty." *Vet Clin North Am Small Anim Pract* 48(5):797–817. doi:10.1016/j.cvsm.2018.05.003.

273. Nantasanti, S., A. de Bruin, J. Rothuizen, L. C. Penning, and B. A. Schotanus. 2016. "Concise review: Organoids are a powerful tool for the study of liver disease and personalized treatment design in humans and animals." *Stem Cells Transl Med* 5(3):325–330. doi:10.5966/sctm.2015-0152.

274. Fieten, H., P. A. Leegwater, A. L. Watson, and J. Rothuizen. 2012. "Canine models of copper toxicosis for understanding mammalian copper metabolism." *Mamm Genome* 23(1–2):62–75. doi:10.1007/s00335-011-9378-7.

275. Miller, E. J., and C. M. Brines. 2018. "Canine diabetes mellitus associated ocular disease." *Top Companion Anim Med* 33(1):29–34. doi:10.1053/j.tcam.2018.03.001.

276. McLellan, G. J., and L. B. Teixeira. 2015. "Feline glaucoma." *Vet Clin North Am Small Anim Pract* 45(6):1307–1333, vii. doi:10.1016/j.cvsm.2015.06.010.

277. Moore, A. S. 1992a. "Chemotherapy for intrathoracic cancer in dogs and cats." *Probl Vet Med* 4(2):351–364.

278. Sande, R. D., and S. A. Bingel. 1983. "Animal models of dwarfism." *Vet Clin North Am Small Anim Pract* 13(1):71–89. doi:10.1016/s0195-5616(83)50005-3.

279. Morris, D. O. 2013. "Ischemic dermatopathies." *Vet Clin North Am Small Anim Pract* 43(1):99–111. doi:10.1016/j.cvsm.2012.09.008.

280. Bonnett, B. N., A. Egenvall, A. Hedhammar, and P. Olson. 2005. "Mortality in over 350,000 insured Swedish dogs from 1995–2000: I. Breed-, gender-, age- and cause-specific rates." *Acta Vet Scand* 46(3):105–120. doi:10.1186/1751-0147-46-105.

281. Kaeberlein, M. 2016. "The biology of aging: Citizen scientists and their pets as a bridge between research on model organisms and human subjects." *Vet Pathol* 53(2):291–298. doi:10.1177/0300985815591082.

282. Swann, J. W., and B. J. Skelly. 2015. "Systematic review of prognostic factors for mortality in dogs with immune-mediated hemolytic anemia." *J Vet Intern Med* 29(1):7–13. doi:10.1111/jvim.12514.

283. Bennett, A. L., L. E. Williams, M. W. Ferguson, M. L. Hauck, S. E. Suter, C. B. Lanier, and P. R. Hess. 2017. "Canine acute leukaemia: 50 cases (1989–2014)." *Vet Comp Oncol* 15(3):1101–1114. doi:10.1111/vco.12251.

284. Bentley, R. T., A. U. Ahmed, A. B. Yanke, A. A. Cohen-Gadol, and M. Dey. 2017. "Dogs are man's best friend: In sickness and in health." *Neuro-Oncology* 19(3):312–322. doi:10.1093/neuonc/now109.

285. Creevy, K. E., S. N. Austad, J. M. Hoffman, D. G. O'Neill, and D. E. L. Promislow. 2016. "The companion dog as a model for the longevity dividend." *Cold Spring Harb Perspect Med* 6(1). doi:ARTN a026633.10.1101/Cshperspect.a026633.

286. Hechler, A. C., and S. A. Moore. 2018. "Understanding and treating Chiari-like malformation and syringomyelia in dogs." *Top Companion Anim Med* 33(1):1–11. doi:10.1053/j.tcam.2018.03.002.

287. Kitz, S., J. G. Thalhammer, U. Glantschnigg, M. Wrzosek, A. Klang, P. Halasz, M. N. Shouse, and A. Pakozdy. 2017. "Feline temporal lobe epilepsy: Review of the experimental literature." *J Vet Intern Med* 31(3):633–640. doi:10.1111/jvim.14699.

288. Galac, S. 2016. "Cortisol-secreting adrenocortical tumours in dogs and their relevance for human medicine." *Mol Cell Endocrinol* 421(C):34–39. doi:10.1016/j.mce.2015.06.026.

289. Hassan, E. A., M. H. Hassan, and F. A. Torad. 2018. "Correlation between clinical severity and type and degree of pectus excavatum in twelve brachycephalic dogs." *J Vet Med Sci* 80(5):766–771. doi:10.1292/jvms.17-0518.

290. Johnston, S. D., and S. Raksil. 1987. "Fetal loss in the dog and cat." *Vet Clin North Am Small Anim Pract* 17(3):535–554. doi:10.1016/s0195-5616(87)50052-3.

291. McEntee, M. C. 2002. "Reproductive oncology." *Clin Tech Small Anim Pract* 17(3):133–149. doi:10.1053/svms.2002.34642.

292. Cunto, M., E. Mariani, E. Anicito Guido, G. Ballotta, and D. Zambelli. 2019. "Clinical approach to prostatic diseases in the dog." *Reprod Domest Anim* 54(6):815–822. doi:10.1111/rda.13437.

293. Lemetayer, J., and S. Taylor. 2014. "Inflammatory joint disease in cats: Diagnostic approach and treatment." *J Feline Med Surg* 16(7):547–562. doi:10.1177/10986 12X14539086.

294. Doerr, K. A., C. A. Outerbridge, S. D. White, P. H. Kass, R. Shiraki, A. T. Lam, and V. K. Affolter. 2013. "Calcinosis cutis in dogs: Histopathological and clinical analysis of 46 cases." *Vet Dermatol* 24(3):355–361, e78–9. doi:10.1111/vde.12026.

295. Subgroup, Iris Canine GN Study Group Standard Therapy, S. Brown, J. Elliott, T. Francey, and D. Polzin, S. Vaden. 2013. "Consensus recommendations for standard therapy of glomerular disease in dogs." *J Vet Intern Med* 27(Suppl 1):S27–43. doi:10.1111/jvim.12230.

296. Rolim, V. M., R. A. Casagrande, A. T. Wouters, D. Driemeier, and S. P. Pavarini. 2016. "Myocarditis caused by feline immunodeficiency virus in five Cats with hypertrophic cardiomyopathy." *J Comp Pathol* 154(1):3–8. doi:10.1016/j.jcpa.2015.10.180.

297. Mueller, R. S. 2012. "An update on the therapy of canine demodicosis." *Compend Contin Educ Vet* 34(4):E1–4.

298. Chetboul, V., I. Pitsch, R. Tissier, V. Gouni, C. Misbach, E. Trehiou-Sechi, A. M. Petit, C. Damoiseaux, J. L. Pouchelon, L. Desquilbet, and E. Bomassi. 2016. "Epidemiological, clinical, and echocardiographic features and survival times of dogs and cats with tetralogy of Fallot: 31 cases (2003–2014)." *J Am Vet Med Assoc* 249(8):909–917. doi:10.2460/javma.249.8.909.

299. Komaromy, A. M., D. Bras, D. W. Esson, R. L. Fellman, S. D. Grozdanic, L. Kagemann, P. E. Miller, S. E. Moroi, C. E. Plummer, J. S. Sapienza, E. S. Storey, L. B. Teixeira, C. B. Toris, and T. R. Webb. 2019. "The future of canine glaucoma therapy." *Vet Ophthalmol* 22(5):726–740. doi:10.1111/vop.12678.

300. Kornegay, J. N. 2017. "The golden retriever model of Duchenne muscular dystrophy." *Skelet Muscle* 7(1). doi:ARTN9.10.1186/s13395-017-0124-z.

301. Duncan, I. D. 1980. "Peripheral nerve disease in the dog and cat." *Vet Clin North Am Small Anim Pract* 10(1):177–211. doi:10.1016/s0195-5616(80)50011-2.

302. Fossum, T. W., and D. A. Hulse. 1992. "Osteomyelitis." *Semin Vet Med Surg Small Anim* 7(1):85–97.

303. Cichocki, B. N., D. R. Dugat, and R. D. Baumwart. 2019. "Pulmonary artery banding in a cat with a perimembranous ventricular septal defect and left-sided congestive heart failure." *J Am Vet Med Assoc* 254(6):723–727. doi:10.2460/javma.254.6.723.

304. Fieten, H., Y. Gill, A. J. Martin, M. Concilli, K. Dirksen, F. G. van Steenbeek, B. Spee, T. S. van den Ingh, E. C. Martens, P. Festa, G. Chesi, B. van de Sluis, R. H. Houwen, A. L. Watson, Y. S. Aulchenko, V. L. Hodgkinson, S. Zhu, M. J. Petris, R. S. Polishchuk, P. A. Leegwater, and J. Rothuizen. 2016. "The Menkes and Wilson disease genes counteract in copper toxicosis in Labrador retrievers: A new canine model for copper-metabolism disorders." *Dis Model Mech* 9(1):25–38. doi:10.1242/dmm.020263.

305. Favier, R. P., B. Spee, L. C. Penning, and J. Rothuizen. 2011. "Copper-induced hepatitis: The COMMD1 deficient dog as a translational animal model for human chronic hepatitis." *Vet Q* 31(1):49–60. doi:10.1080/01652176.2011.563146.

306. Ulrich, S., C. Gottschalk, R. K. Straubinger, K. Schwaiger, and R. Dorfelt. 2020. "Acceleration of the identification of sepsis-inducing bacteria in cultures of dog and cat blood." *J Small Anim Pract* 61(1):42–45. doi:10.1111/jsap.13056.

307. Tabar, M. D., R. G. Maggi, L. Altet, M. Vilafranca, O. Francino, and X. Roura. 2011. "Gammopathy in a Spanish dog infected with Bartonella henselae." *J Small Anim Pract* 52(4):209–212. doi:10.1111/j.1748-5827.2011.01046.x.

308. McIntyre, R. L., J. K. Levy, J. F. Roberts, and R. L. Reep. 2010. "Developmental uterine anomalies in cats and dogs undergoing elective ovariohysterectomy." *J Am Vet Med Assoc* 237(5):542–546. doi:10.2460/javma.237.5.542.

309. Hassan, B. B., S. M. Elshafae, W. Supsavhad, J. K. Simmons, W. P. Dirksen, S. M. Sokkar, and T. J. Rosol. 2017. "Feline mammary cancer." *Vet Pathol* 54(1):32–43. doi:10.1177/0300985816650243.

310. Moriello, K. A., K. Coyner, S. Paterson, and B. Mignon. 2017. "Diagnosis and treatment of dermatophytosis in dogs and cats: Clinical Consensus guidelines of the World Association for Veterinary Dermatology." *Vet Dermatol* 28(3):266-e68. doi:10.1111/vde.12440.

311. Day, M. J. 2010. "Ageing, immunosenescence and inflammageing in the dog and cat." *J Comp Pathol* 141(Suppl 1):S60–69. doi:10.1016/j.jepa.2009.10.011.

312. Hendricks, J. C., and A. R. Morrison. 1981. "Normal and abnormal sleep in mammals." *J Am Vet Med Assoc* 178(2):121–126.

313. Hensel, P., D. Santoro, C. Favrot, P. Hill, and C. Griffin. 2015. "Canine atopic dermatitis: Detailed guidelines for diagnosis and allergen identification." *BMC Vet Res* 11:196. doi:10.1186/s12917-015-0515-5.

314. Houston, D. M., and S. L. Myers. 1993. "A review of Heinz-body anemia in the dog induced by toxins." *Vet Hum Toxicol* 35(2):158–161.

315. Barr, J. W., and M. McMichael. 2012. "Inherited disorders of hemostasis in dogs and cats." *Top Companion Anim Med* 27(2):53–58. doi:10.1053/j.tcam.2012.07.006.

316. Bartges, J., R. F. Kushner, K. E. Michel, R. Sallis, and M. J. Day. 2017. "One health solutions to obesity in people and their pets." *J Comp Pathol* 156(4):326–333. doi:10.1016/j.jcpa.2017.03.008.

317. Scudder, C. J., S. M. Mirczuk, K. M. Richardson, V. J. Crossley, J. T. C. Regan, R. Gostelow, Y. Forcada, K. Hazuchova, N. Harrington, I. M. McGonnell, D. B. Church, P. J. Kenny, M. Korbonits, R. C. Fowkes, and S. J. M. Niessen. 2019. "Pituitary pathology and gene expression in acromegalic cats." *J Endocr Soc* 3(1):181–200. doi:10.1210/js.2018-00226.

318. Jue, T. R., and K. L. McDonald. 2016. "The challenges associated with molecular targeted therapies for glioblastoma." *J Neurooncol* 127(3):427–434. doi:10.1007/s11060-016-2080-6.

319. Egenvall, A., B. N. Bonnett, A. Hedhammar, and P. Olson. 2005. "Mortality in over 350,000 insured Swedish dogs from 1995–2000: II. Breed-specific age and survival patterns and relative risk for causes of death." *Acta Vet Scand* 46(3):121–136. doi:10.1186/1751-0147-46-121.

320. Shakir, S. A., and A. Sundararaj. 1996. "Canine acanthosis nigricans - A report of 3 cases." *Indian Vet J* 73(8):826–828.

321. Tashiro, J., G. A. Rubio, A. H. Limper, K. Williams, S. J. Elliot, I. Ninou, V. Aidinis, A. Tzouvelekis, and M. K. Glassberg. 2017. "Exploring animal models that resemble idiopathic pulmonary fibrosis." *Front Med* 4. doi:ARTN 118.10.3389/fmed.2017.00118.

322. Jacobson, L. S., and R. M. Kirberger. 1996. "Canine multiple cartilaginous exostoses: Unusual manifestations and a review of the literature." *J Am Anim Hosp Assoc* 32(1):45–51. doi:10.5326/15473317-32-1-45.

323. Ruoff, C. M., S. C. Kerwin, and A. R. Taylor. 2018. "Diagnostic imaging of discospondylitis." *Vet Clin North Am Small Anim Pract* 48(1):85–94. doi:10.1016/j.cvsm.2017.08.007.

324. Williams, D. L. 2008. "Immunopathogenesis of keratoconjunctivitis sicca in the dog." *Vet Clin North Am Small Anim Pract* 38(2):251–268, vi. doi:10.1016/j.cvsm.2007.12.002.

325. Young, K. M. 1985. "Myeloproliferative disorders." *Vet Clin North Am Small Anim Pract* 15(4):769–781. doi:10.1016/s0195-5616(85)50035-2.

326. Young, W. M., C. Zheng, M. G. Davidson, and H. D. Westermeyer. 2019. "Visual outcome in cats with hypertensive chorioretinopathy." *Vet Ophthalmol* 22(2):161–167. doi:10.1111/vop.12575.

327. Garden, O. A., D. Pinheiro, and F. Cunningham. 2011. "All creatures great and small: Regulatory T cells in mice, humans, dogs and other domestic animal species." *Int Immunopharmacol* 11(5):576–588. doi:10.1016/j.intimp.2010.11.003.

328. Duncker, D. J., J. Bakkers, B. J. Brundel, J. Robbins, J. C. Tardiff, and L. Carrier. 2015. "Animal and in silico models for the study of sarcomeric cardiomyopathies." *Cardiovasc Res* 105(4):439–448. doi:10.1093/cvr/cvv006.

329. Javadi, S., S. C. Djajadiningrat-Laanen, H. S. Kooistra, A. M. van Dongen, G. Voorhout, F. J. van Sluijs, T. S. G. A. M. van den Ingh, W. H. Boer, and A. Rijnberk. 2005. "Primary hyperaldosteronism, a mediator of progressive renal disease in cats." *Domest Anim Endocrinol* 28(1):85–104. doi:10.1016/j.domaniend.2004.06.010.

330. Estey, C. M. 2016. "Congenital Hydrocephalus." *Vet Clin North Am Small Anim Pract* 46(2):217–229. doi:10.1016/j.cvsm.2015.10.003.

331. Schissler, J. 2019. "Sterile pyogranulomatous dermatitis and panniculitis." *Vet Clin North Am Small Anim Pract* 49(1):27–36. doi:10.1016/j.cvsm.2018.08.003.

332. Xenoulis, P. G., and J. M. Steiner. 2015. "Canine hyperlipidaemia." *J Small Anim Pract* 56(10):595–605. doi:10.1111/jsap.12396.

333. Vischer, A. S., D. J. Connolly, C. J. Coats, V. L. Fuentes, W. J. McKenna, S. Castelletti, and A. A. Pantazis. 2017. "Arrhythmogenic right ventricular cardiomyopathy in Boxer dogs: The diagnosis as a link to the human disease." *Acta Myol* 36(3):135–150.

334. Jaffey, J. A., J. Amorim, and A. E. DeClue. 2018. "Effects of calcitriol on apoptosis, toll-like receptor 4 expression, and cytokine production of endotoxin-primed canine leukocytes." *Am J Vet Res* 79(10):1071–1078. doi:10.2460/ajvr.79.10.1071.

335. Schrank, M., and S. Romagnoli. 2020. "Prostatic neoplasia in the intact and castrated dog: How dangerous is castration?" *Animals (Basel)* 10(1). doi:10.3390/ani10010085.

336. Clavero, S., Y. Ahuja, D. F. Bishop, B. Kwait, M. E. Haskins, U. Giger, and R. J. Desnick. 2013. "Diagnosis of feline acute intermittent porphyria presenting with erythrodontia requires molecular analyses." *Vet J* 198(3):720–722. doi:10.1016/j.tvjl.2013.10.008.

337. Harman, R. M., T. M. Curtis, D. J. Argyle, S. A. Coonrod, and G. R. Van de Walle. 2016. "A comparative study on the *in vitro* effects of the DNA methyltransferase Inhibitor 5-azacytidine (5-AzaC) in breast/mammary cancer of different mammalian species." *J Mammary Gland Biol Neoplasia* 21(1–2):51–66. doi:10.1007/s10911-016-9350-y.

338. Patnaik, A. K., and P. G. Greenlee. 1987. "Canine ovarian neoplasms: A clinicopathologic study of 71 cases, including histology of 12 granulosa cell tumors." *Vet Pathol* 24(6):509–514. doi:10.1177/030098588702400607.

339. Iwasa, N., N. Nishii, S. Takashima, Y. Kobatake, S. Nomura, K. Iwasa, T. Iwasa, T. Suzuki, N. Machida, and H. Kitagawa. 2019. "Long-term management of high-grade atrioventricular block using cilostazol in a cat." *JFMS Open Rep* 5(2):2055116919878913. doi:10.1177/2055116919878913.

340. Milovancev, M., K. Townsend, J. Spina, C. Hurley, S. C. Ralphs, B. Trumpatori, B. Seguin, and K. Jermyn. 2016. "Effect of metoclopramide on the incidence of early postoperative aspiration pneumonia in dogs with acquired idiopathic laryngeal paralysis." *Vet Surg* 45(5):577–581. doi:10.1111/vsu.12491.

341. Adin, C. A., and C. Gilor. 2017. "The diabetic dog as a translational model for human islet transplantation." *Yale J Biol Med* 90(3):509–515.
342. Roman, G. C., R. E. Jackson, R. Gadhia, A. N. Roman, and J. Reis. 2019. "Mediterranean diet: The role of long-chain omega-3 fatty acids in fish; polyphenols in fruits, vegetables, cereals, coffee, tea, cacao and wine; probiotics and vitamins in prevention of stroke, age-related cognitive decline, and Alzheimer disease." *Rev Neurol (Paris)* 175(10):724–741. doi:10.1016/j.neurol.2019.08.005.
343. Kaeberlein, M., K. E. Creevy, and D. E. L. Promislow. 2016. "The dog aging project: Translational geroscience in companion animals." *Mamm Genome* 27(7–8):279–288. doi:10.1007/s00335-016-9638-7.
344. Ueno, H., O. Yamato, T. Sugiura, M. Kohyama, A. Yabuki, K. Miyoshi, K. Matsuda, and T. Uchide. 2016. "GM1 gangliosidosis in a Japanese domestic cat: A new variant identified in Hokkaido, Japan." *J Vet Med Sci* 78(1):91–95. doi:10.1292/jvms.15-0281.
345. Boyce, J. T., S. P. DiBartola, D. J. Chew, and P. W. Gasper. 1984. "Familial renal amyloidosis in Abyssinian cats." *Vet Pathol* 21(1):33–38. doi:10.1177/030098588402100106.
346. Gedon, N. K. Y., and R. S. Mueller. 2018. "Atopic dermatitis in cats and dogs: A difficult disease for animals and owners." *Clin Transl Allergy* 8:41. doi:10.1186/s13601-018-0228-5.
347. Hicks, J., S. Platt, M. Kent, and A. Haley. 2017. "Canine brain tumours: A model for the human disease?" *Vet Comp Oncol* 15(1):252–272. doi:10.1111/vco.12152.
348. Moore, A. R., and P. R. Avery. 2019. "Protein characterization using electrophoresis and immunofixation; a case-based review of dogs and cats." *Vet Clin Pathol* 48(Suppl 1):29–44. doi:10.1111/vcp.12760.
349. van der Gaag, I. 1984. "Hypertrophic gastritis in 21 dogs." *Zentralbl Veterinarmed A* 31(3):161–173. doi:10.1111/j.1439-0442.1984.tb01272.x.
350. Johnson, K. C., and A. Mackin. 2012. "Canine immune-mediated polyarthritis: Part 1: Pathophysiology." *J Am Anim Hosp Assoc* 48(1):12–17. doi:10.5326/JAAHA-MS-5744.
351. Bleakley, S., C. G. Duncan, and E. Monnet. 2015. "Thoracoscopic lung lobectomy for primary lung tumors in 13 dogs." *Vet Surg* 44(8):1029–1035. doi:10.1111/vsu.12411.
352. Saunders, A. B., J. A. Carlson, D. A. Nelson, S. G. Gordon, and M. W. Miller. 2013. "Hybrid technique for ventricular septal defect closure in a dog using an Amplatzer (R) Duct Occluder II." *J Vet Cardiol* 15(3):217–224. doi:10.1016/j.jvc.2013.06.003.
353. Bulman-Fleming, J. 2008. "A rare case of uterine adenomyosis in a Siamese cat." *Can Vet J* 49(7):709–712.
354. Chikazawa, S., and M. D. Dunning. 2016. "A review of anaemia of inflammatory disease in dogs and cats." *J Small Anim Pract* 57(7):348–353. doi:10.1111/jsap.12498.
355. Martinez, I., J. S. Mattoon, K. A. Eaton, D. J. Chew, and S. P. DiBartola. 2003. "Polypoid cystitis in 17 dogs (1978–2001)." *J Vet Intern Med* 17(4):499–509. doi:10.1111/j.1939-1676.2003.tb02471.x.
356. Wu, X., P. A. Leegwater, and H. Fieten. 2016. "Canine models for copper homeostasis disorders." *Int J Mol Sci* 17(2):196. doi:10.3390/ijms17020196.
357. Stalin, C., R. Gutierrez-Quintana, K. Faller, J. Guevar, C. Yeamans, and J. Penderis. 2015. "A review of canine atlantoaxial joint subluxation." *Vet Comp Orthop Traumatol* 28(1):1–8. doi:10.3415/VCOT-14-05-0064.
358. Tamada, H., N. Kawate, T. Inaba, T. Kuwamura, M. Maeda, T. Kajikawa, and T. Sawada. 2005. "Adenomyosis with severe inflammation in the uterine cervix in a dog." *Can Vet J* 46(4):333–334.

359. Bartges, J. W. 2012. "Chronic kidney disease in dogs and cats." *Vet Clin North Am Small Anim Pract* 42(4):669–692, vi. doi:10.1016/j.cvsm.2012.04.008.

360. Castillo, V. A., and M. F. Gallelli. 2010. "Corticotroph adenoma in the dog: Pathogenesis and new therapeutic possibilities." *Res Vet Sci* 88(1):26–32. doi:10.1016/j.rvsc.2009.07.005.

361. Carlos, G., F. P. dos Santos, and P. E. Froehlich. 2020. "Canine metabolomics advances." *Metabolomics* 16(2). doi:ARTN 16. 10.1007/s11306-020-1638-7.

362. Rozanski, E. 2020. "Canine chronic bronchitis: An update." *Vet Clin North Am Small Anim Pract* 50(2):393–404. doi:10.1016/j.cvsm.2019.10.003.

363. Clark, L. A., and M. L. Cox. 2012. "Current status of genetic studies of exocrine pancreatic insufficiency in dogs." *Top Companion Anim Med* 27(3):109–112. doi:10.1053/j.tcam.2012.04.001.

364. Moore, S. A., N. Granger, N. J. Olby, I. Spitzbarth, N. D. Jeffery, A. Tipold, Y. S. Nout-Lomas, R. C. da Costa, V. M. Stein, L. J. Noble-Haeusslein, A. R. Blight, R. G. Grossman, D. M. Basso, and J. M. Levine. 2017. "Targeting translational successes through CANSORT-SCI: Using pet dogs to identify effective treatments for spinal cord injury." *J Neurotrauma* 34(12):2007–2018. doi:10.1089/neu.2016.4745.

365. Charalambous, M., D. Brodbelt, and H. A. Volk. 2014. "Treatment in canine epilepsy - A systematic review." *BMC Vet Res* 10. doi:ARTN 257.10.1186/s12917-014-0257-9.

366. Bertoy, R. W. 2002. "Megacolon in the cat." *Vet Clin North Am Small Anim Pract* 32(4):901–915. doi:10.1016/s0195-5616(02)00020-7.

367. Bergman, P. J. 2012. "Paraneoplastic hypercalcemia." *Top Companion Anim Med* 27(4):156–158. doi:10.1053/j.tcam.2012.09.003.

368. DeClue, A. E., C. R. Sharp, R. L. Cohen, E. F. Leverenz, and C. R. Reinero. 2010. "Cysteinyl-leukotriene receptor antagonism blunts the acute hypotensive response to endotoxin in cats." *J Feline Med Surg* 12(10):754–759. doi:10.1016/j.jfms.2010.05.012.

369. Yu, X. R., B. Bao, Y. Echigoya, and T. Yokota. 2015. "Dystrophin-deficient large animal models: Translational research and exon skipping." *Am J Transl Res* 7(8):1314–1331.

370. Spycher, M., A. Bauer, V. Jagannathan, M. Frizzi, M. De Lucia, and T. Leeb. 2018. "A frameshift variant in the COL5A1 gene in a cat with Ehlers-Danlos syndrome." *Anim Genet* 49(6):641–644. doi:10.1111/age.12727.

371. Hoppe, A., T. Denneberg, J. O. Jeppsson, and B. Kagedal. 1993. "Canine cystinuria: An extended study on the effects of 2-mercaptopropionylglycine on cystine urolithiasis and urinary cystine excretion." *Br Vet J* 149(3):235–251. doi:10.1016/S0007-1935(05)80170-8.

372. Donzel, E., L. Arti, and S. Chahory. 2017. "Epidemiology and clinical presentation of canine cataracts in France: A retrospective study of 404 cases." *Vet Ophthalmol* 20(2):131–139. doi:10.1111/vop.12380.

373. Goggs, R., and J. A. Letendre. 2019. "Evaluation of the host cytokine response in dogs with sepsis and noninfectious systemic inflammatory response syndrome." *J Vet Emerg Crit Care (San Antonio)* 29(6):593–603. doi:10.1111/vec.12903.

374. Fiani, N., F. J. Verstraete, and B. Arzi. 2016. "Reconstruction of congenital nose, cleft primary palate, and lip disorders." *Vet Clin North Am Small Anim Pract* 46(4):663–675. doi:10.1016/j.cvsm.2016.02.001.

375. Bonnett, B. N., and A. Egenvall. 2010. "Age patterns of disease and death in insured Swedish dogs, cats and horses." *J Comp Pathol* 141(Suppl 1):S33–38. doi:10.1016/j.jcpa.2009.10.008.

376. Simpson, S., J. Edwards, T. F. N. Ferguson-Mignan, M. Cobb, N. P. Mongan, and C. S. Rutland. 2015. "Genetics of human and canine dilated cardiomyopathy." *Int J Genomics*. doi:ARTN 204823.10.1155/2015/204823.

377. Taylor, M. A. 2001. "Recent developments in ectoparasiticides." *Vet J* 161(3):253–268. doi:10.1053/tvjl.2000.0549.

378. Sanders, K., H. S. Kooistra, and S. Galac. 2018. "Treating canine Cushing's syndrome: Current options and future prospects." *Vet J* 241:42–51. doi:10.1016/j.tvjl.2018.09.014.

379. Strain, G. M. 1999. "Congenital deafness and its recognition." *Vet Clin North Am Small Anim Pract* 29(4):895–907, vi. doi:10.1016/s0195-5616(99)50079-x.

380. Urfer, S. R., T. L. Kaeberlein, S. Mailheau, P. J. Bergman, K. E. Creevy, D. E. Promislow, and M. Kaeberlein. 2017. "Asymptomatic heart valve dysfunction in healthy middle-aged companion dogs and its implications for cardiac aging." *GeroScience* 39(1):43–50. doi:10.1007/s11357-016-9956-4.

381. Zaragoza, C., C. Gomez-Guerrero, J. L. Martin-Ventura, L. Blanco-Colio, B. Lavin, B. Mallavia, C. Tarin, S. Mas, A. Ortiz, and J. Egido. 2011. "Animal models of cardiovascular diseases." *J Biomed Biotechnol*. doi:ARTN.497841.10.1155/2011/497841.

382. Simpson, S., M. D. Dunning, S. de Brot, L. Grau-Roma, N. P. Mongan, and C. S. Rutland. 2017. "Comparative review of human and canine osteosarcoma: Morphology, epidemiology, prognosis, treatment and genetics." *Acta Vet Scand* 59(1). doi:ARTN 71.10.1186/s13028-017-0341-9.

383. Lackner, P. A. 2001. "Techniques for surgical correction of adnexal disease." *Clin Tech Small Anim Pract* 16(1):40–50. doi:10.1053/svms.2001.22805.

384. Dimakopoulos, A. C., and R. J. Mayer. 2002. "Aspects of neurodegeneration in the canine brain." *J Nutr* 132(6):1579S–182S. doi:10.1093/jn/132.6.1579S.

385. Shmuel, D. L., and Y. Cortes. 2013. "Anaphylaxis in dogs and cats." *J Vet Emerg Crit Care (San Antonio)* 23(4):377–394. doi:10.1111/vec.12066.

386. Simpson, K. W. 2015. "Pancreatitis and triaditis in cats: Causes and treatment." *J Small Anim Pract* 56(1):40–49. doi:10.1111/jsap.12313.

387. Daure, E., L. Ross, and C. R. L. Webster. 2017a. "Gastroduodenal ulceration in small animals: Part 1. Pathophysiology and epidemiology." *J Am Anim Hosp Assoc* 53(1):1–10. doi:10.5326/Jaaha-Ms-6635.

388. Ohl, K., K. Tenbrock, and M. Kipp. 2016. "Oxidative stress in multiple sclerosis: Central and peripheral mode of action." *Exp Neurol* 277:58–67. doi:10.1016/j.expneurol.2015.11.010.

389. Nardone, R., Y. Holler, A. C. Taylor, P. Lochner, F. Tezzon, S. Golaszewski, F. Brigo, and E. Trinka. 2016. "Canine degenerative myelopathy: A model of human amyotrophic lateral sclerosis." *Zoology* 119(1):64–73. doi:10.1016/j.zool.2015.09.003.

390. Egenvall, A., B. N. Bonnett, B. Haggstrom, B. S. Holst, L. Moller, and A. Nodtvedt. 2010. "Morbidity of insured Swedish cats during 1999–2006 by age, breed, sex, and diagnosis." *J Feline Med Surg* 12(12):948–959. doi:10.1016/j.jfms.2010.08.008.

391. Nishiya, A. T., C. O. Massoco, C. R. Felizzola, E. Perlmann, K. Batschinski, M. V. Tedardi, J. S. Garcia, P. P. Mendonca, T. F. Teixeira, and M. L. Zaidan Dagli. 2016. "Comparative aspects of canine melanoma." *Vet Sci* 3(1). doi:10.3390/vetsci3010007.

392. Butler, J. R., and J. Gambino. 2017. "Canine hip dysplasia diagnostic imaging." *Vet Clin North Am Small Anim Pract* 47(4):777–793. doi:10.1016/j.cvsm.2017.02.002.

393. Reinero, C. R. 2011. "Advances in the understanding of pathogenesis, and diagnostics and therapeutics for feline allergic asthma." *Vet J* 190(1):28–33. doi:10.1016/j.tvjl.2010.09.022.

394. Foutz, A. S., M. M. Mitler, and W. C. Dement. 1980. "Narcolepsy." *Vet Clin North Am Small Anim Pract* 10(1):65–80. doi:10.1016/s0195-5616(80)50004-5.

395. Klein, S. C., and M. E. Peterson. 2010b. "Canine hypoadrenocorticism: Part II." *Can Vet J Rev Vet Canadienne* 51(2):179–184.

396. Loughin, C. A. 2016. "Chiari-like malformation." *Vet Clin North Am Small Anim Pract* 46(2):231–242. doi:10.1016/j.cvsm.2015.10.002.

397. Lin Blache, J., K. Ryan, and K. Arceneaux. 2011. "Histoplasmosis." *Compend Contin Educ Vet* 33(3):E1–10; quiz E11.

398. Pretzer, S. D. 2008. "Medical management of canine and feline dystocia." *Theriogenology* 70(3):332–336. doi:10.1016/j.theriogenology.2008.04.031.

399. Buddington, R. K., and P. T. Sangild. 2011. "Companion animals symposium: Development of the mammalian gastrointestinal tract, the resident microbiota, and the role of diet in early life." *J Anim Sci* 89(5):1506–1519. doi:10.2527/jas.2010-3705.

400. Daure, E., L. Ross, and C. R. L. Webster. 2017b. "Gastroduodenal ulceration in small animals: Part 2. Proton pump inhibitors and Histamine-2 receptor antagonists." *J Am Anim Hosp Assoc* 53(1):11–23. doi:10.5326/Jaaha-Ms-6634.

401. Guilford, W. G. 1990. "Megaesophagus in the dog and cat." *Semin Vet Med Surg Small Anim* 5(1):37–45.

402. Johnson, L. R., E. G. Johnson, W. Vernau, P. H. Kass, and B. A. Byrne. 2016. "Bronchoscopy, imaging, and concurrent diseases in dogs with bronchiectasis: (2003–2014)." *J Vet Intern Med* 30(1):247–254. doi:10.1111/jvim.13809.

403. Boydell, P. 2010. "Coonhound paralysis in South Yorkshire?" *Vet Rec* 167(9):351. doi:10.1136/vr.c4510.

404. Coates, J. R., and F. A. Wininger. 2010. "Canine degenerative myelopathy." *Vet Clin North Am Small Anim Pract* 40(5):929–920. doi:10.1016/j.cvsm.2010.05.001.

405. Goebel, K., and N. D. Merner. 2017. "A monograph proposing the use of canine mammary tumours as a model for the study of hereditary breast cancer susceptibility genes in humans." *Vet Med Sci* 3(2):51–62. doi:10.1002/vms3.61.

406. Whitney, M. S. 1992. "Evaluation of hyperlipidemias in dogs and cats." *Semin Vet Med Surg Small Anim* 7(4):292–300.

407. Podell, M., H. A. Volk, M. Berendt, W. Loscher, K. Munana, E. E. Patterson, and S. R. Platt. 2016. "2015 ACVIM small animal consensus statement on seizure management in dogs." *J Vet Intern Med* 30(2):477–490. doi:10.1111/jvim.13841.

408. Hinney, B., M. Gottwald, J. Moser, B. Reicher, B. J. Schafer, R. Schaper, A. Joachim, and F. Kunzel. 2017. "Examination of anonymous canine faecal samples provides data on endoparasite prevalence rates in dogs for comparative studies." *Vet Parasitol* 245:106–115. doi:10.1016/j.vetpar.2017.08.016.

409. Hargis, A. M., and P. E. Ginn. 1999. "Feline herpesvirus 1-associated facial and nasal dermatitis and stomatitis in domestic cats." *Vet Clin North Am Small Anim Pract* 29(6):1281–1290. doi:10.1016/s0195-5616(99)50126-5.

410. Hamelin, A., D. Begon, F. Conchou, M. Fusellier, and M. Abitbol. 2017. "Clinical characterisation of polydactyly in Maine Coon cats." *J Feline Med Surg* 19(4):382–393. doi:10.1177/1098612X16628920.

411. Egenvall, A., A. Nodtvedt, J. Haggstrom, B. S. Holst, L. Moller, and B. N. Bonnett. 2009. "Mortality of life-insured Swedish cats during 1999–2006: Age, breed, sex, and diagnosis." *J Vet Intern Med* 23(6):1175–1183. doi:10.1111/j.1939-1676.2009.0396.x.

412. Galac, S., and E. Korpershoek. 2017. "Pheochromocytomas and paragangliomas in humans and dogs." *Vet Comp Oncol* 15(4):1158–1170. doi:10.1111/vco.12291.

413. Gosselin, S. J., C. C. Capen, S. L. Martin, and S. Krakowka. 1982. "Autoimmune lymphocytic thyroiditis in dogs." *Vet Immunol Immunopathol* 3(1–2):185–201. doi:10.1016/0165-2427(82)90035-6.

414. Petrakovsky, J., A. Bianchi, H. Fisun, P. Najera-Aguilar, and M. M. Pereira. 2014. "Animal leptospirosis in Latin America and the Caribbean countries: Reported outbreaks and literature review (2002–2014)." *Int J Environ Res Public Health* 11(10):10770–10789. doi:10.3390/ijerph111010770.

415. Park, Y. W., J. Y. Kim, M. B. Jeong, S. H. Kim, J. Yoon, and K. Seo. 2015. "A Retrospective study on the association between vitreous degeneration and cataract in dogs." *Vet Ophthalmol* 18(4):304–308. doi:10.1111/vop.12230.

416. Hill, R. C. 2009. "Conference on "Multidisciplinary approaches to nutritional problems". Symposium on "Nutrition and health". Nutritional therapies to improve health: Lessons from companion animals." *Proc Nutr Soc* 68(1):98–102. doi:10.1017/S0029665108008835.

417. Kiviranta, A. M., A. K. Lappalainen, K. Hagner, and T. Jokinen. 2011. "Dermoid sinus and spina bifida in three dogs and a cat." *J Small Anim Pract* 52(6):319–324. doi:10.1111/j.1748-5827.2011.01062.x.

418. Ewing, G. O. 1969. "Familial nonspherocytic hemolytic anemia of Basenji dogs." *J Am Vet Med Assoc* 154(5):503–507.

419. Blonk, M., I. Van de Maele, A. Combes, B. Stablay, H. De Cock, I. Polis, G. Rybachuk, and H. de Rooster. 2017. "Congenital lobar emphysema in a kitten." *J Small Anim Pract* 58(11):659–663. doi:10.1111/jsap.12668.

420. Schmidt, M. K., and A. H. Estrada. 2010. "ECG of the month. Respiratory sinus arrhythmia." *J Am Vet Med Assoc* 237(9):1045–1047. doi:10.2460/javma.237.9.1045.

3 Specific Diseases of Large Animals and Man

Timothy Lescun

CONTENTS

INTRODUCTION

Specific diseases of man which occur in large animal species are numerous. The similarity of disease and possible translation value varies considerably and in some circumstances multiple animal species may provide a more robust approach to the study of a particular disease than focusing on a single species model. Large animals considered in this chapter will include those which are called 'large' within the veterinary profession, rather than 'large' by the research community, and includes horses, cattle, sheep, goats, and swine. It is not possible to address all of the diseases of these species which could serve as a source of naturally occurring animal disease similar to man in a single chapter. Therefore, a select group of diseases will be covered to highlight some of the advantages and limitations which arise when using these animal diseases as models, and resources will be provided for further exploration by the reader into other diseases where similarities exist between man and animals. The diseases covered in this chapter will also focus on those diseases which are naturally occurring at a high enough prevalence to be plausible for a researcher to establish the number of cases necessary to study within a reasonable time frame. It will include only non-infectious diseases, although clearly a large and ever expanding group of both zoonotic, potentially zoonotic, and comparable etiologic diseases (such as influenza) have great potential in advancing our understanding of these diseases in both humans and animals. In addition, while large animal models have been used for the study of cellular, tissue, and whole animal level processes such as fracture and wound healing, endotoxemia and the systemic inflammatory response, sepsis, blood loss, disseminated intravascular coagulation, response to injury and implants, along with many others, these will not be covered in this chapter of naturally occurring large animal diseases seen in man. A systematic approach of presenting comparable diseases of large animals and man will be made mainly by organ system (see Table 3.1). As an introduction, some background information on the large animal species of interest will be presented to familiarize the researcher with some of the advantages and disadvantages of actually working with each animal species.

HORSES

As a domesticated species, horses have lived with humans in society in at least as many ways as any other animal. From agriculture and transport, to leisure activities, equestrian sports, and as companions, horses continue to have a wide variety of roles in society. Horses, and other equids such as donkeys and mules, can have different roles in a particular society that are largely dependent upon the development status of the country. In developing countries, equids (horses, mules, and donkeys) are primarily used as working animals. This accounts for close to 90% of the global population of equids. In developed countries, such as the United States, far fewer equids are used for work supporting human livelihood and agriculture. There are approximately 10 million horses in the United States according to the Food and Agriculture Organization of the United Nations and over 60

TABLE 3.1
Common Naturally Occurring Models of Human Disease Seen in Large Animals

Disease or System	Large Animal Species	Reference
Musculoskeletal		
Osteoarthritis	Horse	(Cantley et al. 1999) (McCoy 2015)
Osteochondrosis	Horse, Pig	(Mccoy et al. 2013) (McCoy et al. 2016) (Weeren 2016)
Stress Fracture	Horse	(O'Sullivan and Lumsden 2003) (Whitton et al. 2019)
Muscular Dystrophy	Pig	(Klymiuk et al. 2013) (Yu et al. 2016)
Malignant Hyperthermia	Pig	(Nelson 2002) (Kim et al. 2019)
Polysaccharide Storage Myopathy	Horse	(Mickelson and Valberg 2015)
Tendinopathy	Horse	(Smith 2008)
Respiratory		
Asthma	Horse	(Aun et al. 2017; Bond et al. 2018; Williams and Roman 2016)
Progressive Ethmoid Hematoma	Horse	(Head and Dixon 1999)
Gastrointestinal		
Gastric Ulcer	Horse, Swine, Cattle	(Burkitt et al. 2017; Gottardo et al. 2017) (Jones et al. 2014)
Nervous		
Hydrocephalus	Pig, Cattle, Horse	(Leech, Hauges, and Christoferson 1978; Leipold and Dennis 1987; Smith and Stevenson 1973)
Neuronal Ceroid Lipofuscinosis	Sheep, Cattle, Goat, Horse	(Cook et al. 2002)
Ophthalmologic		
Recurrent Uveitis	Horse	(Deeg et al. 2008; Witkowski et al. 2016)
Integument		
Connective Tissue Disorders		(Brinkman et al. 2017; Halper 2014; Malfait and De Paepe 2014)
Urinary		
Urolithiasis	Sheep, Goat, Pig, Horse, Cattle	(Van Metre et al. 2014)
Hematopoietic		
Hemophilia A	Sheep	(Lozier and Nichols 2013)
Von Willebrand	Pig	(Denis and Wagner 1999)
Age		
Neonatal Health	Horse	(Marr 2015)
Aging	Horse	(Kampf et al. 2019)

million worldwide (www.fao.org/faostat/en/#data/QA). Approximately 25% of the horse population in the United States resides on ranches and farms, while over 50% of horses are used for pleasure (USDA:APHIS:VS 2016). An estimate of the total number of equids worldwide in 2017 was 116 million animals. Consideration of the use of horses as a species to study naturally occurring diseases that are seen in man should include the variety of roles that horses play in people's lives and the different perspectives that owners will have of their animal (companion, pleasure, racing, or working horse). The health status of domesticated horses is typically closely monitored as they are an intensively managed species. Horses are generally amenable to some diagnostic and even surgical procedures being performed standing with sedation and local anesthesia without the need for general anesthesia. Many diseases in horses have been studied in detail and characterized with the ongoing advancements in equine medicine.

Cattle

Similar to the horse, cattle have long been a domesticated species in human society providing meat, milk, and hide production. Generally, cattle are divided into dairy and beef breeds, and management practices are vastly different between these groups. Dairy cattle are managed intensively during lactation, and milking is performed 2–3 times per day. Beef cattle are often managed extensively on large acreage farmland, although intensive management in feedlots is used in some regions for the final stage of growing cattle before slaughter for meat. There are estimated to be approximately 1.5 billion cattle worldwide and almost 94 million cattle in the United States. Specialized facilities for handling cattle are essential for personnel safety and many diagnostic procedures can be performed in the conscious or sedated animal with the aid of these handling facilities. As herbivores, cattle are ruminants and have a method of digestion in their rumen that relies on the microbial breakdown of plant material to molecules that can be absorbed and utilized for energy and other nutritional needs.

Sheep/Goats

Similar to cattle, sheep and goats are ruminants. Handling sheep and goats is less physically demanding than cattle and as such there is less need for specialized handling facilities for these species. There are over 1.2 billion sheep worldwide and just over 5 million in the United States. There are over 1 billion goats worldwide, with 2.6 million in the United States. Sheep are utilized for their wool and meat, while goats are divided into dairy and meat breeds similar to cattle.

Swine

There are almost 1 billion pigs worldwide with over 73 million in the United States. In addition to the larger domestic breeds used for commercial pork production, there are a number of miniature swine breeds, some which have been purposely developed for biomedical research. Pigs are omnivorous and monogastric animals having a gastrointestinal tract most similar to humans. Housing and handling of pigs require specialized equipment and facilities. Pigs are less tolerant than the other large animal species of having procedures performed while conscious and so often heavy sedation or general anesthesia is required. The immune system and body size of pigs is similar to people, at least when they are young and growing. Skeletally mature commercial pigs can weigh over 1,000 pounds, while special minipigs are closer to human bodyweights when they are fully grown.

A COMPARISON BY ORGAN SYSTEM OF DISEASES SEEN IN BOTH MAN AND ANIMALS

MUSCULOSKELETAL SYSTEM

Osteoarthritis

Naturally occurring osteoarthritis (OA) is a common disease in horses and other large animal species. Horses develop osteoarthritis both in their domesticated and wild environments (McCoy 2015; Cantley et al. 1999). Similarities between human and large animal joint structures, such as thickness of articular cartilage, as well as the relative size of joints, make study of the naturally occurring disease in these species comparable to the human condition (McCoy 2015). In addition, the larger relative size of joints in the horse compared to small animal species or rodents allows serial collection of synovial fluid for analysis, performance of clinical diagnostic techniques including arthroscopic examination, lameness and pain scoring, diagnostic imaging, and evaluations of histologic, biochemical, and biomechanical properties. The common athletic use of the horse allows for the assessment of rehabilitation and exercise programs on the progression of disease or in response to an intervention.

Osteoarthritis related to athletic use in horses often occurs at predictable sites and with consistent lesion locations, similar to human occupational and sports-related OA (McCoy 2015; Vina and Kwoh 2018; McIlwraith 2016). In racehorses, the carpus is one of two joints commonly affected by osteochondral fragmentation, and the progression of concurrent OA is predictable (Kawcak and Barrett 2016). This naturally occurring disease has been developed into an induced model of OA in the horse by creating the osteochondral fragmentation in a controlled manner arthroscopically (McIlwraith, Frisbie, and Kawcak 2012). This simulates the spontaneous disease in the horse and has been used for the evaluation of a range of therapeutics in controlled studies from corticosteroids, to biologics, and chondroprotective agents. Other joints commonly affected by posttraumatic OA due to athletic use in the horse are the metacarpophalangeal joint and the stifle (femorotibial joints) (McIlwraith 2016).

Spontaneous OA is uncommon in sheep and goats. However, due to the anatomic similarities to the human knee of the sheep or goat stifle, these species are used in induced models of OA despite the relatively low incidence of naturally occurring disease (McCoy 2015; Proffen et al. 2012). Pigs and cattle also do not develop spontaneous OA as commonly as the horse (or dog); however, cattle managed intensively can suffer from cranial cruciate ligament rupture in the stifle joint as a result of traumatic injury and develop secondary OA due to joint instability. The size of the animal makes repair of the ligament or prosthetic reconstruction challenging and not consistently successful (Crawford 1990). In addition, with better management conditions in cattle farming, a lower incidence of naturally occurring cruciate ligament injuries is likely over time as economic losses aim to be minimized by commercial operations.

Osteochondrosis

Osteochondrosis (OC) is a commonly recognized and relatively well-studied disease in large animal species, particularly horses and pigs. The economic consequences of the disease in these species and its relatively high prevalence has prompted ongoing investigation into its pathogenesis and potential therapeutic or preventative interventions. The underlying pathology of the disease is a failure of endochondral ossification in the articular-epiphyseal cartilage complex resulting in an area of thickened and necrotic cartilage at a location that focally prevents the advancement of secondary ossification toward the articular surface (McCoy et al. 2013; van Weeren 2016). These changes in the articular-epiphyseal cartilage complex may remain sub-clinical and go undetected, resolving over time as the animal matures. Alternatively, these lesions produce clinical disease due to a defect or cleft developing in the articular cartilage. The cartilage defect may progress and manifest as a partially detached flap or an osteochondral fragment. The articular pathology results in secondary synovial inflammation and joint effusion, mild joint pain, or lameness. These lesions are characteristically seen in specific joints and locations in the horse and the pig, including but not limited to the hock joint (human ankle), the stifle (human knee), and the fetlock (metacarpo- and metatarsophalangeal joints) in the horse, and the elbow, stifle, and hock joint in the pig (McCoy et al. 2013; Etterlin et al. 2014; Ytrehus et al. 2004; Toth et al. 2016). Until recently, the strong underlying associations between OC seen in animals and the disease in children and adolescents were not fully recognized (McCoy et al. 2013; Ytrehus, Carlson, and Ekman 2007). However, OC in humans, also termed osteochondritis dissecans or juvenile osteochondritis dissecans, has been shown to have strong similarities with the animal disease in terms of the underlying pathology at the articular epiphyseal cartilage complex. The discovery of identical lesions to those seen in animals at predilection sites of the femoral condyle in cadavers (Tóth et al. 2018) and the recognition that the pattern of disease development seen across the spectrum of different lesion locations, joints, and age groups, makes appealing the similarities between the animal disease and that found in man. Radiographic (horses) and postmortem (pigs) surveys found a high prevalence of OC in these species with most lesions being asymptomatic. Radiographic surveys of young horses generally found a prevalence of between 10 and 25% of study populations, varying by breed, joint location, and method of evaluation (van Weeren 2016). Postmortem surveys in pigs have similarly found a high prevalence. Interestingly, while up to 100% of pigs have microscopic OC lesions at an early age, the majority of these lesions resolve during maturation and do not manifest clinical disease (Toth et al. 2016). A postmortem and computed tomography study evaluating the hock joints of domestic pigs and wild boars found a prevalence of only 13% in the wild boars and 100% in the domestic pigs, highlighting that either genetic or environmental factors play a role in the prevalence of disease (Etterlin et al. 2017). In horses and pigs, heritability estimates can be as high as 0.52, again illustrating the potential role of genetics in the development of disease (McCoy et al. 2013; McCoy et al. 2016). Conversely in humans, low prevalence rates from 0.03% and up to 4.1% have been reported for symptomatic and radiographic disease, respectively (McCoy et al. 2013; Kida et al. 2014). One of the peculiarities of the human condition has been the reporting of each joint or joint location as a distinct disease. This specificity has led to multiple disease descriptions, many of which may have the common underlying pathology of OC but vary in their clinical presentation due to age of onset, joint involved, and prognosis for treatment. Examples of these human diseases include Thiemann's disease, Panner's disease, osteochondritis dissecans of the elbow, knee, or ankle, and Freiberg's disease (McCoy et al. 2013). Differing theories regarding the underlying pathology of these diseases may have resulted not only from the varied clinical presentations but also the information gained from studying lesions following surgical removal for treatment. The healing of osteochondral fragments in what are typically end-stage lesions resulted in an unclear picture of the underlying pathogenesis of OC in humans (McCoy et al. 2013). In addition, healing of radiographic juvenile osteochondritis dissecans lesions is reported to occur in human patients, which is similar to results of longitudinal radiographic monitoring in horses and postmortem surveys in pigs (McCoy et al. 2013; van Weeren 2016; Toth et al. 2016). Overall, spontaneously occurring OC in horses and pigs provides an excellent model for studying the human disease.

Stress Fracture

Stress fractures account for up to 20% of athletic injuries (Moreira and Bilezikian 2017) and are prominent in military recruits, ballet dancers, and competitive athletes and runners. Military recruits suffer stress fractures at a rate of approximately 7% (Davey et al. 2015). Stress fractures develop at specific sites in the skeleton as a result of repetitive physical activity that loads the affected area of bone beyond its elastic limits in such a way that it sustains repeated focal microdamage without complete bone failure. Maintenance of healthy bone tissue requires a balance between removal and replacement of damaged tissue. Over time with ongoing repetitive exercise, attempts at remodeling the area of damaged bone are insufficient to keep up with the accumulated focal damage and a stress injury or stress fracture results (Saunier and Chapurlat 2018; Moreira and Bilezikian 2017; Whitton et al. 2019; Entwistle et al. 2009). The remodeling process itself, through the creation of bone porosity during osteoclastic resorption of damaged tissue, may also contribute to a focal susceptibility to injury and temporary weakness in the bone (Entwistle et al. 2009; Stover 2017). There are many features of stress fractures seen in horses, predominantly racehorses, which are consistent with the disease in man. As a naturally occurring disease model, the condition as it exists in the racehorse offers several advantages for the researcher to utilize it as an investigative model. Stress fractures are relatively common in racehorses and they cover a broad range of injuries, both in terms of severity and specific locations. Similar to the disease in people, there are a number of common predilection sites, including the tibia (Whitton et al. 2019; O'Sullivan and Lumsden 2003), third metacarpal (Jalim et al. 2010; Powell 2012), and third metatarsal bones (Powell 2012), humerus (Whitton et al. 2019; O'Sullivan and Lumsden 2003), scapula (Vallance, Lumsden, and O'Sullivan 2009; Vallance, Spriet, and Stover 2011), pelvis and vertebrae (Haussler and Stover 1998). All racehorses undergo some degree of modeling and remodeling of their bones in response to the repeated activity of training and racing and the majority of skeletal injuries in racehorses are related to stress remodeling of bone. Unfortunately, an all too often consequence of stress fracture in the racehorse is its propagation into a complete fracture. These high energy injuries are often unable to be treated successfully, for a range of reasons, and in those cases euthanasia of the animal occurs on humane grounds (Vallance, Spriet, and Stover 2011; Estberg et al. 1998; 1996; Parkin et al. 2006). The result of this current reality is that there is a lot of postmortem information available from the bones of these horses. Many racing jurisdictions mandate performance of a necropsy on euthanized or deceased animals to maintain the integrity of racing by investigating for foul play, and to understand the cause of injury and/or death in each case (Stover and Murray 2008). Through these postmortem examinations a spectrum of the disease process has been identified, from mild periosteal callus formation and microscopic cortical bone damage at typical predilection sites through to complete or incomplete fractures of the same location in the opposite limb to the original fracture.

There are many similarities in the clinical presentation and risk factors for stress fracture in racehorses when compared to that seen in man. The distribution of injuries in military recruits and runners are predominantly in the lower limbs (Saunier and Chapurlat 2018) and in racehorses the majority of catastrophic stress-related injuries occur below the carpus and tarsus (Stover and Murray 2008). In runners, the tibia is the most common site of stress fracture (Saunier and Chapurlat 2018) while in horses, stress fractures of the tibia occur in younger racehorses and are more commonly diagnosed before complete fracture, compared to other sites such as the humerus (Whitton et al. 2019). Training features that increase the risk of stress fracture in people include an increase in intensity, duration, or frequency of the activity, with sudden increases in training often preceding a stress fracture (Saunier and Chapurlat 2018). Similar relationships have been found for some stress-related injuries in the horse when examining exercise intensity and training and racing distances galloped relative to the injury occurrence (Parkin 2008; Hill et al. 2004). Hard surface training results in a higher risk of stress fracture in people and surface features of racetracks have also been found to influence the occurrence and type of stress fracture observed in racehorses (Parkin 2008; MacKinnon et al. 2015). A change of footwear increases the risk of a stress fracture in human athletes (Saunier and Chapurlat 2018; Moreira and Bilezikian 2017), and the effect of shoeing characteristics have similarly been examined in racehorses and found to influence stress-related injury occurrence (Hill et al. 2004; Hernandez et al. 2005; Kane et al. 1996). While there are several similarities, there are also some differences of note. Women are 2–10 times more likely to suffer a stress fracture in the military than men (Saunier and Chapurlat 2018; Moreira and Bilezikian 2017). However, in racehorses a higher incidence of stress fractures has more commonly been seen in males if there is a difference at all (Parkin 2008). This difference may reflect an underlying lack of hormonal influence in female horses on the pathogenesis of stress fracture when compared to the influence in women. There are potentially confounding features of women that are not as prominent in female horses, which could make determining a difference between sexes in horses less likely. Female horses cycle seasonally, during the spring and summer, and most transition into a winter anestrous period based on day length. In contrast, a lot of women athletes who suffer from stress fractures are found to have irregular menstrual function (Moreira and Bilezikian 2017). Female racehorses have a similar body mass and bone mass to their male counterparts, again in contrast to the differences between women and men (Saunier and Chapurlat 2018; Moreira and Bilezikian 2017). There is also no documented difference in dietary energy availability for female racehorses compared to males. Therefore, the female athlete triad of irregular menstrual function, reduced bone mineral density, and low energy availability (Moreira and Bilezikian 2017), referenced as a significant risk factor in women athletes, would not appear to be present in the horse, which also supports the finding that female horses are not seen to be at higher risk of stress fracture than male horses. Low calcium intake and low vitamin D serum levels are present in human athletes at higher risk for stress fracture, though it is unknown what role nutrition may play in the equine athlete (Saunier and Chapurlat 2018; Moreira and Bilezikian 2017). Another notable difference between human athletes and their equine counterparts is anatomical. While on the surface this may appear to be a disadvantage of using this naturally occurring disease as a model for the disease in man, there is information to be gained by interpreting findings across a broader anatomical and physiological range. An example of this is the occasional finding that a specific type of stress-related injury occurs more frequently on one side of the body of a racehorse than the other, presumably due to the direction of racing around a circular or oval track. Specifically, for Australian Thoroughbred racehorses racing counterclockwise, tibial stress fractures of the caudolateral aspect of the bones midshaft occurred in the left limb compared to the right limb at a ratio of 10:3 (Whitton et al. 2019). Examining these and other examples can give insight into disease mechanism in a broader sense than studying man alone.

Similar to people, radiographs are often normal in equine athletes with a stress fracture, though there are some occasions where radiographs can be diagnostic, particularly in the lower limb. Bone scintigraphy is currently the most sensitive imaging modality used in horses to identify stress fractures (Whitton et al. 2019; O'Sullivan and Lumsden 2003). While scintigraphy was the gold standard for stress fracture diagnosis in people, with 100% sensitivity but low specificity, magnetic resonance imaging has become the gold standard diagnostic in people with 100% sensitivity and 85% specificity (Matcuk et al. 2016). Magnetic resonance imaging allows for grading of stress injuries from stress syndrome (termed stress reaction in horses) to stress fracture in people (Matcuk et al. 2016), and has also been introduced for the detection of lower limb injuries including stress fractures in the horse (Powell 2012). Additional advantages in using the equine athlete as a model of naturally occurring stress fractures in people include the ability to strictly control or monitor high-speed exercise activity or diet. Disadvantages of this naturally occurring disease model in horses are primarily related to the size of the animal, the challenge of tracking specific horses over time to follow disease progression, and the inability currently to perform advanced imaging such as MRI routinely on all areas of the limb, or on some areas of the limb without general anesthesia (Powell 2012).

Muscular Dystrophy

Duchenne muscular dystrophy is a fatal muscle disorder for which two induced or genetically modified models in pigs have been developed for study of the human condition. In addition to the spontaneously occurring disease in dogs discussed in the previous chapter, the pig models were developed by manipulating the DMD gene (Yu et al. 2016; Klymiuk et al. 2013). While these are not naturally occurring diseases, they do add to the tools a researcher can use in terms of evaluating the effect of therapeutics and the progression of the disease itself in an animal species that has a body size, diet, and immune system comparable to man (Perleberg, Kind, and Schnieke 2018; Wells 2018).

Malignant Hyperthermia

Malignant hyperthermia (MH) is an example of a human disease that our understanding of has benefited greatly from the existence of a similar, naturally occurring disease in the pig. The occurrence of MH in the pig contributed greatly to the understanding of the etiology, treatment effectiveness, and inheritance of the human disease. While advances have been made in the management of MH in humans (and pigs), it remains a clinical concern in various affected families in which the disease is present (Nelson 2002; Kim, Kriss, and Tautz 2019). The disease has also been reported in the dog and the horse (Nelson 2002; Mickelson and Valberg 2015). The underlying defect in MH is a mutation within the ryanodine receptor protein (RyR1), which forms the major calcium release channel from the sarcoplasmic reticulum following excitation-contraction coupling of the skeletal muscle cell. There are genetic differences between the human and pig diseases; however, each of them result in a RyR1 protein defect which results in a very similar disease phenotype (Nelson 2002). The disease manifests most commonly as an inappropriate yet unpredictable response to general anesthesia with a halogenated anesthetic agent. At the cellular level, during an MH episode, there is uncontrolled calcium release from the sarcoplasmic reticulum through the RyR1 calcium release channel. The return of calcium via a sarcolemmal sodium-calcium pump is an energy-dependent process, which is overwhelmed by the uncontrolled calcium release (Kim, Kriss, and Tautz 2019). The clinical consequence of these cellular events is a hypermetabolic state that includes tachycardia, a five-fold increase in oxygen consumption, hyperthermia, rhabdomyolysis, metabolic and respiratory acidosis, and electrolyte disturbances. In the absence of treatment, acidosis and electrolyte disturbances result in cardiac arrhythmias and death (Nelson 2002; Kim, Kriss, and Tautz 2019).

Stress syndrome in pigs and MH were initially linked at around the same time that MH was recognized in people in the 1960s (Nelson 2002). The link between the pig and human disease was eventually made by observing similar abnormal muscle biopsy contracture sensitivity to caffeine and halothane (Nelson 2002). Prior to the development of definitive treatments for MH, mortality rates of up to 70% were reported in affected people undergoing anesthesia with halogenated anesthetic agents. The discovery of MH in pigs allowed for the testing of candidate drugs to treat the disease. Dantrolene blocks release of calcium from skeletal muscle cells by binding to the RyR1 calcium release channel and causes relaxation in the muscle. The discovery and testing of this drug in pigs to ameliorate the clinical signs of MH was a major step forward in treating the human disease and resulted in dramatic reductions in mortality from MH episodes. Dantrolene is also currently used for prophylaxis and treatment of malignant hyperthermia in pigs and horses.

The MH story is an excellent example of a naturally occurring animal disease providing complementary and essential information to help improve the clinical outcomes in human patients. In the other direction, greater research resources available to study the human disease in pigs, considering its human health impact, have provided veterinarians with a better understanding of the underlying pathophysiology and treatments for both affected pigs and horses. The other aspect to this animal model example is that the genetic mutations are not the same, but they do result in essentially the same disease expression between species, which is a recurring theme in many naturally occurring animal models of disease in man.

Polysaccharide Storage Myopathy

Polysaccharide storage myopathy (PSSM) is a relatively common condition found in horses, typically in well-muscled breeds such as the Quarter Horse and Draft breeds (Mickelson and Valberg 2015). The hallmark signs of the disease, stiffness, firm muscles, pain, and reluctance to move, are due to the accumulation of glycogen within muscle cells which results in the development of myopathy during or after exercise. Type 1 PSSM in horses is due to a mutation in the glycogen synthase gene, which differs from most glycogen storage diseases in man. However, glycogen synthase deficiency is a disease which causes exercise-related arrhythmia and exercise intolerance in man (Tarnopolsky 2018; Akman, Raghavan, and Craigen 2011).

Tendinopathy

Similar to other musculoskeletal injuries in human athletes in which a spontaneous animal disease model may be utilized to advance the understanding of disease, tendinopathy occurs in the equine athlete at a relatively high rate. The most commonly injured tendon in the athletic horse is the superficial digital flexor tendon (SDFT), and tendon overstrain injuries can account for up to half of the racetrack limb injuries that occur during racing (Smith 2008). The types of injuries seen in the SDFT can vary from focal or core lesions located in the central region of the tendon, to generalized lesions with tendon thickening and minor fiber disruption, to peripheral injuries directly associated with surrounding peritendinous tissues, and finally, complete rupture. Similar to tendinopathy in man, injury recurrence is also common in the horse. There is evidence that repetitive loading of the tendon may result in degenerative changes within the tendon, or at least impaired healing of microdamage within the tendon substance (Smith 2008; Lui et al. 2011). Tendinopathy in horses has similarities to Achilles tendinopathy in man (Lui et al. 2011). The SDFT and Achilles tendons both function to store large amounts of energy during locomotion and reach strains during athletic use that are very close to their functional strain limits (Bogers and Barrett 2019). Both tendons are prone to overstrain injury associated with cumulative load of the tendon and have high re-injury rates (Smith 2008; Bogers and Barrett 2019). Histologically, fiber disruption, collagen fragmentation, and loss of matrix organization is observed along with hypercellularity, hypervascularity, and potential rounding of cells nuclei into a chondrocyte phenotype, are seen as a result of chronic injury (Lui et al. 2011).

As a result of the high occurrence of injury and the high recurrence rate in equine tendinopathy, an area of active research has been the application of regenerative therapies for treatment (Colbath et al. 2017). The regulatory constraints on veterinary use of these products has allowed some therapies to be adopted into common practice relatively quickly (Bogers and Barrett 2019). Regenerative therapies have evolved from an exploration of the potential of various cells, blood products, proteins, or extracellular matrix from within the body to provide anti-inflammatory and/or regenerative properties within an injured tissue (Bogers and Barrett 2019). The most commonly utilized therapies are platelet-rich plasma, autologous conditioned serum, and mesenchymal stem cells. These products are currently produced by commercially sold kits; however, the growth factor and cytokine profiles of these preparations can vary due to both patient and preparation factors. Early clinical trials reporting the use of mesenchymal stem cells for the treatment of tendinopathy in horses show promising results; however, a lack of randomized clinical trials with long-term follow-up and a comparable control group weakens the evidence that is currently available (Godwin et al. 2012). There are also many unanswered questions at this time regarding the best methods of application of many of these treatments. Timing relative to injury, optimum dosing, repeat treatments, and rehabilitation approaches combined with treatment are all approached in a somewhat empirical manner at this time. Further efforts to answer the effect of some of these variables may benefit both human and equine athletes in the future.

RESPIRATORY SYSTEM

Equine Asthma

Asthma is a significant human disease which affects over 300 million people worldwide (Aun et al. 2017). Asthma is a disease characterized by chronic inflammation of the lower airway, but it is heterogeneous in nature having a range of different phenotypes (Aun et al. 2017; Bond et al. 2018). Pathologic features of the disease include airway remodeling, mucus hypersecretion, epithelial fibrosis, metaplasia/hyperplasia of mucus-secreting cells, hypertrophy of airway smooth muscle, and bronchoconstriction (Aun et al. 2017; Bond et al. 2018; Williams and Roman 2016). Laboratory animal models of asthma lack the ability to perform long-term studies of this chronic disease (Kirschvink and Reinhold 2008). There are two naturally occurring diseases that serve as relevant animal models of asthma; these are feline and equine asthma (Aun et al. 2017; Williams and Roman 2016).

Recently, a realignment of terminology has been proposed for conditions which fall under the broader definition of equine asthma (Bond et al. 2018). There are a range of previously used terms that described these conditions in the horse, including heaves, equine chronic obstructive pulmonary disease, inflammatory airway disease (IAD), recurrent airway obstruction (RAO), and summer pasture associated obstructive pulmonary disease, to name but a few (Bond et al. 2018). However, efforts to consolidate and simplify terminology into one broad grouping of equine asthma now include the descriptive and previously well-accepted terms of IAD and RAO, while acknowledging that these descriptions fall within a spectrum of asthma disease seen in the horse. The key distinguishing feature between these two phenotypes of asthma in the horse is the clinical presence of increased respiratory effort at rest in cases of RAO (Bond et al. 2018). The mild and moderate forms of equine asthma are described as IAD, while more severe disease is described as RAO. An excellent review is available on equine asthma highlighting which features of human asthma phenotypes are most suited to using the naturally occurring disease in the horse as an appropriate model (Bond et al. 2018). Notably, both allergic and non-allergic asthma in humans have a range of similar features seen in the horse, although limitations exist and are discussed.

There are several advantages to using an equine model to study asthma. Diagnostic procedures such as bronchoalveolar lavage to study airway cytology are well tolerated in the horse and results have been previously well characterized. Lung function testing can be performed over a longitudinal study design to assess therapeutic interventions or disease progression. The disease can be induced in horses with exposure to an antigen and similarly ameliorated by removal of that exposure. Horses are tolerant of the disease in most cases, even when RAO is present, and clinical signs can be relieved using standard therapies of inhaled corticosteroids, bronchodilators, and removal of exposure to known antigens. These aspects of the disease, and the fact that the use of horses as a preclinical model for human asthma does not require euthanasia, make it a unique and ethical approach (Bullone and Lavoie 2019). Also of note in considering advantages and disadvantages of the equine asthma model is the range of predominant cell types which can occur in the different manifestations of the naturally occurring disease. In humans, in allergic asthma the predominant cell type appears to be eosinophils in the airway. In horses, an eosinophilic response can be seen in young horses, but overall a neutrophilic response is more common. Exposure to certain allergens such as dust and mold spores can also invoke a mixed granulocytic inflammation in horses. As with many models of disease, certain aspects of a disease will be suited to a naturally occurring model such as the equine asthma model, providing a more robust appreciation of the underlying disease processes than can be attained from induced and laboratory models of disease alone.

Progressive Ethmoid Hematoma

The progressive ethmoid hematoma of the horse is a non-neoplastic mass that has an unknown etiology and originates predominantly from the ethmoid labyrinth, though it is possible to find them in the maxillary, frontal, or sphenopalatine sinuses (Head and Dixon 1999). The lesions have a characteristic smooth surface and a range of colors reflecting the breakdown products of a hematoma in various stages, such as red, purple, green, and yellow. The typical clinical presentation in the horse is mild epistaxis or blood tinged nasal discharge from the affected side of the nasal passage. The mass is covered by a pseudostratified columnar epithelium and a fibrous tissue capsule develops with chronicity, although complete fibrosis and resolution of the entire mass of hemorrhage is not reported to occur. Surgical removal, chemical ablation, cryotherapy, and laser ablation of the mass are the most common treatment approaches; however, recurrence is a known and relatively common complication and may occur in up to 67% of cases (Tremaine and Dixon 2001b). In a survey of sinonasal disease treated at a single referral center over a 12-year period, progressive ethmoid hematoma comprised 7.6% of the cases diagnosed (Tremaine and Dixon 2001a).

Organized hematoma is an uncommon, benign lesion described in man that occurs primarily in the maxillary sinus, but is also observed in the sphenoid and frontal sinus, and in the nasal cavity (Pang et al. 2016; Kim, Oh, and Kwon 2016). The condition has many similarities to progressive ethmoid hematoma seen in horses; however, it occurs less commonly, comprising only 0.4% of cases undergoing endoscopic sinus surgery at a single surgery center over a 20-year period (Kim, Oh, and Kwon 2016). The clinical presentation of organized hematoma in humans involves epistaxis and nasal obstruction in over half of patients. The primary concern in making an accurate diagnosis in these cases is to ensure that the mass is not a form of malignancy. Often organized hematomas are incorrectly diagnosed at initial examination (Kim, Oh, and Kwon 2016). Histologically these lesions are an accumulation of hemorrhage within a fibrous capsule. The lesions can grow slowly and compress bony structures of the paranasal sinuses causing bony resorption to be seen on advanced imaging in approximately half the cases (Pang et al. 2016; Kim, Oh, and Kwon 2016). Endoscopic surgery is successful in the removal of organized hematoma, although one large case series had a recurrence rate of 6% at a mean of 23 months following the initial surgery (Pang et al. 2016). Given that the etiology of both progressive ethmoid hematoma of horses and organized hematoma of man are unknown, and that the clinical presentation, imaging, and pathological findings are similar, the use of progressive ethmoid hematoma as a model of this human disease may shed light on an etiology of both diseases and alternative treatment options that could reduce the recurrence rate following surgery (Tessier et al. 2013).

GASTROINTESTINAL SYSTEM

Gastric Ulcer Disease

Gastric ulceration has been described in several large animal species and is a clinically significant disease which can impair performance, quality of life, and farm animal productivity (Jones and Smith 2014; Gottardo et al. 2017; Burkitt et al. 2017). The primary large animal species affected with naturally occurring gastric ulceration are horses, swine, and cattle. The disease in each of these large animals has slightly different clinical presentations and unique features as well as some common risk factors both between these species and with peptic ulcer disease in man.

The pig was the first large animal to be considered as a potential model for gastric ulceration in people. In man, the two primary factors in the development of ulcer disease are the use of non-steroidal anti-inflammatory drugs and *Helicobacter pylori* infection. Pigs have been shown to harbor their own Helicobacter species, *H. suis*, which has been associated with the occurrence of gastritis, although a true cause and effect relationship is far from clear. Stress, feeding, and farm management practices have been shown to be associated with a higher risk of more severe and chronic forms of gastric ulceration in pigs (Gottardo et al. 2017).

Gastric ulceration in horses has recently been subdivided into two distinctly different disease manifestations based upon the anatomic location in which it occurs (Jones and Smith 2014). The equine stomach has a prominent squamous portion and a glandular portion and ulceration of each of these regions appears to have a different set of risk factors and expected response to therapy. Endoscopy of the horse's stomach can be performed to assess the gastric mucosa and scoring systems have been established to characterize ulceration and assess response to therapy. Horses are constant secretors of gastric acid due to their natural constant grazing tendencies. Ulceration of the squamous portion of the stomach is largely a disease of imposed management practices, with greater than 70% of Thoroughbred racehorses exhibiting evidence of ulceration while they are in race training (Jones and Smith 2014). Other breeds also show a high prevalence of visible ulcers in the stomach, though the clinical significance of mild ulcerations has certainly been questioned. However, it is possible to induce a high incidence of the disease by imposing a set of risk factors on the horse, such as a lack of grazing time, high concentrate diets, and high intensity exercise. By distinguishing differences between ulceration of the squamous and glandular regions of the stomach in the horse, it has become apparent that these two areas comprise different diseases with different risk factors. Prevalence of ulceration of the gastric region of the stomach is lower than the squamous region. Glandular ulceration is less responsive to omeprazole therapy than squamous region ulceration, leading some to suspect that there may be other as yet unknown factors involved in these cases, such as Helicobacter infection or anti-inflammatory drug use, similar to the disease in man.

Cattle are the other large animal species in which 'gastric' ulceration occurs. The forestomachs (rumen, reticulum, and omasum) precede the abomasum in ruminants. The abomasum is the equivalent of the monogastric stomach and abomasal ulceration is a distinct disease in this species. However, definitive ulcer diagnosis can be more challenging in cattle since endoscopy of the abomasum is not possible with the anatomical arrangement of the ruminant forestomachs. Clinical signs such as melena and anemia may provide a degree of suspicion of a bleeding ulcer. In contrast to the other species, ulcers in cattle perforate at a higher rate leading to either localized or generalized peritonitis. This may be due to the non-distinct clinical signs that are associated with ulcer disease in cattle and a failure to recognize the disease before significant progression. The prevalence of ulcers is reported as being up to 76% in calves and up to 20% in adult cattle at slaughter. As with the horse, pig, and humans, stress, diet, and NSAID use are involved in the pathogenesis of abomasal ulcers in cattle. A disease which crosses species such as gastric ulcer disease provides a unique comparative aspect to understanding the strong underlying causes of the disease in the different species and in man. Clearly, stress, diet, and NSAID drug use are common to each; however, at this time only the pig appears to have a strong relationship with Helicobacter infection in the pathogenesis of ulcer disease.

NERVOUS SYSTEM

Hydrocephalus

Congenital hydrocephalus has been reported in pigs, cattle, and the horse (Smith and Stevenson 1973; Leipold and Dennis 1987; Leech, Hauges, and Christoferson 1978). The condition has been reported as a recessive inherited trait in pigs and cattle, with most affected individuals not living longer than a few days if they were born alive (Smith and Stevenson 1973; Leech, Hauges, and Christoferson 1978). Several cattle breeds have been associated with the disease including Hereford, Shorthorn, Ayrshire, Holstein-Friesian, Jersey, and Angus (Leech, Hauges, and Christoferson 1978). In pigs, both purebred and crossbred animals have been reported with hydrocephalus (Smith and Stevenson 1973). The clinical features of some of these naturally occurring cases of congenital hydrocephalus have been described, including cerebellar hypoplasia, microphthalmia, and retinal dysplasia. The pathological basis of these diseases has been reported as a compressive or obstructive lesion in the ventricular system most commonly (Leech, Hauges, and Christoferson 1978). Another form of hydrocephalus observed in cattle is a result of intrauterine infection with viral agents, including bovine viral diarrhea virus, Schmallenberg virus, and blue tongue virus (Agerholm et al. 2015). Considering the complex array of potential causes of congenital hydrocephalus in humans and the lack of detailed knowledge of these naturally occurring diseases in large animals, it is an area that would require further background work to identify a suitable model of the disease in children (McAllister 2012). Our understanding of multifactorial diseases such as hydrocephalus can benefit from having a broad number of animal models to work with and follow up on mechanistically. Two features of cattle may assist in producing a model which can be studied. First, farmers are usually very willing to remove affected animals from their breeding stock, as with many heritable diseases; consequently, collection of both genetic and postmortem material can be readily achieved (Leech, Hauges, and Christoferson 1978). Secondly, the common use of advanced reproductive technology in modern cattle breeding, such as superovulation and embryo transfer, could make generating stock for genetic testing and disease characterization more feasible than in other species.

Neuronal Ceroid Lipofuscinosis (Batten Disease)

The neuronal ceroid lipofuscinoses (NCL) are a group of diseases in humans and animals in which lipopigment accumulates, predominantly within neurons, resulting in neurodegenerative changes to the brain and retina. Effects on other tissues outside the nervous system are also reported (Cooper and Mole 2020). A range of specific disorders have been identified in people based on clinical phenotype, properties of the storage material, and genetic analysis (Cook et al. 2002; Cooper and Mole 2020). There are reports of the disease in sheep, cattle, goats, and horses (Cook et al. 2002). More commonly for research purposes, models in rodents, cats, and dogs have been described. However, as various treatments have been developed over time, there has been the realization that animal model systems beyond rodents are required to fully explore therapeutic delivery and response before entering into human trials. For example, this includes promising new therapeutic areas such as virus associated gene delivery (Cooper and Mole 2020). Large animal models such as those seen in Merino and South Hampshire sheep have been characterized with the goal of providing these types of tools for the researcher (Cook et al. 2002; Tammen et al. 2001; Cronin et al. 2016).

OPHTHALMOLOGIC

Equine Recurrent Uveitis

While there are multiple examples of ophthalmologic diseases in large animal species that could serve as models for human disease, equine recurrent uveitis (ERU) has been shown to have a strong similarity to human autoimmune uveitis in clinical, pathological, and immunological aspects of the disease (Witkowski et al. 2016; Deeg et al. 2008). In horses, naturally occurring ERU is a common disease, with a prevalence of around 10% in the general equine population (Witkowski et al. 2016; Deeg et al. 2008). Clinical features of ERU include a cycle of remission and relapse with inflammatory changes present in the uveal tract of the eye. It should be distinguished from primary uveitis, which is less common than the recurring disease and may not involve an immune-mediated source of inflammation. An insidious form of ERU occurs in which the intraocular inflammation is mild but persistent, resulting in destructive changes to the eye without obvious clinical signs of pain or acute episodes (Witkowski et al. 2016). Acute episodes with signs of anterior uveitis are painful and may worsen with repeat bouts of disease. End stage disease occurs when sufficient damage has occurred to cause blindness (Witkowski et al. 2016). Genetic influences in the disease are evidenced by the high prevalence of disease in Appaloosas as well as the prevalence of bilateral disease within this breed compared to the general population (80% vs. 40%) (Witkowski et al. 2016). The local immune-mediated process of ocular inflammation involves both humoral and cellular mechanisms in ERU. There are several candidate autoantigens that are shared between horses and humans and ongoing investigations into these features of the disease are likely to yield mutually beneficial findings (Deeg et al. 2008; Kleinwort et al. 2016). Leptospira spp. infection and seropositivity have been established in the horse as a risk factor for ERU, although a Leptospiral etiology appears to be somewhat dependent on geographic location (Witkowski et al. 2016). The features of ERU that make it an attractive naturally occurring model of disease for autoimmune uveitis in people include: 1) the high prevalence of the disease in horses; 2) the availability of specialist veterinary ophthalmologists to collaborate, examine, and characterize the disease in horses; 3) the similar autoimmune features of ERU, including some specific autoantigens identified in both humans and horses; 4) the long life span of the horse which enables monitoring of disease progression over time and specific hypothesis testing trials to be performed; 5) the highly domesticated nature of most horses which makes ocular examination a routine veterinary procedure; and 6) the general willingness of horse owners to pursue clinical trials that may benefit both people and their horse.

INTEGUMENT

Connective Tissue Disorders

There are a number of connective tissue disorders seen in large animal species that have similarity with human diseases. Ehlers-Danlos syndromes (EDS) are a group of diseases which display soft connective tissue fragility clinically affecting skin, ligaments, joints, organs, and blood vessels in people. There are a number of subtypes described within EDS and these are based on the phenotype, inheritance, and the underlying molecular or biochemical defect (Malfait and De Paepe 2014). Heritable equine regional dermal asthenia (HERDA) is a disorder of horses in which loose and fragile skin are the hallmark clinical signs (Brinkman et al. 2017; Halper 2014). This is an autosomal recessive disorder that has been well described in Quarter Horse breeds, with some estimates of an increasing incidence of heterozygotes in certain sub-populations (Rashmir-Raven and Spier 2015). The disease is due to a mutation in the gene that encodes cyclophilin B, which acts in the processing of procollagen and is required to form the triple helix of fibrillar collagen (Brinkman et al. 2017). Cyclophilin B also has functions of trafficking, processing, and chain association during collagen synthesis. The HERDA phenotype is most closely aligned with the EDS subtype VI, known as the kyphoscoliotic form (Brinkman et al. 2017; Rashmir-Raven and Spier 2015). Another subtype of EDS is type VIIC, dermatosparaxis, which is characterized by fragile skin. This condition has been described in sheep and cattle and is due to mutations of the ADAMTS2 gene or of the procollagen I N-proteinase gene in cattle (Halper 2014).

Urinary System

Urolithiasis

Urolithiasis is a disease that occurs in large animal species including sheep, goats, pigs, horses, and cattle (Van Metre and Dawson Soto 2014). It is also a disease that is seen worldwide in the human population (Yasui et al. 2017). Urolithiasis is a multifactorial disease in both animals and humans. Some common contributing factors include genetics and environmental factors such as diet, lifestyle, gender, time of year, and dehydration (Yasui et al. 2017; Van Metre and Dawson Soto 2014). Following the establishment of a nidus, such as mucoproteins, cellular debris, urinary casts or bacteria, mineral precipitation, and crystal formation are dependent on the mineral content of the urine and the urine pH, and in herbivores such as horses and ruminants urine pH tends to be higher than animals on meat-based diets. In ruminants, early castration as part of herd management practice has been shown to have a negative effect on the urethral diameter and may predispose to urinary obstruction from calculi passing along the urethra (Videla and van Amstel 2016; Van Metre and Dawson Soto 2014). This should be considered when examining the incidence of disease in these species if they are considered as a model of human disease. Diet has a major influence on the type of calculi that may be present in large animals. Silicates are common in pasture-grazing animals, particularly on rangelands in western North America (Van Metre and Dawson Soto 2014; Videla and van Amstel 2016). Phosphate-based calculi are more common with high-concentrate grain feeding in farm animals as the calcium-to-phosphorus ratio in the diet may be less than 2:1. Struvite (magnesium ammonium phosphate) and apatite (calcium phosphate) uroliths are the most commonly observed in these circumstances, although for struvite uroliths the role of magnesium, potassium, and phosphorus cycling from saliva has also been implicated in an increased incidence of disease (Van Metre and Dawson Soto 2014; Robinson et al. 2008). In the small ruminant species of sheep and goats, calcium carbonate stones are common, although this can vary with geographic location and pasture or forage availability (Videla and van Amstel 2016). In people, calcium oxalate stones are common and these have been recorded in most animal species, typically associated with consuming oxalate-containing plants (Videla and van Amstel 2016; Robinson et al. 2008); however, a thorough understanding of the dietary and metabolic factors which influence their occurrence in ruminants is not available (Van Metre and Dawson Soto 2014). Urolithiasis is most commonly diagnosed in large animal species as a result of urethral obstruction, which can precipitate a life-threatening crisis if it is not alleviated. Nephrolithiasis and ureterolithiasis do occur but are often not detected in large animal species due to vague clinical signs and difficulty in obtaining sensitive diagnostic imaging of these locations. Depending on the species and the location of the obstruction, there is an extensive list of surgical options for relieving urethral obstruction (Videla and van Amstel 2016). The array of urolith types occurring naturally in the range of large animal species presented gives rise to opportunities to further the understanding of this disease for both man and animals. An opportunity exists to control diets and other environmental factors in research trial settings to uncover a more complete understanding of pathophysiology and treatment of urolithiasis in man and animals.

HEMATOPOIETIC SYSTEM

Bleeding Disorders

Hemophilia A has been studied in sheep based on a severe factor VIII deficiency (Lozier and Nichols 2013). The genetics of the initial line of sheep that were studied had to be reestablished through advanced breeding technologies as the original animals were not maintained. This was achieved through cryopreservation of semen, intracytoplasmic sperm injection, and embryo transfer. The result of this effort was an ability to further characterize the genetic basis for the lack of factor VIII activity. Unfortunately, this line of sheep suffers severe bleeding and so are difficult to maintain without serious consequences and therefore are a difficult animal model to study (Lozier and Nichols 2013). Hemophilia A has also been reported in the horse, but it is rare.

Von Willebrand disease, due to a lack of von Willebrand factor (VWF), is naturally occurring in pigs and dogs, and has many similarities to the human disease. The VWF is found in platelets, endothelial cells, and megakaryocytes in both pigs and humans and there is a high degree of homology between VWF across the species which results in cross reactivity and function in binding platelets, collagen, and factor VIII. Von Willebrand disease is not fully characterized in pigs as the gene mutation responsible has not been identified as yet; however, many other details of the disease in pigs are known and have been well documented, including similar levels of VWF relative to that seen in humans, and the presence of low levels of VWF in affected individuals (Denis and Wagner 1999). The disease in pigs is transmitted as an autosomal recessive trait (Lozier and Nichols 2013; Denis and Wagner 1999).

AGE-RELATED HEALTH COMPARISONS

Neonatal Health

There are many similarities in neonatal care that span across species including man. Common issues include lung maturity and surfactant properties at birth, true congenital anomalies, neurological development and the effects of prolonged or difficult parturition, skeletal, and muscular development in terms of normal joint and limb formation and growth, and the impact of placental abnormalities or infectious agents. The list is long and the differences between animals and man are many; however, in some cases the comparative aspects to these areas of challenge may provide insights that are not apparent with a tunnel vision approach to the study of one species.

Aging

Study of the effects of aging is suited to utilizing species such as the horse and the dog. Horses have an expected life span of up to 40 years and the equine population is getting older as a result of improved health care, diets, and owners' attitudes towards equine 'retirement'. Some of the challenges of caring for older horses are being recognized by both owners and their veterinarians. Information regarding immune function, nervous system changes, gastrointestinal health and disease, respiratory disease susceptibility, quality of life issues including lameness, and musculoskeletal health, as they relate to aging will be important for equine health care moving forward, but may also provide insights into the aging process in people.

REFERENCES

1. Agerholm, Jorgen S., Marion Hewicker-Trautwein, Klaas Peperkamp, and Peter A. Windsor. 2015. "Virus-Induced Congenital Malformations in Cattle." *Acta Veterinaria Scandinavica* 57(September): 54. doi:10.1186/s13028-015-0145-8.
2. Akman, H. Orhan, Adithya Raghavan, and William J. Craigen. 2011. "Animal Models of Glycogen Storage Disorders." *Progress in Molecular Biology and Translational Science* 100: 369–88. Elsevier. doi:10.1016/B978-0-12-384878-9.00009-1.
3. Aun, Marcelo, Rafael Bonamichi-Santos, Fernanda Magalhães Arantes-Costa, Jorge Kalil, and Pedro Giavina-Bianchi. 2017. "Animal Models of Asthma: Utility and Limitations." *Journal of Asthma and Allergy* 10(November): 293–301. doi:10.2147/JAA.S121092.
4. Bogers, Sophie H., and Jennifer G. Barrett. 2019. "Chapter 4: Veterinary Medicine's Advances in Regenerative Orthopedics." In: *Metabolic Therapies in Orthopedics*, 2nd ed., edited by Ingrid Kohlstadt and Kenneth Cintron, 57–89. Boca Raton, FL: CRC Press.
5. Bond, Stephanie, Renaud Léguillette, Eric A. Richard, Laurent Couetil, Jean-Pierre Lavoie, James G. Martin, and R. Scott Pirie. 2018. "Equine Asthma: Integrative Biologic Relevance of a Recently Proposed Nomenclature." *Journal of Veterinary Internal Medicine* 32(6): 2088–98. doi:10.1111/jvim.15302.
6. Brinkman, Erin L., Benjamin C. Weed, Sourav S. Patnaik, Bryn L. Brazile, Ryan M. Centini, Robert W. Wills, Bari Olivier, et al. 2017. "Cardiac Findings in Quarter Horses with Heritable Equine Regional Dermal Asthenia." *Journal of the American Veterinary Medical Association* 250(5): 538–47. doi:10.2460/javma.250.5.538.
7. Bullone, Michela, and Jean-Pierre Lavoie. 2019. "The Equine Asthma Model of Airway Remodeling: From a Veterinary to a Human Perspective." *Cell and Tissue Research*, November. doi:10.1007/s00441-019-03117-4.
8. Burkitt, Michael D., Carrie A. Duckworth, Jonathan M. Williams, and D. Mark Pritchard. 2017. "Helicobacter pylori-Induced Gastric Pathology: Insights from *In Vivo* and *Ex Vivo* Models." *Disease Models and Mechanisms* 10(2): 89–104. doi:10.1242/dmm.027649.
9. Cantley, C. E., E. C. Firth, J. W. Delahunt, D. U. Pfeiffer, and K. G. Thompson. 1999. "Naturally Occurring Osteoarthritis in the Metacarpophalangeal Joints of Wild Horses." *Equine Veterinary Journal* 31(1): 73–81. doi:10.1111/j.2042-3306.1999. tb03794.x.
10. Colbath, Aimée C., David D. Frisbie, Steven W. Dow, John D. Kisiday, C. Wayne McIlwraith, and Laurie R. Goodrich. 2017. "Equine Models for the Investigation of Mesenchymal Stem Cell Therapies in Orthopaedic Disease." *Operative Techniques in Sports Medicine*, Update on Orthobiologics 25(1): 41–9. doi:10.1053/j. otsm.2016.12.007.

11. Cook, R. W., R. D. Jolly, D. N. Palmer, I. Tammen, M. F. Broom, and R. McKinnon. 2002. "Neuronal Ceroid Lipofuscinosis in Merino Sheep." *Australian Veterinary Journal* 80(5): 292–97. doi:10.1111/j.1751-0813.2002.tb10847.x.

12. Cooper, Jonathan D., and Sara E. Mole. 2020. "Future Perspectives: What Lies Ahead for Neuronal Ceroid Lipofuscinosis Research?" *Biochimica et Biophysica Acta (BBA). Molecular Basis of Disease*, January, 165681. doi:10.1016/j.bbadis.2020.165681.

13. Crawford, W. H. 1990. "Intra-Articular Replacement of Bovine Cranial Cruciate Ligaments with an Autogenous Fascial Graft." *Veterinary Surgery: VS* 19(5): 380–88. doi:10.1111/j.1532-950x.1990.tb01213.x.

14. Cronin, Greg M., Danai F. Beganovic, Amanda L. Sutton, J. Palmer David, Peter C. Thomson, and Imke Tammen. 2016. "Manifestation of Neuronal Ceroid Lipofuscinosis in Australian Merino Sheep: Observations on Altered Behaviour and Growth." *Applied Animal Behaviour Science* 175(February): 32–40. doi:10.1016/j.applanim.2015.11.012.

15. Davey, Trish, Susan A. Lanham-New, Anneliese M. Shaw, Rosalyn Cobley, Adrian J. Allsopp, Mark O. R. Hajjawi, Timothy R. Arnett, Pat Taylor, Cyrus Cooper, and Joanne L. Fallowfield. 2015. "Fundamental Differences in Axial and Appendicular Bone Density in Stress Fractured and Uninjured Royal Marine Recruits--A Matched Case-Control Study." *Bone* 73(April): 120–26. doi:10.1016/j.bone.2014.12.018.

16. Deeg, Cornelia A., Stefanie M. Hauck, Barbara Amann, Dirk Pompetzki, Frank Altmann, Albert Raith, Thomas Schmalzl, Manfred Stangassinger, and Marius Ueffing. 2008. "Equine Recurrent Uveitis--A Spontaneous Horse Model of Uveitis." *Ophthalmic Research* 40(3–4): 151–53. doi:10.1159/000119867.

17. Denis, C. V., and D. D. Wagner. 1999. "Insights from Von Willebrand Disease Animal Models." *Cellular and Molecular Life Sciences: CMLS* 56(11–12): 977–90. doi:10.1007/s000180050487.

18. Entwistle, Rachel C., Sara C. Sammons, Robert F. Bigley, Scott J. Hazelwood, David P. Fyhrie, Jeffery C. Gibeling, and Susan M. Stover. 2009. "Material Properties Are Related to Stress Fracture Callus and Porosity of Cortical Bone Tissue at Affected and Unaffected Sites." *Journal of Orthopaedic Research* 27(10): 1272–79. doi:10.1002/jor.20892.

19. Estberg, L., S. M. Stover, I. A. Gardner, C. M. Drake, B. Johnson, and A. Ardans 1996. "High-Speed Exercise History and Catastrophic Racing Fracture in Thoroughbreds." *American Journal of Veterinary Research* 57(11): 1549–55.

20. Estberg, L., S. M. Stover, I. A. Gardner, B. J. Johnson, R. A. Jack, J. T. Case, A. Ardans, et al. 1998. "Relationship between Race Start Characteristics and Risk of Catastrophic Injury in Thoroughbreds: 78 Cases (1992)." *Journal of the American Veterinary Medical Association* 212(4): 544–49.

21. Etterlin, P. E., S. Ekman, R. Strand, K. Olstad, and C. J. Ley. 2017. "Osteochondrosis, Synovial Fossae, and Articular Indentations in the Talus and Distal Tibia of Growing Domestic Pigs and Wild Boars." *Veterinary Pathology* 54(3): 445–56. doi:10.1177/0300985816688743.

22. Etterlin, Pernille Engelsen, Bjørnar Ytrehus, Nils Lundeheim, Eva Heldmer, Julia Österberg, and Stina Ekman. 2014. "Effects of Free-Range and Confined Housing on Joint Health in a Herd of Fattening Pigs." *BMC Veterinary Research* 10(September): 208. doi:10.1186/s12917-014-0208-5.

23. Godwin, E. E., N. J. Young, J. Dudhia, I. C. Beamish, and R. K. W. Smith. 2012. "Implantation of Bone Marrow-Derived Mesenchymal Stem Cells Demonstrates Improved Outcome in Horses with Overstrain Injury of the Superficial Digital Flexor Tendon." *Equine Veterinary Journal* 44(1): 25–32. doi:10.1111/j.2042-3306.2011.00363.x.

24. Gottardo, F., A. Scollo, B. Contiero, M. Bottacini, C. Mazzoni, and S. A. Edwards. 2017. "Prevalence and Risk Factors for Gastric Ulceration in Pigs Slaughtered at 170 Kg." *Animal: An International Journal of Animal Bioscience* 11(11): 2010–18. doi:10.1017/S1751731117000799.

25. Halper, Jaroslava. 2014. "Chapter 14: Connective Tissue Disorders in Domestic Animals." *Progress in Heritable Soft Connective Tissue Diseases*, 231–40. Advances in Experimental Medicine and Biology 802. Dordrecht; New York: Springer.

26. Haussler, K. K., and S. M. Stover. 1998. "Stress Fractures of the Vertebral Lamina and Pelvis in Thoroughbred Racehorses." *Equine Veterinary Journal* 30(5): 374–81. doi:10.1111/j.2042-3306.1998.tb04504.x.

27. Head, K. W., and P. M. Dixon. 1999. "Equine Nasal and Paranasal Sinus Tumours. Part 1: Review of the Literature and Tumour Classification." *Veterinary Journal* 157(3): 261–78. doi:10.1053/tvjl.1998.0370.

28. Hernandez, Jorge A., Mary C. Scollay, Dan L. Hawkins, Julie A. Corda, and Traci M. Krueger. 2005. "Evaluation of Horseshoe Characteristics and High-Speed Exercise History as Possible Risk Factors for Catastrophic Musculoskeletal Injury in Thoroughbred Racehorses." *American Journal of Veterinary Research* 66(8): 1314–20.

29. Hill, Ashley E., Ian A. Gardner, Tim E. Carpenter, and Susan M. Stover. 2004. "Effects of Injury to the Suspensory Apparatus, Exercise, and Horseshoe Characteristics on the Risk of Lateral Condylar Fracture and Suspensory Apparatus Failure in Forelimbs of Thoroughbred Racehorses." *American Journal of Veterinary Research* 65(11): 1508–17.

30. Jalim, S. L., C. W. McIlwraith, N. L. Goodman, and G. A. Anderson. 2010. "Lag Screw Fixation of Dorsal Cortical Stress Fractures of the Third Metacarpal Bone in 116 Racehorses." *Equine Veterinary Journal* 42(7): 586–90. doi:10.1111/j.2042-3306.2010.00071.x.

31. Jones, Samuel L., and Bradford P. Smith, eds. 2014. "Chapter 32: Diseases of the Alimentary Tract." *Large Animal Internal Medicine*, 5th ed., 638–842. Saint Louis, MI: Elsevier.

32. Kane, A. J., S. M. Stover, I. A. Gardner, J. T. Case, B. J. Johnson, D. H. Read, and A. A. Ardans. 1996. "Horseshoe Characteristics as Possible Risk Factors for Fatal Musculoskeletal Injury of Thoroughbred Racehorses." *American Journal of Veterinary Research* 57(8): 1147–52.

33. Kawcak, Christopher E., and Myra F. Barrett. 2016. "22 - Carpus." In: *Joint Disease in the Horse*, 2nd ed., edited by C. Wayne McIlwraith, David D. Frisbie, Christopher E. Kawcak, and P. René van Weeren, 318–31. Edinburgh: W.B. Saunders. doi:10.1016/B978-1-4557-5969-9.00022-X.

34. Kida, Y., T. Morihara, Y. Kotoura, T. Hojo, H. Tachiiri, T. Sukenari, Y. Iwata, et al. 2014. "Prevalence and Clinical Characteristics of Osteochondritis Dissecans of the Humeral Capitellum among Adolescent Baseball Players." *American Journal of Sports Medicine* 42(8): 1963–71. doi:10.1177/0363546514536843.

35. Kim, J. S., J. S. Oh, and S. H. Kwon. 2016. "The Increasing Incidence of Paranasal Organizing Hematoma: A 20-Year Experience of 23 Cases at a Single Center." *Rhinology Journal* 54(2): 176–82. doi:10.4193/Rhin15.158.

36. Kim, Kyeong Seon M., Robert Scott Kriss, and Timothy J. Tautz. 2019. "Malignant Hyperthermia." *Advances in Anesthesia* 37(December): 35–51. doi:10.1016/j.aan.2019.08.003.

37. Kirschvink, Nathalie, and Petra Reinhold. 2008. "Use of Alternative Animals as Asthma Models." *Current Drug Targets* 9(6): 470–84. doi:10.2174/138945008784533525.

38. Kleinwort, Kristina J. H., Barbara Amann, Stefanie M. Hauck, Regina Feederle, Walter Sekundo, and Cornelia A. Deeg. 2016. "Immunological Characterization of Intraocular Lymphoid Follicles in a Spontaneous Recurrent Uveitis Model." *Investigative Opthalmology and Visual Science* 57(10): 4504. doi:10.1167/iovs.16-19787.

39. Klymiuk, Nikolai, Andreas Blutke, Alexander Graf, Sabine Krause, Katinka Burkhardt, Annegret Wuensch, Stefan Krebs, et al. 2013. "Dystrophin-Deficient Pigs Provide New Insights into the Hierarchy of Physiological Derangements of Dystrophic Muscle." *Human Molecular Genetics* 22(21): 4368–82. doi:10.1093/hmg/ddt287.

40. Leech, R. W., C. N. Hauges, and L. A. Christoferson. 1978. "Hydrocephalus, Congenital Hydrocephalus. Aminal Model: Bovine Hydrocephalus, Congenital Internal Hydrocephalus, Aqueductal Stenosis." *The American Journal of Pathology* 92(2): 567–70.

41. Leipold, H. W., and S. M. Dennis. 1987. "Congenital Defects of the Bovine Central Nervous System." *The Veterinary Clinics of North America. Food Animal Practice* 3(1): 159–77. doi:10.1016/s0749-0720(15)31188-9.

42. Lozier, Jay N., and Timothy C. Nichols. 2013. "Animal Models of Hemophilia and Related Bleeding Disorders." *Seminars in Hematology* 50(2): 175–84. doi:10.1053/j.seminhematol.2013.03.023.

43. Lui, P. P. Y., N. Maffulli, C. Rolf, and R. K. W. Smith. 2011. "What Are the Validated Animal Models for Tendinopathy?" *Scandinavian Journal of Medicine and Science in Sports* 21(1): 3–17. doi:10.1111/j.1600-0838.2010.01164.x.

44. MacKinnon, M. C., D. Bonder, R. C. Boston, and M. W. Ross. 2015. "Analysis of Stress Fractures Associated with Lameness in Thoroughbred Flat Racehorses Training on Different Track Surfaces Undergoing Nuclear Scintigraphic Examination: Stress Fractures and Training Surface." *Equine Veterinary Journal* 47(3): 296–301. doi:10.1111/evj.12285.

45. Malfait, Fransiska, and Anne De Paepe. 2014. "Chapter 9: The Ehlers-Danlos Syndrome." *Progress in Heritable Soft Connective Tissue Diseases*, 129–43. Advances in Experimental Medicine and Biology 802. Dordrecht; New York: Springer.

46. Matcuk, George R., Scott R. Mahanty, Matthew R. Skalski, Dakshesh B. Patel, Eric A. White, and Christopher J. Gottsegen. 2016. "Stress Fractures: Pathophysiology, Clinical Presentation, Imaging Features, and Treatment Options." *Emergency Radiology* 23(4): 365–75. doi:10.1007/s10140-016-1390-5.

47. McAllister, James P. 2012. "Pathophysiology of Congenital and Neonatal Hydrocephalus." *Seminars in Fetal and Neonatal Medicine*, Fetal Neurology: Volume 1 17(5): 285–94. doi:10.1016/j.siny.2012.06.004.

48. McCoy, A. M. 2015. "Animal Models of Osteoarthritis: Comparisons and Key Considerations." *Veterinary Pathology* 52(5): 803–18. doi:10.1177/0300985815588611.

49. McCoy, A. M., F. Toth, N. I. Dolvik, S. Ekman, J. Ellermann, K. Olstad, B. Ytrehus, and C. S. Carlson. 2013. "Articular Osteochondrosis: A Comparison of Naturally-Occurring Human and Animal Disease." *Osteoarthritis and Cartilage* 21(11): 1638–47. doi:10.1016/j.joca.2013.08.011.

50. McCoy, Annette M., Samantha K. Beeson, Rebecca K. Splan, Sigrid Lykkjen, Sarah L. Ralston, James R. Mickelson, and Molly E. McCue. 2016. "Identification and Validation of Risk Loci for Osteochondrosis in Standardbreds." *BMC Genomics* 17(January): 41. doi:10.1186/s12864-016-2385-z.

51. McIlwraith, C. W., D. D. Frisbie, and C. E. Kawcak. 2012. "The Horse as a Model of Naturally Occurring Osteoarthritis." *Bone and Joint Research* 1(11): 297–309. doi:10.1302/2046-3758.111.2000132.

52. McIlwraith, C. Wayne. 2016. "3 - Traumatic Arthritis and Posttraumatic Osteoarthritis in the Horse." In: *Joint Disease in the Horse*, 2nd ed., edited by C. Wayne McIlwraith, David D. Frisbie, Christopher E. Kawcak, and P. René van Weeren, 33–48. Edinburgh: W.B. Saunders.

53. Mickelson, James R., and Stephanie J. Valberg. 2015. "The Genetics of Skeletal Muscle Disorders in Horses." *Annual Review of Animal Biosciences* 3: 197–217. doi:10.1146/annurev-animal-022114-110653.

54. Moreira, Carolina A., and John P. Bilezikian. 2017. "Stress Fractures: Concepts and Therapeutics." *The Journal of Clinical Endocrinology and Metabolism* 102(2): 525–34. doi:10.1210/jc.2016-2720.

55. Nelson, Thomas E. 2002. "Malignant Hyperthermia: A Pharmacogenetic Disease of Ca++ Regulating Proteins." *Current Molecular Medicine* 2(4): 347–69. doi:10.2174/1566524023362429.

56. O'Sullivan, Christopher B., and Jonathan M. Lumsden. 2003. "Stress Fractures of the Tibia and Humerus in Thoroughbred Racehorses: 99 Cases (1992–2000)." *Journal of the American Veterinary Medical Association* 222(4): 491–98. doi:10.2460/javma.2003.222.491.

57. Pang, Wenhui, Li Hu, Huan Wang, Yan Sha, Na Ma, Shuyi Wang, Quan Liu, Xicai Sun, and Dehui Wang. 2016. "Organized Hematoma: An Analysis of 84 Cases with Emphasis on Difficult Prediction and Favorable Management." *Otolaryngology– Head and Neck Surgery* 154(4): 626–33. doi:10.1177/0194599815625956.

58. Parkin, T. D. H., P. D. Clegg, N. P. French, C. J. Proudman, C. M. Riggs, E. R. Singer, P. M. Webbon, and K. L. Morgan. 2006. "Catastrophic Fracture of the Lateral Condyle of the Third Metacarpus/Metatarsus in UK Racehorses - Fracture Descriptions and Pre-Existing Pathology." *Veterinary Journal (London, England: 1997)* 171(1): 157–65. doi:10.1016/j.tvjl.2004.10.009.

59. Parkin, Tim D. H. 2008. "Epidemiology of Racetrack Injuries in Racehorses." *The Veterinary Clinics of North America. Equine Practice* 24(1): 1–19. doi:10.1016/j.cveq.2007.11.003.

60. Perleberg, Carolin, Alexander Kind, and Angelika Schnieke. 2018. "Genetically Engineered Pigs as Models for Human Disease." *Disease Models and Mechanisms* 11(1): UNSP dmm030783. doi:10.1242/dmm.030783.

61. Powell, S. E. 2012. "Low-Field Standing Magnetic Resonance Imaging Findings of the Metacarpo/Metatarsophalangeal Joint of Racing Thoroughbreds with Lameness Localised to the Region: A Retrospective Study of 131 Horses." *Equine Veterinary Journal* 44(2): 169–77. doi:10.1111/j.2042-3306.2011.00389.x.

62. Proffen, Benedikt L., Megan McElfresh, Braden C. Fleming, and Martha M. Murray. 2012. "A Comparative Anatomical Study of the Human Knee and Six Animal Species." *The Knee* 19(4): 493–99. doi:10.1016/j.knee.2011.07.005.

63. Rashmir-Raven, A. M., and S. J. Spier. 2015. "Hereditary Equine Regional Dermal Asthenia (HERDA) in Quarter Horses: A Review of Clinical Signs, Genetics and Research." *Equine Veterinary Education* 27(11): 604–11.

64. Robinson, Marnie R., Regina D. Norris, Roger L. Sur, and Glenn M. Preminger. 2008. "Urolithiasis: Not Just a 2-Legged Animal Disease." *The Journal of Urology* 179(1): 46–52. doi:10.1016/j.juro.2007.08.123.

65. Saunier, Jordane, and Roland Chapurlat. 2018. "Stress Fracture in Athletes." *Joint Bone Spine* 85(3): 307–10. doi:10.1016/j.jbspin.2017.04.013.

66. Smith, H.J., and R.G. Stevenson. 1973. "Congenital Hydrocephalus in Swine." *Canadian Veterinary Journal-Revue Veterinaire Canadienne* 14(12): 311–12.

67. Smith, Roger K. W. 2008. "Mesenchymal Stem Cell Therapy for Equine Tendinopathy." *Disability and Rehabilitation* 30(20–22): 1752–58. doi:10.1080/09638280701788241.
68. Stover, S. M. 2017. "Nomenclature, Classification, and Documentation of Catastrophic Fractures and Associated Preexisting Injuries in Racehorses." *Journal of Veterinary Diagnostic Investigation* 29(4): 396–404. doi:10.1177/1040638717692846.
69. Stover, Susan M., and Amanda Murray. 2008. "The California Postmortem Program: Leading the Way." *The Veterinary Clinics of North America. Equine Practice* 24(1): 21–36. doi:10.1016/j.cveq.2007.11.009.
70. Tammen, I., R. W. Cook, F. W. Nicholas, and H. W. Raadsma. 2001. "Neuronal Ceroid Lipofuscinosis in Australian Merino Sheep: A New Animal Model." *European Journal of Paediatric Neurology* 5(Suppl A): 37–41. doi:10.1053/ejpn.2000.0432.
71. Tarnopolsky, Mark A. 2018. "Myopathies Related to Glycogen Metabolism Disorders." *Neurotherapeutics: The Journal of the American Society for Experimental Neurotherapeutics* 15(4): 915–27. doi:10.1007/s13311-018-00684-2.
72. Tessier, Caroline, Andreas Brühschwein, Johann Lang, Martin Konar, Markus Wilke, Walter Brehm, and Patrick Kircher. 2013. "Magnetic Resonance Imaging Features of Sinonasal Disorders in Horses." *Veterinary Radiology and Ultrasound* 54(1): 54–60. doi:10.1111/j.1740-8261.2012.01975.x.
73. Toth, F., J. L. Torrison, L. Harper, D. Bussieres, M. E. Wilson, T. D. Crenshaw, and C. S. Carlson. 2016. "Osteochondrosis Prevalence and Severity at 12 and 24 Weeks of Age in Commercial Pigs with and without Organic-Complexed Trace Mineral Supplementation." *Journal of Animal Science* 94(9): 3817–25. doi:10.2527/jas.2015-9950.
74. Tóth, Ferenc, Marc A. Tompkins, Kevin G. Shea, Jutta M. Ellermann, and Cathy S. Carlson. 2018. "Identification of Areas of Epiphyseal Cartilage Necrosis at Predilection Sites of Juvenile Osteochondritis Dissecans in Pediatric Cadavers." *The Journal of Bone and Joint Surgery. American Volume* 100(24): 2132–39. doi:10.2106/JBJS.18.00464.
75. Tremaine, W. H., and P. M. Dixon. 2001a. "A Long-Term Study of 277 Cases of Equine Sinonasal Disease. Part 1: Details of Horses, Historical, Clinical and Ancillary Diagnostic Findings." *Equine Veterinary Journal* 33(3): 274–82.
76. Tremaine, W. H., and P. M. Dixon. 2001b. "A Long-Term Study of 277 Cases of Equine Sinonasal Disease. Part 2: Treatments and Results of Treatments." *Equine Veterinary Journal* 33(3): 283–89.
77. USDA:APHIS:VS. 2016. "Equine 2015, Part I: Baseline Reference of Equine Health and Management in the United States, 2015." Survey N451-1006. National Animal Health Monitoring System. Fort Collins, CO: United States Department of Agriculture.
78. Vallance, S. A., J. M. Lumsden, and C. B. O'Sullivan. 2009. "Scapula Stress Fractures in Thoroughbred Racehorses: Eight Cases (1997–2006)." *Equine Veterinary Education* 21(10): 554–59. doi:10.2746/095777309X472514.
79. Vallance, S. A., M. Spriet, and S. M. Stover. 2011. "Catastrophic Scapular Fractures in Californian Racehorses: Pathology, Morphometry and Bone Density." *Equine Veterinary Journal* 43(6): 676–85. doi:10.1111/j.2042-3306.2010.00346.x.
80. Van Metre, David C., and Dominic R. Dawson Soto, eds.. 2014. "Chapter 34: Diseases of the Renal System." *Large Animal Internal Medicine*, 5th ed., 873–916. Saint Louis, MI: Elsevier.
81. Videla, Ricardo, and Sarel van Amstel. 2016. "Urolithiasis." *The Veterinary Clinics of North America. Food Animal Practice* 32(3): 687–700. doi:10.1016/j.cvfa.2016.05.010.

82. Vina, Ernest R., and C. Kent Kwoh. 2018. "Epidemiology of Osteoarthritis: Literature Update." *Current Opinion in Rheumatology* 30(2): 160–67. doi:10.1097/BOR.0000000000000479.

83. Weeren, P. René van. 2016. "5 - Osteochondritis Dissecans." In: *Joint Disease in the Horse*, 2nd ed., edited by C. Wayne McIlwraith, David D. Frisbie, Christopher E. Kawcak, and P. René van Weeren, 57–84. Edinburgh: W.B. Saunders.

84. Wells, Dominic J. 2018. "Tracking Progress: An Update on Animal Models for Duchenne Muscular Dystrophy." *Disease Models and Mechanisms* 11(6): UNSP dmm035774. doi:10.1242/dmm.035774.

85. Whitton, R. C., E. A. Walmsley, A. S. M. Wong, S. M. Shannon, E. J. Frazer, N. J. Williams, J. F. Guerow, and P. L. Hitchens. 2019. "Associations between Pre-Injury Racing History and Tibial and Humeral Fractures in Australian Thoroughbred Racehorses." *Veterinary Journal* 247(May): 44–9. doi:10.1016/j.tvjl.2019.03.001.

86. Williams, Kurt, and Jesse Roman. 2016. "Studying Human Respiratory Disease in Animals - Role of Induced and Naturally Occurring Models." *Journal of Pathology* 238(2): 220–32. doi:10.1002/path.4658.

87. Witkowski, Lucjan, Anna Cywinska, Katarzyna Paschalis-Trela, Mark Crisman, and Jerzy Kita. 2016. "Multiple Etiologies of Equine Recurrent Uveitis--A Natural Model for Human Autoimmune Uveitis: A Brief Review." *Comparative Immunology, Microbiology and Infectious Diseases* 44(February): 14–20. doi:10.1016/j.cimid.2015.11.004.

88. Yasui, Takahiro, Atsushi Okada, Shuzo Hamamoto, Ryosuke Ando, Kazumi Taguchi, Keiichi Tozawa, and Kenjiro Kohri. 2017. "Pathophysiology-Based Treatment of Urolithiasis." *International Journal of Urology* 24(1): 32–8. doi:10.1111/iju.13187.

89. Ytrehus, B., C. S. Carlson, and S. Ekman. 2007. "Etiology and Pathogenesis of Osteochondrosis." *Veterinary Pathology* 44(4): 429–48. doi:10.1354/vp.44-4-429.

90. Ytrehus, B., E. Grindflek, J. Teige, E. Stubsjoen, T. Grondalen, C. S. Carlson, and S. Ekman. 2004. "The Effect of Parentage on the Prevalence, Severity and Location of Lesions of Osteochondrosis in Swine." *Journal of Veterinary Medicine. Series A* 51(4): 188–95. doi:10.1111/j.1439-0442.2004.00621.x.

91. Yu, Hong-Hao, Heng Zhao, Yu-Bo Qing, Wei-Rong Pan, Bao-Yu Jia, Hong-Ye Zhao, Xing-Xu Huang, and Hong-Jiang Wei. 2016. "Porcine Zygote Injection with Cas9/SgRNA Results in DMD-Modified Pig with Muscle Dystrophy." *International Journal of Molecular Sciences* 17(10): 1668. doi:10.3390/ijms17101668.

92. Aun, M. V., R. Bonamichi-Santos, F. M. Arantes-Costa, J. Kalil, and P. Giavina-Bianchi. 2017. "Animal models of asthma: Utility and limitations." *Journal of Asthma and Allergy* 10:293–301. doi:10.2147/JAA.S121092.

93. Bond, S., R. Leguillette, E. A. Richard, L. Couetil, J. P. Lavoie, J. G. Martin, and R. S. Pirie. 2018. "Equine asthma: Integrative biologic relevance of a recently proposed nomenclature." *Journal of Veterinary Internal Medicine* 32(6):2088–2098. doi:10.1111/jvim.15302.

94. Brinkman, E. L., B. C. Weed, S. S. Patnaik, B. L. Brazile, R. M. Centini, R. W. Wills, B. Olivier, D. G. Sledge, J. Cooley, J. Liao, and A. M. Rashmir-Raven. 2017. "Cardiac findings in Quarter Horses with heritable equine regional dermal asthenia." *JAVMA-Journal of the American Veterinary Medical Association* 250(5):538–547.

95. Burkitt, M. D., C. A. Duckworth, J. M. Williams, and D. M. Pritchard. 2017. "Helicobacter pylori-induced gastric pathology: Insights from *in vivo* and *ex vivo* models." *Disease Models and Mechanisms* 10(2):89–104. doi:10.1242/dmm.027649.

96. Cantley, C. E. L., E. C. Firth, J. W. Delahunt, D. U. Pfeiffer, and K. G. Thompson. 1999. "Naturally occurring osteoarthritis in the metacarpophalangeal joints of wild horses." *Equine Veterinary Journal* 31(1):73–81. doi:10.1111/j.2042-3306.1999.tb03794.x.

97. Cook, R. W., R. D. Jolly, D. N. Palmer, I. Tammen, M. F. Broom, and R. McKinnon. 2002. "Neuronal ceroid lipofuscinosis in Merino sheep." *Australian Veterinary Journal* 80(5):292–297. doi:10.1111/j.1751-0813.2002.tb10847.x.

98. Deeg, C. A., S. M. Hauck, B. Amann, D. Pompetzki, F. Altmann, A. Raith, T. Schmalzl, M. Stangassinger, and M. Ueffing. 2008. "Equine recurrent uveitis - A spontaneous horse model of uveitis." *Ophthalmic Research* 40(3–4):151–153. doi:10.1159/000119867.

99. Denis, C. V., and D. D. Wagner. 1999. "Insights from von Willebrand disease animal models." *Cellular and Molecular Life Sciences: CMLS* 56(11–12):977–990. doi:10.1007/s000180050487.

100. Gottardo, F., A. Scollo, B. Contiero, M. Bottacini, C. Mazzoni, and S. A. Edwards. 2017. "Prevalence and risk factors for gastric ulceration in pigs slaughtered at 170 kg." *Animal: An International Journal of Animal Bioscience* 11(11):2010–2018. doi:10.1017/S1751731117000799.

101. Halper, J. 2014. "Connective tissue disorders in domestic animals." *Progress in Heritable Soft Connective Tissue Diseases* 802:231–240. doi:10.1007/978-94-007-7893-1_14.

102. Head, K. W., and P. M. Dixon. 1999. "Equine nasal and paranasal sinus tumours. Part 1: Review of the literature and tumour classification." *Veterinary Journal* 157(3):261–278. doi:10.1053/tvjl.1998.0370.

103. Kampf, S., E. Seiler, J. Bujok, R. Hofmann-Lehmann, B. Riond, A. Makhro, and A. Bogdanova. 2019. "Aging markers in equine red blood cells." *Frontiers in Physiology* 10:893. doi:10.3389/fphys.2019.00893.

104. Kim, M., Kyeong Seon, Robert Scott Kriss, and Timothy J. Tautz. 2019. "Malignant hyperthermia: A clinical review." *Advances in Anesthesia* 37(December):35–51. doi:10.1016/j.aan.2019.08.003.

105. Klymiuk, N., A. Blutke, A. Graf, S. Krause, K. Burkhardt, A. Wuensch, S. Krebs, B. Kessler, V. Zakhartchenko, M. Kurome, E. Kemter, H. Nagashima, B. Schoser, N. Herbach, H. Blum, R. Wanke, A. Aartsma-Rus, C. Thirion, H. Lochmuller, M. C. Walter, and E. Wolf. 2013. "Dystrophin-deficient pigs provide new insights into the hierarchy of physiological derangements of dystrophic muscle." *Human Molecular Genetics* 22(21):4368–4382. doi:10.1093/hmg/ddt287.

106. Leech, R. W., C. N. Hauges, and L. A. Christoferson. 1978. "Hydrocephalus, congenital hydrocephalus. Aminal model: Bovine hydrocephalus, congenital internal hydrocephalus, aqueductal stenosis." *American Journal of Pathology* 92(2):567–570.

107. Leipold, H. W., and S. M. Dennis. 1987. "Congenital defects of the bovine central nervous system." *Veterinary Clinics of North America. Food Animal Practice* 3(1):159–177. doi:10.1016/s0749-0720(15)31188-9.

108. Lozier, J. N., and T. C. Nichols. 2013. "Animal models of hemophilia and related bleeding disorders." *Seminars in Hematology* 50(2):175–184. doi:10.1053/j.seminhematol.2013.03.023.

109. Malfait, F., and A. De Paepe. 2014. "The Ehlers-Danlos syndrome." *Progress in Heritable Soft Connective Tissue Diseases* 802:129–143. doi:10.1007/978-94-007-7893-1_9.

110. Marr, C. M. 2015. "The equine neonatal cardiovascular system in health and disease." *Veterinary Clinics of North America. Equine Practice* 31(3):545–565. doi:10.1016/j.cveq.2015.09.005.

111. McCoy, A. M. 2015. "Animal models of osteoarthritis: Comparisons and key considerations." *Veterinary Pathology* 52(5):803–818. doi:10.1177/0300985815588611.

112. McCoy, A. M., S. K. Beeson, R. K. Splan, S. Lykkjen, S. L. Ralston, J. R. Mickelson, and M. E. McCue. 2016. "Identification and validation of risk loci for osteochondrosis in standardbreds." *BMC Genomics* 17. ARTN 41. doi:10.1186/s12864-016-2385-z.

113. McCoy, A. M., F. Toth, N. I. Dolvik, S. Ekman, J. Ellermann, K. Olstad, B. Ytrehus, and C. S. Carlson. 2013. "Articular osteochondrosis: A comparison of naturally-occurring human and animal disease." *Osteoarthritis and Cartilage* 21(11):1638–1647. doi:10.1016/j.joca.2013.08.011.

114. Mickelson, J. R., and S. J. Valberg. 2015. "The genetics of skeletal muscle disorders in horses." *Annual Review of Animal Biosciences* 3:197–217. doi:10.1146/annurev-animal-022114-110653.

115. Nelson, T. E. 2002. "Malignant hyperthermia: A pharmacogenetic disease of Ca++ regulating proteins." *Current Molecular Medicine* 2(4):347–369. doi:10.2174/1566524023362429.

116. O'Sullivan, C. B., and J. M. Lumsden. 2003. "Stress fractures of the tibia and humerus in thoroughbred racehorses: 99 cases (1992–2000)." *Journal of the American Veterinary Medical Association* 222(4):491–498. doi:10.2460/javma.2003.222.491.

117. Smith, H. J., and R. G. Stevenson. 1973. "Congenital hydrocephalus in swine." *Canadian Veterinary Journal = la Revue Veterinaire Canadienne* 14(12):311–312.

118. Smith, R. K. 2008. "Mesenchymal stem cell therapy for equine tendinopathy." *Disability and Rehabilitation* 30(20–22):1752–1758. doi:10.1080/09638280701788241.

119. Van Metre, David C., and Dominic R. Dawson eds. 2014. "Chapter 34: Diseases of the renal system." *Large Animal Internal Medicine*, 5th ed., 873–916. Saint Louis: Elsevier.

120. Weeren, P. René van. 2016. "5 - Osteochondritis Dissecans." In: *Joint Disease in the Horse*, 2nd ed., edited by, C. Wayne McIlwraith, David D. Frisbie, Christopher E. Kawcak, and P. René van Weeren, 57–84. Edinburgh: W.B. Saunders.

121. Whitton, R. C., E. A. Walmsley, A. S. M. Wong, S. M. Shannon, E. J. Frazer, N. J. Williams, J. F. Guerow, and P. L. Hitchens. 2019. "Associations between pre-injury racing history and tibial and humeral fractures in Australian Thoroughbred racehorses." *Veterinary Journal* 247:44–49. doi:10.1016/j.tvjl.2019.03.001.

122. Williams, K., and J. Roman. 2016. "Studying human respiratory disease in animals - Role of induced and naturally occurring models." *Journal of Pathology* 238(2):220–232. doi:10.1002/path.4658.

123. Witkowski, L., A. Cywinska, K. Paschalis-Trela, M. Crisman, and J. Kita. 2016. "Multiple etiologies of equine recurrent uveitis - A natural model for human auto-immune uveitis: A brief review." *Comparative Immunology, Microbiology and Infectious Diseases* 44:14–20. doi:10.1016/j.cimid.2015.11.004.

124. Yu, H. H., H. Zhao, Y. B. Qing, W. R. Pan, B. Y. Jia, H. Y. Zhao, X. X. Huang, and H. J. Wei. 2016. "Porcine zygote injection with Cas9/sgRNA results in DMD-modified pig with muscle dystrophy." *International Journal of Molecular Sciences* 17(10). doi:10.3390/ijms17101668.

4 Cancer Research Is Leading the Way

Diane Peters

CONTENTS

GENERAL OVERVIEW OF COMPARATIVE ONCOLOGY AND THE UNIQUE BENEFITS OF THIS APPROACH

With a clinical approval rate lower than 8%, it is widely recognized that there are significant hurdles to the development of therapeutic agents in oncology (Hay et al. 2014, Wong, Siah, and Lo 2019). While a multitude of factors contribute to this staggering failure rate, a primary culprit is the limited predictive value of efficacy data obtained using conventional animal models of cancer (Johnson et al. 2001). The heterogenous nature of human cancers, paired with their often complex polygenic pathobiologies and reliance on an intact immune system to regulate growth and progression, make human neoplasia exceedingly difficult to model in a laboratory setting.

Comparative oncology, or the study of spontaneously occurring veterinary cancers with translational relevance to human disease, presents an exciting opportunity to generate relevant biologic and pharmacologic data in a disease state sharing the complexities of human cancer, with the added benefit of accelerating therapeutic development for both veterinary and human cancer patients.

Comparative oncology offers many unique benefits relative to conventional animal models of cancer, including:

1. Pets develop spontaneous heterogenous disease. Many cancer types exhibit conserved tumor biology, behavior, and response to treatment when compared to human cancers (Gardner, Fenger, and London 2016). In other words, these tumor characteristics are maintained or preserved between pets and humans.
2. Cancer is common in pets. According to the National Cancer Institute, an estimated 6 million new canine cancer diagnoses are made annually in the United States. Cancer is a leading cause of death in dogs accounting for >40% of mortality in dogs over 10 years old (Bronson 1982).
3. Pet owners are highly motivated to treat cancers and are often willing to consider experimental interventions when conventional treatments have failed or are inaccessible (Paoloni and Khanna 2008).
4. Pets have comparable exposures to environmental risk factors (Kelsey, Moore, and Glickman 1998).
5. *The canine genome has higher homology with the human genome than the mouse genome* (Lindblad-Toh et al. 2005, Hoeppner et al. 2014).
6. Veterinary patients have intact immune systems, enabling the study of prospective therapeutics in an environment where the immunologic impacts on cancer growth and metastasis remain present (Khanna et al. 2006).
7. Patient size often permits serial sampling for blood and/or tumor tissues with minimal discomfort (Khanna et al. 2006).
8. *Cancers that are common in dogs and rare in humans can provide a platform to accelerate clinical discovery for orphan diseases* (Garden et al. 2018).
9. The shortened lifespan and relatively rapid progression of cancer in pets enables completion of long-term efficacy studies more quickly than comparable human studies (Paoloni and Khanna 2008).

Although both comparative oncology trials and traditional pharmacology/toxicology animal studies are performed during the preclinical phase of therapeutic development, the goals of these studies are distinct. Comparative oncology studies are most commonly utilized to address questions that would be difficult, or impossible, to evaluate using conventional animal models and are thus adjunctive to traditional studies defining the basic pharmacologic and toxicologic properties of investigative therapeutic agents. Comparative oncology trials can be designed to probe environmental risk factors for cancer in both pet and human populations, to explore the genetic profiles of cancer across neoplasia subtypes, across breeds, and/or across species, to develop and optimize translationally relevant imaging modalities, to evaluate novel therapeutics for efficacy at an earlier phase of development than would be possible through the standard drug development pipeline, to validate biomarkers and/or pharmacodynamic assays when targets are conserved, to inform first-in-human clinical trials, and to promote the co-development of pharmacologic agents for the management of veterinary and human cancers.

Importantly, resources exist to encourage and facilitate active collaboration between clinical veterinarians, biomedical researchers, and pharmaceutical companies. In 2003 the National Cancer Institute (NCI) Comparative Oncology Program (COP) was founded, which currently forms a network of 24 academic veterinary oncology centers in the United States and Canada (Table 4.1), providing infrastructure facilitating the design and execution of clinical trials of novel cancer therapeutics in canine patients. Trials conducted through the NCI-COP are designed to generate clinical and biologic data of immediate relevance to human Phase I/II clinical trial design (Gordon et al. 2009). To further support these translational efforts, in 2007 the NCI also established the Comparative Oncology Trials Consortium Pharmacodynamic Core (COTC PD); a multidisciplinary network of laboratories with capabilities in pathology, genomics, proteomics, pharmacokinetics, etc., to facilitate the timely analysis of study samples generated across trial sites in quality-controlled settings (Paoloni and Lana et al. 2010).

TABLE 4.1

Academic Veterinary Oncology Centers That Form the Comparative Oncology Program

University	City and State
University of Saskatchewan	Saskatoon, Saskatchewan, Canada
Tufts University	North Grafton, Massachusetts
University of Pennsylvania	Philadelphia, Pennsylvania
Cornell University	Ithaca, New York
University of Guelph	Guelph, Ontario, Canada
Ohio State University	Columbus, Ohio
Virginia-Maryland College of Veterinary Medicine	Blacksburg, Virginia
North Carolina State University	Raleigh, North Carolina
University of Tennessee	Knoxville, Tennessee
University of Georgia	Athens, Georgia
Auburn University	Auburn, Alabama
University of Florida	Gainesville, Florida
Texas A&M University	College Station, Texas
Purdue University	West Lafayette, Indiana
University of Illinois	Urbana, Illinois
University of Missouri	Columbia, Missouri
Iowa State University	Ames, Iowa
University of Wisconsin	Madison, Wisconsin
University of Minnesota	St. Paul, Minnesota
Kansas State University	Manhattan, Kansas
Colorado State University	Ft. Collins, Colorado
Washington State University	Pullman, Washington
Oregon State University	Corvallis, Oregon
University of California	Davis, California

Another relevant resource to consider is the Pfizer-Canine Comparative Oncology and Genomics Consortium (CCOGC) Biospecimen Repository. This was established in 2006 following the initial sequencing of the canine genome. Their initial objective was to acquire clinical specimens from 3,000 canine patients with common malignancies of high translational relevance including: osteosarcoma, lymphoma, melanoma, hemangiosarcoma, soft tissue sarcoma, mast cell tumor, and pulmonary tumor (Mazcko and Thomas 2015). In 2013, the Pfizer-CCOGC Biospecimen Repository was opened to the biomedical research community where, following an application process, clinical specimens (such as tumor, plasma, whole blood, and urine) could be purchased for experimental purposes. The CCOGC has six approved tissue collection sites (Table 4.2) located at academic veterinary oncology centers and continued collaboration between veterinary oncologists, pet owners, and referring veterinarians is essential to promote maintenance of this valuable archive.

The above resources provide a platform enabling all veterinarians and biomedical researchers access to samples and resources with the capacity to transform oncology drug discovery research. There are numerous published examples of comparative oncology studies that have advanced our understanding of cancer biology and/or that have contributed to the development of FDA-approved

---

TABLE 4.2
List of Canine Comparative Oncology and Genomics Consortium That Collect Tissue and Fluid

University	Contact
Colorado State University	Lynelle Lopez Phone: 970.297.5000 Email: lynelle.lopez@colostate.edu
Ohio State University	Dr. Holly Borghese Phone: 614.247.2044 Email: borghese.19@osu.edu
University of Wisconsin	Ilene Kurzman Phone: 608.263.9754 Email: kurzmani@svm.vetmed.wisc.edu
Tufts University	Dr. Kristine Burgess Phone: 508.887.4251 Email: kristine.burgess@tufts.edu Diane Welsh & Sarah Cass Phone: 508.887.4441
University of California, Davis	Teri Guerrero Phone: 530.752.01251 Email: tguerrero@ucdavis.edu
University of Missouri	

TABLE 4.3

Examples of Investigational Therapeutics That Were Evaluated in Phase II Comparative Oncology Trials and Are Now Being Evaluated, or Are Approved for, Human Clinical Use

Indication	Drug Name	Stage of Development	References for Comparative Oncology Trial(s)
Osteosarcoma	ADXS-HER2	Phase I	(Mason et al. 2016)
	SPI-77	Phase II	(Vail et al. 2002)
	Mifamurtide	Phase II, approved for use in Europe	(MacEwen et al. 1989, Kurzman et al. 1995)
	Auranofin	FDA approved for other indications	(Endo-Munoz et al. 2019)
	Rapamycin	FDA approved for other indications	(Paoloni et al. 2010)
Lymphoma	LMP744	Phase I	(Burton et al. 2018)
	Hydroxychloroquine	Phase I	(Barnard et al. 2014)
	GS-9219	Phase II	(Vail et al. 2009)
	Verdinexor	Phase II	(Sadowski et al. 2018)
	Ibrutinib	FDA approved	(Honigberg et al. 2010)
Glioblastoma	PAC-1	Phase I	(Joshi et al. 2017)
Malignant Melanoma	Tyrosinase Vaccine	Phase II, FDA approved for vet use	(Bergman et al. 2006, Liao et al. 2006)
Epithelial Tumors	NHS-IL12	Phase I	(Paoloni et al. 2015)

oncology therapeutics. Some of these successes are highlighted in Table 4.3 and selected examples in lymphoma and osteosarcoma are further enumerated below.

EXAMPLES OF THE TRANSLATIONAL IMPACT OF COMPARATIVE ONCOLOGY STUDIES

LYMPHOMA

Non-Hodgkin's lymphoma (NHL) is a disease occurring in both dogs and humans with similar rates of incidence reported across species (15.5–29.9 per 100,000 in people; 15–30 per 100,000 in dogs) (Gardner, Fenger, and London 2016). In both humans and dogs, the majority of NHL diagnoses are B-cell lymphomas, with diffuse large B-cell lymphoma being the most common subtype (Gardner, Fenger, and London 2016). Response to chemotherapeutic agents is highly conserved between canine and human NHL. They are sensitive to agents including vincristine, cyclophosphamide, doxorubicin, and mitoxantrone, while exhibiting reduced sensitivity to the chemotherapeutics gemcitabine, cisplatin, and carbo-platin (Paoloni and Khanna 2007). Given its prevalence and biologic similarity to human disease, canine NHL has been widely utilized in the evaluation of pro-spective therapeutics for both human and canine NHL as is exemplified below for non-camptothecin topoisomerase 1 inhibitors and Bruton's tyrosine kinase inhibitors.

Indenoisoquinoline Topoisomerase 1 (TOP1) Inhibitors

DNA topoisomerase 1 (TOP1) is an enzyme that induces single strand breaks in supercoiled DNA permitting relaxation and remodeling, which is essential for transcription, replication, and repair. TOP1 is dysregulated in a variety of cancers. Two TOP1 inhibitors, irinotecan and topotecan, have been FDA approved for use in ovarian, small cell-lung, cervical, colorectal, and/or gastric cancers (Pommier 2006). Both FDA-approved TOP1 inhibitors are in the camptothecin class, and these compounds have significant limitations including chemical instability, short half-life, susceptibility to efflux mediated drug-resistance, and dose-limiting diarrhea (Burton et al. 2018). To bypass these limitations, novel chemical classes of TOP1 inhibitors have been developed. The indenoisoquinoline class of TOP1 inhibitors is one alternate class of compounds which displays nanomolar potency and has enhanced chemical stability and drug efflux properties (Burton et al. 2018). Three indenoisoquinoline TOP1 inhibitors with varying pharmacokinetic properties were examined in a comparative oncology trial in dogs with NHL. While all three compounds displayed objective therapeutic activity, a single com-pound was identified as having significantly enhanced tumor accumulation and retention relative to the others (Burton et al. 2018). This trial demonstrated not only that indenoisoquinoline TOP1 inhibitors may be therapeutically relevant in the treatment of canine NHL, but importantly also allowed for identification of a clinical lead compound, LMP744, that is currently under evaluation in human clinical trials (Burton et al. 2018).

Bruton's Tyrosine Kinase (BTK) Inhibitors

Bruton's tyrosine kinase (BTK) is a crucial enzyme for B-cell differentiation, proliferation, and survival (Pal Singh, Dammeijer, and Hendriks 2018). In the context of B-cell malignancies, including NHL, inhibition of BTK alters cytokine signaling resulting in decreased proliferation and impaired cell migration (Pal Singh, Dammeijer, and Hendriks 2018). The earliest evidence in support of clini-cal efficacy of BTK inhibitors was generated in a comparative oncology trial in canines with spontaneous lymphoma (Honigberg et al. 2010). This particular trial was unique in that there were no suitable mouse models to utilize for preclinical efficacy evaluation, as mouse models of B-cell lymphoma had impaired B-cell receptor signaling that was dissimilar to humans and canines (Thamm 2019). Thus, the canine lymphoma trial was the first *in vivo* study to demonstrate proof-of-concept that BTK inhibition could lead to measurable antitumor responses in lymphoma (Honigberg et al. 2010). Additionally, this study was critical for the development of pharmacodynamic assays used in subsequent human clinical trials to ensure adequate drug exposures (Honigberg et al. 2010). The results of this canine oncology trial directly informed human clinical trials, leading to FDA approval for ibrutinib use in several B-cell malignancies (Thamm 2019).

OSTEOSARCOMA

Osteosarcoma (OSA) is the most common primary bone tumor of dogs, with an incidence as high as 8.9% reported for predisposed breeds (Anfinsen et al. 2011). In contrast, OSA is a rare disease in humans with fewer than 1,000 cases diagnosed annually in the United States (Paoloni et al. 2009). Although rare, OSA is the most common primary bone cancer of adolescents where it is a significant source of morbidity and mortality (Paoloni et al. 2009). Despite the estimation that OSA occurs with 27 times higher frequency in dogs than in humans, from a biological perspective there are striking similarities in this disease across species (Simpson et al. 2017). The majority of primary tumors occur in the appendicular skeleton accounting for 80% of canine primary tumors and 90% of human primary tumors (Morello, Martano, and Buracco 2011). There are known genetic abnormalities occurring at high frequency in both canine and human OSA including mutations or copy number alterations in critical players including: *TP53*, *RB1*, *PTEN*, and *MYC* (Gardner et al. 2019). Further, a recent study comparing the gene expression signatures of OSA in canines and humans found that the global gene expression profiles are largely conserved across species (Paoloni et al. 2009). As the 5-year survival time for non-metastatic OSA in humans has remained stagnant at 70%, and the 1-year survival rate for canines of 35%, there is clear clinical need for novel therapeutics in both human and veterinary medicine (Paoloni et al. 2009, Moore et al. 2007). Canine OSA patients can contribute significantly to the advancement of drug development for OSA. This is clearly evidenced in the comparative oncology evaluations of L-MTP-PE and rapamycin for use as adjunctive OSA therapeutics as detailed below.

Liposome Encapsulated Muramyl Tripeptide-Phosphatidylethanolamine (L-MTP-PE)

L-MTP-PE is a synthetic molecule mimicking a bacterial cell wall that has the potent ability to activate host monocytes/macrophages and to trigger the selective killing of tumor cells (Kleinerman, Maeda, and Jaffe 1993). As one-third of human OSA patients develops chemotherapy-refractory pulmonary metastases following standard-of-care treatment, there is significant interest in developing an adjunctive therapeutic to activate the patient's immune system and attenuate tumor resistance (Nardin et al. 2006). Over the course of its development, three comparative oncology trials were performed evaluating L-MTP-PE in canines with OSA. These studies found that administering L-MTP-PE following standard OSA treatments (limb amputation +/– cisplatin chemotherapy) significantly increased median survival times (MacEwen et al. 1989, Kurzman et al. 1995). These encouraging results were translated to trials in human pediatric patients with OSA, which also demonstrated significantly improved long-term survival rates (Meyers et al. 2008). In 2009, L-MTP-PE (mifamurtide, Mepact™) received approval in Europe for use as an adjuvant agent in the treatment of high-grade non-metastatic osteosarcoma.

Rapamycin

Rapamycin was the first clinically approved inhibitor of the mTOR pathway; a pathway whose dysregulation is associated with many human diseases including: cancer, diabetes, obesity, neurological diseases, such as epilepsy and autism, and various genetic disorders (Li, Kim, and Blenis 2014). Rapamycin is FDA approved for use as an immunosuppressive agent in organ and bone marrow transplantation and several of its analogs, commonly referred to as "rapalogs", have been evaluated for efficacy in various solid state tumors and lymphomas. The rapalog temsirolimus has received FDA approval for use in the treatment of advanced renal cell carcinoma (Kwitkowski et al. 2010). There is significant preclinical biological evidence to support that inhibition of the mTOR pathway may have positive benefit in the treatment of OSA. Given the challenges of studying rapamycin in a limited pediatric patient population, studies to optimize dosing and to identify safe and pharmacokinetically/pharmacodynamically relevant treatment regimens were first completed in canines (Paoloni and Mazcko et al. 2010). Further Phase II efficacy studies of rapamycin in canine OSA remain in progress. Since this time, pediatric clinical trials evaluating the rapalog, ridaforolimus, have also been performed for human OSA (Chawla et al. 2012, Demetri et al. 2013).

CONCLUSION

The above examples illustrate the impact that comparative oncology trials can have on our understanding of disease biology and on drug development. While lymphoma and osteosarcoma were discussed as specific examples, it is important to note that many other cancers share strong resemblance to human disease and would also be of high translational relevance. The success of comparative oncology trials requires the interplay of many experts: those with thorough understanding of the biological pathway being explored, those with knowledge of the veterinary and human disease states, those with access to recruit and treat appropriate patients, those with the ability to analyze samples from non-human species, those with access to well-characterized investigational therapeutics, etc. The degree of collaboration required to facilitate a successful trial can be daunting. There is no doubt, however, that the culmination of this effort has led to remarkable discoveries that have aided veterinary and human patients and that will continue to accelerate drug discovery in areas where there is unmet clinical need.

REFERENCES

Anfinsen, K. P., T. Grotmol, O. S. Bruland, and T. J. Jonasdottir. 2011. "Breed-specific incidence rates of canine primary bone tumors--A population based survey of dogs in Norway." *Can J Vet Res* 75(3):209–15.

Barnard, R. A., L. A. Wittenburg, R. K. Amaravadi, D. L. Gustafson, A. Thorburn, and D. H. Thamm. 2014. "Phase I clinical trial and pharmacodynamic evaluation of combination hydroxychloroquine and doxorubicin treatment in pet dogs treated for spontaneously occurring lymphoma." *Autophagy* 10(8):1415–25. doi: 10.4161/auto.29165.

Bergman, P. J., M. A. Camps-Palau, J. A. McKnight, N. F. Leibman, D. M. Craft, C. Leung, J. Liao, I. Riviere, M. Sadelain, A. E. Hohenhaus, P. Gregor, A. N. Houghton, M. A. Perales, and J. D. Wolchok. 2006. "Development of a xenogeneic DNA vaccine program for canine malignant melanoma at the Animal Medical Center." *Vaccine* 24(21):4582–5. doi: 10.1016/j.vaccine.2005.08.027.

Bronson, R. T. 1982. "Variation in age at death of dogs of different sexes and breeds." *Am J Vet Res* 43(11):2057–9.

Burton, J. H., C. Mazcko, A. LeBlanc, J. M. Covey, J. Ji, R. J. Kinders, R. E. Parchment, C. Khanna, M. Paoloni, S. Lana, K. Weishaar, C. London, W. Kisseberth, E. Krick, D. Vail, M. Childress, J. N. Bryan, L. Barber, E. J. Ehrhart, M. Kent, T. Fan, K. Kow, N. Northup, H. Wilson-Robles, J. Tomaszewski, J. L. Holleran, M. Muzzio, J. Eiseman, J. H. Beumer, J. H. Doroshow, and Y. Pommier. 2018. "NCI comparative oncology program testing of non-camptothecin indenoisoquinoline topoisomerase I inhibitors in naturally occurring canine lymphoma." *Clin Cancer Res* 24(23):5830–40. doi: 10.1158/1078-0432.CCR-18-1498.

Chawla, S. P., A. P. Staddon, L. H. Baker, S. M. Schuetze, A. W. Tolcher, G. Z. D'Amato, J. Y. Blay, M. M. Mita, K. K. Sankhala, L. Berk, V. M. Rivera, T. Clackson, J. W. Loewy, F. G. Haluska, and G. D. Demetri. 2012. "Phase II study of the mammalian target of rapamycin inhibitor Ridaforolimus in patients with advanced bone and soft tissue sarcomas." *J Clin Oncol* 30(1):78–84. doi: 10.1200/JCO.2011.35.6329.

Demetri, G. D., S. P. Chawla, I. Ray-Coquard, A. Le Cesne, A. P. Staddon, M. M. Milhem, N. Penel, R. F. Riedel, B. Bui-Nguyen, L. D. Cranmer, P. Reichardt, E. Bompas, T. Alcindor, D. Rushing, Y. Song, R. M. Lee, S. Ebbinghaus, J. E. Eid, J. W. Loewy, F. G. Haluska, P. F. Dodion, and J. Y. Blay. 2013. "Results of an international randomized phase III trial of the mammalian target of rapamycin inhibitor Ridaforolimus versus placebo to control metastatic sarcomas in patients after benefit from prior chemotherapy." *J Clin Oncol* 31(19):2485–92. doi: 10.1200/JCO.2012.45.5766.

Endo-Munoz, L., T. C. Bennett, E. Topkas, S. Y. Wu, D. H. Thamm, L. Brockley, M. Cooper, S. Sommerville, M. Thomson, K. O'Connell, A. Lane, G. Bird, A. Peaston, N. Matigian, R. C. Straw, and N. A. Saunders. 2019. "Auranofin improves overall survival when combined with standard of care in a pilot study involving dogs with osteosarcoma." *Vet Comp Oncol.* doi: 10.1111/vco.12533.

Garden, O. A., S. W. Volk, N. J. Mason, and J. A. Perry. 2018. "Companion animals in comparative oncology: One Medicine in action." *Vet J* 240:6–13. doi: 10.1016/j. tvjl.2018.08.008.

Gardner, H. L., J. M. Fenger, and C. A. London. 2016. "Dogs as a model for cancer." *Annu Rev Anim Biosci* 4:199–222. doi: 10.1146/annurev-animal-022114-110911.

Gardner, H. L., K. Sivaprakasam, N. Briones, V. Zismann, N. Perdigones, K. Drenner, S. Facista, R. Richholt, W. Liang, J. Aldrich, J. M. Trent, P. G. Shields, N. Robinson, J. Johnson, S. Lana, P. Houghton, J. Fenger, G. Lorch, K. A. Janeway, C. A. London, and W. P. D. Hendricks. 2019. "Canine osteosarcoma genome sequencing identifies recurrent mutations in DMD and the histone methyltransferase gene SETD2." *Commun Biol* 2:266. doi: 10.1038/s42003-019-0487-2.

Gordon, I., M. Paoloni, C. Mazcko, and C. Khanna. 2009. "The Comparative Oncology Trials Consortium: Using spontaneously occurring cancers in dogs to inform the cancer drug development pathway." *PLoS Med* 6(10):e1000161. doi: 10.1371/journal. pmed.1000161.

Hay, M., D. W. Thomas, J. L. Craighead, C. Economides, and J. Rosenthal. 2014. "Clinical development success rates for investigational drugs." *Nat Biotechnol* 32(1):40–51. doi: 10.1038/nbt.2786.

Hoeppner, M. P., A. Lundquist, M. Pirun, J. R. Meadows, N. Zamani, J. Johnson, G. Sundstrom, A. Cook, M. G. FitzGerald, R. Swofford, E. Mauceli, B. T. Moghadam, A. Greka, J. Alfoldi, A. Abouelleil, L. Aftuck, D. Bessette, A. Berlin, A. Brown, G. Gearin, A. Lui, J. P. Macdonald, M. Priest, T. Shea, J. Turner-Maier, A. Zimmer, E. S. Lander, F. di Palma, K. Lindblad-Toh, and M. G. Grabherr. 2014. "An improved canine genome and a comprehensive catalogue of coding genes and non-coding transcripts." *PLoS One* 9(3):e91172. doi: 10.1371/journal.pone.0091172.

Honigberg, L. A., A. M. Smith, M. Sirisawad, E. Verner, D. Loury, B. Chang, S. Li, Z. Pan, D. H. Thamm, R. A. Miller, and J. J. Buggy. 2010. "The Bruton tyrosine kinase inhibitor PCI-32765 blocks B-cell activation and is efficacious in models of autoimmune disease and B-cell malignancy." *Proc Natl Acad Sci U S A* 107(29):13075–80. doi: 10.1073/pnas.1004594107.

Johnson, J. I., S. Decker, D. Zaharevitz, L. V. Rubinstein, J. M. Venditti, S. Schepartz, S. Kalyandrug, M. Christian, S. Arbuck, M. Hollingshead, and E. A. Sausville. 2001. "Relationships between drug activity in NCI preclinical *in vitro* and *in vivo* models and early clinical trials." *Br J Cancer* 84(10):1424–31. doi: 10.1054/bjoc.2001.1796.

Joshi, A. D., R. C. Botham, L. J. Schlein, H. S. Roth, A. Mangraviti, A. Borodovsky, B. Tyler, S. Joslyn, J. S. Looper, M. Podell, T. M. Fan, P. J. Hergenrother, and G. J. Riggins. 2017. "Synergistic and targeted therapy with a procaspase-3 activator and temozolomide extends survival in glioma rodent models and is feasible for the treatment of canine malignant glioma patients." *Oncotarget* 8(46):80124–38. doi: 10.18632/oncotarget.19085.

Kelsey, J. L., A. S. Moore, and L. T. Glickman. 1998. "Epidemiologic studies of risk factors for cancer in pet dogs." *Epidemiol Rev* 20(2):204–17. doi: 10.1093/oxfordjournals.epirev.a017981.

Khanna, C., K. Lindblad-Toh, D. Vail, C. London, P. Bergman, L. Barber, M. Breen, B. Kitchell, E. McNeil, J. F. Modiano, S. Niemi, K. E. Comstock, E. Ostrander, S. Westmoreland, and S. Withrow. 2006. "The dog as a cancer model." *Nat Biotechnol* 24(9):1065–6. doi: 10.1038/nbt0906-1065b.

Kleinerman, E. S., M. Maeda, and N. Jaffe. 1993. "Liposome-encapsulated muramyl tripeptide: A new biologic response modifier for the treatment of osteosarcoma." *Cancer Treat Res* 62:101–7. doi: 10.1007/978-1-4615-3518-8_14.

Kurzman, I. D., E. G. MacEwen, R. C. Rosenthal, L. E. Fox, E. T. Keller, S. C. Helfand, D. M. Vail, R. R. Dubielzig, B. R. Madewell, C. O. Rodriguez, Jr. et al. 1995. "Adjuvant therapy for osteosarcoma in dogs: Results of randomized clinical trials using combined liposome-encapsulated muramyl tripeptide and cisplatin." *Clin Cancer Res* 1(12):1595–601.

Kwitkowski, V. E., T. M. Prowell, A. Ibrahim, A. T. Farrell, R. Justice, S. S. Mitchell, R. Sridhara, and R. Pazdur. 2010. "FDA approval summary: Temsirolimus as treatment for advanced renal cell carcinoma." *Oncologist* 15(4):428–35. doi: 10.1634/theoncologist.2009-0178.

Li, J., S. G. Kim, and J. Blenis. 2014. "Rapamycin: One drug, many effects." *Cell Metab* 19(3):373–9. doi: 10.1016/j.cmet.2014.01.001.

Liao, J. C., P. Gregor, J. D. Wolchok, F. Orlandi, D. Craft, C. Leung, A. N. Houghton, and P. J. Bergman. 2006. "Vaccination with human tyrosinase DNA induces antibody responses in dogs with advanced melanoma." *Cancer Immun* 6:8.

Lindblad-Toh, K., C. M. Wade, T. S. Mikkelsen, E. K. Karlsson, D. B. Jaffe, M. Kamal, M. Clamp, J. L. Chang, E. J. Kulbokas, 3rd, M. C. Zody et al. 2005. "Genome sequence, comparative analysis and haplotype structure of the domestic dog." *Nature* 438(7069):803–19. doi: 10.1038/nature04338.

MacEwen, E. G., I. D. Kurzman, R. C. Rosenthal, B. W. Smith, P. A. Manley, J. K. Roush, and P. E. Howard. 1989. "Therapy for osteosarcoma in dogs with intravenous injection of liposome-encapsulated muramyl tripeptide." *J Natl Cancer Inst* 81(12):935–8. doi: 10.1093/jnci/81.12.935.

Mason, N. J., J. S. Gnanandarajah, J. B. Engiles, F. Gray, D. Laughlin, A. Gaurnier-Hausser, A. Wallecha, M. Huebner, and Y. Paterson. 2016. "Immunotherapy with a HER2-targeting Listeria Induces HER2-specific immunity and demonstrates potential therapeutic effects in a Phase I trial in canine osteosarcoma." *Clin Cancer Res* 22(17):4380–90. doi: 10.1158/1078-0432.CCR-16-0088.

Mazcko, C., and R. Thomas. 2015. "The establishment of the Pfizer-canine comparative oncology and genomics consortium biospecimen repository." *Vet Sci* 2(3):127–30. doi: 10.3390/vetsci2030127.

Meyers, P. A., C. L. Schwartz, M. D. Krailo, J. H. Healey, M. L. Bernstein, D. Betcher, W. S. Ferguson, M. C. Gebhardt, A. M. Goorin, M. Harris, E. Kleinerman, M. P. Link, H. Nadel, M. Nieder, G. P. Siegal, M. A. Weiner, R. J. Wells, R. B. Womer, H. E. Grier, and Group Children's Oncology. 2008. "Osteosarcoma: The addition of muramyl tripeptide to chemotherapy improves overall survival--A report from the Children's Oncology Group." *J Clin Oncol* 26(4):633–8. doi: 10.1200/JCO.2008.14.0095.

Moore, A. S., W. S. Dernell, G. K. Ogilvie, O. Kristal, R. Elmslie, B. Kitchell, S. Susaneck, R. Rosenthal, M. K. Klein, J. Obradovich, A. Legendre, T. Haddad, K. Hahn, B. E. Powers, and D. Warren. 2007. "Doxorubicin and BAY 12-9566 for the treatment of osteosarcoma in dogs: A randomized, double-blind, placebo-controlled study." *J Vet Intern Med* 21(4):783–90. doi: 10.1892/0891-6640(2007)21[783:dabftt]2.0.co;2.

Morello, E., M. Martano, and P. Buracco. 2011. "Biology, diagnosis and treatment of canine appendicular osteosarcoma: Similarities and differences with human osteosarcoma." *Vet J* 189(3):268–77. doi: 10.1016/j.tvjl.2010.08.014.

Nardin, A., M. L. Lefebvre, K. Labroquere, O. Faure, and J. P. Abastado. 2006. "Liposomal muramyl tripeptide phosphatidylethanolamine: Targeting and activating macrophages for adjuvant treatment of osteosarcoma." *Curr Cancer Drug Targets* 6(2):123–33. doi: 10.2174/156800906776056473.

Pal Singh, S., F. Dammeijer, and R. W. Hendriks. 2018. "Role of bruton's tyrosine kinase in B cells and malignancies." *Mol Cancer* 17(1):57. doi: 10.1186/s12943-018-0779-z.

Paoloni, M., S. Davis, S. Lana, S. Withrow, L. Sangiorgi, P. Picci, S. Hewitt, T. Triche, P. Meltzer, and C. Khanna. 2009. "Canine tumor cross-species genomics uncovers targets linked to osteosarcoma progression." *BMC Genomics* 10:625. doi: 10.1186/1471-2164-10-625.

Paoloni, M., and C. Khanna. 2008. "Translation of new cancer treatments from pet dogs to humans." *Nat Rev Cancer* 8(2):147–56. doi: 10.1038/nrc2273.

Paoloni, M., S. Lana, D. Thamm, C. Mazcko, and S. Withrow. 2010. "The creation of the comparative oncology trials consortium pharmacodynamic core: Infrastructure for a virtual laboratory." *Vet J* 185(1):88–9. doi: 10.1016/j.tvjl.2010.04.019.

Paoloni, M., C. Mazcko, K. Selting, S. Lana, L. Barber, J. Phillips, K. Skorupski, D. Vail, H. Wilson, B. Biller, A. Avery, M. Kiupel, A. LeBlanc, A. Bernhardt, B. Brunkhorst, R. Tighe, and C. Khanna. 2015. "Defining the pharmacodynamic profile and therapeutic index of NHS-IL12 immunocytokine in dogs with malignant melanoma." *PLoS One* 10(6):e0129954. doi: 10.1371/journal.pone.0129954.

Paoloni, M. C., and C. Khanna. 2007. "Comparative oncology today." *Vet Clin North Am Small Anim Pract* 37(6):1023–32; v. doi: 10.1016/j.cvsm.2007.08.003.

Paoloni, M. C., C. Mazcko, E. Fox, T. Fan, S. Lana, W. Kisseberth, D. M. Vail, K. Nuckolls, T. Osborne, S. Yalkowsy, D. Gustafson, Y. Yu, L. Cao, and C. Khanna. 2010. "Rapamycin pharmacokinetic and pharmacodynamic relationships in osteosarcoma: A comparative oncology study in dogs." *PLoS One* 5(6):e11013. doi: 10.1371/journal.pone.0011013.

Pommier, Y. 2006. "Topoisomerase I inhibitors: Camptothecins and beyond." *Nat Rev Cancer* 6(10):789–802. doi: 10.1038/nrc1977.

Sadowski, A. R., H. L. Gardner, A. Borgatti, H. Wilson, D. M. Vail, J. Lachowicz, C. Manley, A. Turner, M. K. Klein, A. Waite, A. Sahora, and C. A. London. 2018. "Phase II study of the oral selective inhibitor of nuclear export (SINE) KPT-335 (verdinexor) in dogs with lymphoma." *BMC Vet Res* 14(1):250. doi: 10.1186/s12917-018-1587-9.

Simpson, S., M. D. Dunning, S. de Brot, L. Grau-Roma, N. P. Mongan, and C. S. Rutland. 2017. "Comparative review of human and canine osteosarcoma: Morphology, epidemiology, prognosis, treatment and genetics." *Acta Vet Scand* 59(1):71. doi: 10.1186/s13028-017-0341-9.

Thamm, D. H. 2019. "Canine cancer: Strategies in experimental therapeutics." *Front Oncol* 9:1257. doi: 10.3389/fonc.2019.01257.

Vail, D. M., I. D. Kurzman, P. C. Glawe, M. G. O'Brien, R. Chun, L. D. Garrett, J. E. Obradovich, R. M. Fred, 3rd, C. Khanna, G. T. Colbern, and P. K. Working. 2002. "STEALTH liposome-encapsulated cisplatin (SPI-77) versus carboplatin as adjuvant therapy for spontaneously arising osteosarcoma (OSA) in the dog: A randomized multicenter clinical trial." *Cancer Chemother Pharmacol* 50(2):131–6. doi: 10.1007/s00280-002-0469-8.

Vail, D. M., D. H. Thamm, H. Reiser, A. S. Ray, G. H. Wolfgang, W. J. Watkins, D. Babusis, I. N. Henne, M. J. Hawkins, I. D. Kurzman, R. Jeraj, M. Vanderhoek, S. Plaza, C. Anderson, M. A. Wessel, C. Robat, J. Lawrence, and D. B. Tumas. 2009. "Assessment of GS-9219 in a pet dog model of non-Hodgkin's lymphoma." *Clin Cancer Res* 15(10):3503–10. doi: 10.1158/1078-0432.CCR-08-3113.

Wong, C. H., K. W. Siah, and A. W. Lo. 2019. "Estimation of clinical trial success rates and related parameters." *Biostatistics* 20(2):273–86. doi: 10.1093/biostatistics/kxx069.

5 Investment Dynamics in the World of Pharma

Bryan Jones

CONTENTS

INTRODUCTION

The development of new pharmaceuticals is expensive; constantly at risk due to scientific, regulatory, and market forces; and driven by the willingness of companies and/or investors to invest in a given program, whether the target market is for humans or animals. The Food and Drug Administration (FDA) regulates drugs for both industries, so there are overlapping elements in the steps to drug approval, but macroeconomic forces drive where investment is focused [for ease of reference, in this chapter, *human = Food and Drug Administration (FDA), animal = Center for Veterinary Medicine (CVM)*].*

---

* The human market is regulated by the FDA-CDER (drugs) and the FDA-CBER (biologics and vaccines); the animal market is regulated by the FDA-CVM (drugs) and USDA-APHIS-CVB (most biologics/vaccines). Some cell-based and large molecule products are directed through the CVM. There is a CVM/CVB jurisdiction panel that decides which agency regulates a particular product. The Jurisdiction Committee is organized according to APHIS Agreement # 04-9100-0859-MU; FDA Serial # 225-05-7000.

Historically, large pharmaceutical companies have not developed a new compound for both humans and animals in parallel. This philosophy was driven by the simple fact that human drugs have much larger markets, so companies were nervous that a side effect discovered in animals might adversely impact the perception of the drug's safety in humans. Additionally, human drugs can typically support higher price points than a veterinary drug, so having the identical compound in both markets comes with strategic challenges in how to support differential pricing.

In the past, human drug companies were focused on medical indications that affected large populations such as essential hypertension, whereas veterinary companies concentrated on parasite medications (e.g., flea treatment and prophylaxis, heartworm prevention, etc.), diagnostics and supportive products (e.g., food, supplies). Human drugs were either used "off- label" (i.e., extra-label) in animals, or a similar compound, usually a related compound to the proprietary human compound, was developed for animals. But the shift of the human pharmaceutical industry toward smaller populations, more refined indications and typically higher price points, particularly with biologics (e.g., antibody, protein) therapies, and the increasing willingness of pet owners to pay more for treatments for their pets, are major macroeconomic forces that have dramatically influenced investment paradigms (Kleinman 2012). For example, the total spent on pets in the United States has more than doubled in the past two decades from $28.5 billion in 2001 to $58 billion in 2014 to $72.56 billion in 2018 (2019).

According to the Animal Health Institute (AHI), the foremost animal health trade association in the field, the US animal health market comprises roughly 2% of the total US pharmaceutical market ($9.9 billion animal compared to $450 billion human medicines) (2020). The US animal health market is approximately one-third of the global market (2020), with roughly 60% of animal health sales in the United States for companion animal products and 40% for products for food-producing animals (2020).

This chapter will compare and contrast human and veterinary drug development requirements, explore changing business models in the pharmaceutical industry and how that is likely to impact future investment in veterinary drugs. Note that the focus will be on drugs for disease treatment and largely ignores a huge component of the veterinary industry that was built on animal food and supplies, veterinary diagnostics, and anti-parasitic/flea treatment products.

NET PRESENT VALUE

The pharmaceutical industry is no exception to businesses and investors that use the concept of net present value (NPV) to quantitate the attractiveness of an opportunity, but the term is not as commonly used by scientists, researchers, or clinicians. The basic premise is that if an investment in a new drug does not have the potential to generate a return on the investment that is more than a certain rate of return, such as could be obtained by investing in another vehicle or project within the company, or perhaps in another company (such as the investment involved in making an acquisition), a more generalized investment in the market such as an index fund, or in the least risky investments of a bond or a savings account, there is no incentive to risk the investment required to get the new drug approved.

Many articles and books have been written on the details of establishing an NPV (Svennebring 2013), but for the purpose of this chapter, there are four components to keep in mind:

1. Expense of development
2. Time required to achieve a return on the investment
3. Risk that the activities will be successful
4. Potential return achieved if the drug is successful

Without getting into the mechanics, the fundamentals are likely to be intuitive: if the program expenses are higher, or it takes longer to return the investment (which also increases the cost), the higher the potential payoff must be to justify the investment. In the comparison of human to animal drug development (Figure 5.1), the market sizes of animal products are significantly lower, but the timelines are often shorter and certain development costs (such as those involved with establishing target animal safety and effectiveness) can be considerably less, while others (like manufacturing), may be no different. Risk is a variable that has many layers of complicated analysis, but tends to favor the animal product. More specifics of each of these variables are explained in the following sections.

SUMMARY OF THE COMPARISON OF HUMAN AND VETERINARY PROGRAMS

Figure 5.1 shows a schematic of the major activities required to get a drug approved for a typical novel compound, i.e., New Chemical Entity (NCE). There are many exceptions to this base case, but the general directionality of the discussion below is the same. What is clear at a glance is that human drugs require more toxicology and clinical information and by necessity it takes longer to complete all the required steps. The increase in the number of activities required, expense of coordinating those activities, and the length of time to complete the activities directly inflates the expense of a human development program. This concept applies to medical resources and the human resources needed to drive the projects. The increased complexity can be exponential in expense. In contrast, the content of the Chemistry and Manufacturing Controls (CMC) portion of the programs for both humans and animals is essentially the same and can often be the rate-limiting step to drug approval. However, like the other technical information that is required from a drug sponsor, a product's manufacturing technical section will be reviewed by different divisions within the agency, even if the product for use in humans and animals is identical.

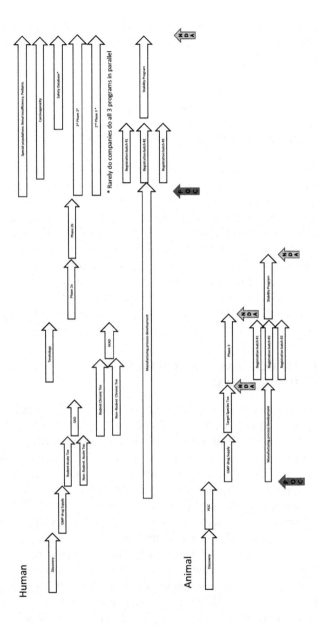

FIGURE 5.1 Comparison of the major buckets of development activities between human and animal. The arrows are intended to show the typical sequence of activities but are not meant to be accurate for relative timelines. There are several key conclusions: (1) human programs require significantly more investment; (2) the two required Phase 3 studies and the total number of safety exposures are rarely done in parallel, which significantly increases the total length of time for the human program. The time and the amount of investment required to obtain Proof of Concept (POC) data is significantly less for veterinary products.

VETERINARY SAFETY STUDIES ARE LESS EXPENSIVE

Studies designed to establish the safety of the new compound, expressed as a consideration of risk and benefit, are an essential component that drives the execution of drug development activities.

Human development programs typically require toxicology studies in two animal species before human testing can begin (one rodent and one non-rodent species). It is very common for the two species to be rats (or mice) and dogs. Primate studies are discouraged, but some new drugs may be viewed as requiring primates to accurately assess the drugs toxicological potential.

1. To get into the clinic rapidly, most companies begin with an evaluation of acute toxicology. However, most acute exposure programs only allow the company to perform a Single Ascending Dose (SAD) or Phase 1a study in humans.
2. Assuming the drug is not intended for a single use, companies are required to complete 9-month repeat dosing toxicology studies to assess a drug's chronic toxicological liability and study drug accumulation, again, typically in two species. The chronic toxicology is required prior to a Multiple Ascending Dose (MAD) study, or Phase 1b, in humans. It should be noted that this is a common risk-gating activity for companies. Larger companies can more easily afford to perform the 9-month repeat dose toxicology study prior to initiating the human SAD study to de-risk the program. In contrast, and depending on the company's funding situation, smaller companies tend to do the longer (and more expensive) toxicology studies in parallel or even sometimes subsequent to the SAD study.

   The major purposes of these toxicology studies are three-fold: (i) to determine the starting dose for testing in humans, (ii) to elucidate any safety issues that are of particular interest for human studies, and (iii) although not always possible, to establish a pharmacokinetic to pharmacodynamic ratio or indices (PK/PD), (i.e., the activity of the drug as dependent on dose over time). The PK/PD helps establish a therapeutic dose range to be targeted in future human effectiveness studies and, in the best case, surrogate endpoints for dose ranging studies.
3. The next steps in establishing the safety of a human drug are to perform two dose ranging studies, typically in healthy volunteers. A Phase 1a study (SAD) is used to determine the upper dose range of safety and to determine if there are any differences in the safety profile as compared to what was seen in the animal toxicology studies. Next, the Phase 1b (MAD) study is designed to determine if there is any drug accumulation, novel safety signals, or the amplification of the safety signals seen in the SAD study.

In addition to the acute and chronic toxicology studies, there are many additional safety studies required for approval, such as teratology and carcinogenicity, that may or may not be required for veterinary drugs. It is also necessary to develop and validate a pharmacokinetic assay for each of the different animal species and for humans. The total cost of all the toxicology and supporting studies can be several million dollars. Note that in Figure 5.1, the carcinogenicity study was drawn in parallel to Phase 3. This is another common risk-gating item because of its cost (in the millions of dollars) and duration (several years), so many companies don't take the risk of this step and delay this investment until the compound has been shown to be safe in the Phase 1, or even the Phase 2, portions of the program.

Animal development programs differ from their human drug counterparts in that the toxicology requirement has been replaced by a 1X, 3X, 5X margin of safety study (or multiples thereof). This safety study is completed only in the target animal species (although sponsors are encouraged to reference supplemental data in other species, if available), and replaces the studies that would be defined as the Phase 1a/b series in human drug programs. This work serves to create a "dosage justification" that is presented to the CVM. Validated PK assays are required, but only for the target species. Depending on the species and dosing mechanism, these programs are likely to cost significantly less than those to meet the human requirements. Statistics from a 2015 study of the US domestic market cited by AHI found that on average, when developing a drug with a new active ingredient, it takes 6.5 years and $22.5 million to bring a new companion animal pharmaceutical to market and 8.5 years and $30.5 million for a new pharmaceutical product for livestock (Institute 2020).

VETERINARY CLINICAL WORK IS LESS EXPENSIVE

Clinical drug development activities include studies designed to establish the effectiveness of the new compound, but more importantly, the risk/benefit ratio (i.e., safety/efficacy).

1. *For a new human drug*, the expense of doing the clinical effectiveness studies varies widely depending on the disease indication for which the drug is being developed and how long it takes to measure the primary efficacy endpoint. Recent estimates are that an entire development program, including toxicology and manufacturing, taken through approval costs between $2–3 billion; a significant portion of those costs is the clinical program (Moore et al. 2018). Note that this number has increased significantly and perhaps as much as doubled in recent years, partially influenced by smaller patient populations as indications are more narrowly defined with advanced diagnostics. Newer biological drugs also have a more complicated and expensive manufacturing process than organic chemicals (small molecules).

For human clinical programs, often multiple Phase 2 studies are conducted to identify the target dose range and dosing frequency, as well as to clarify and refine the exact definition of the target population. Once the dosing regimen is identified, two well-controlled Phase 3 (pivotal) trials are needed for approval. In the United States, these studies are typically of the active compound compared with placebo, whereas in the European Union, an active comparator arm is used (when available) instead of a placebo arm. Pivotal studies are required to be powered to a p value of less than 0.05. For a new chemical entity, a mean of 1,700 total exposures was required to establish a broad safety database (Duijnhoven et al. 2013). In addition, separate clinical trials may be required depending on the target patient population, such as individuals with renal impairment or pediatric populations.

2. *For a new veterinary drug*, the requirements are more streamlined. A single well-controlled study, typically at least 100 animals with the disease receiving the investigational product and a corresponding number of placebo controls, depending on the study design, is required for approval. While a study may be powered to reach significance with fewer subjects, 100 treated animals has been the default number used to allow for inference across different breeds and across presentations of the disease that fit within the indication. It is worth noting that while owners make the final decision to put their pets in a clinical trial following a rigorous process of informed consent, for many indications, enrollment is easier for animals than recruiting subjects for human trials. Roughly 80% of all human studies have been reported to miss enrollment projections (Lopienski 2017, CBInsights 2018). This challenge with enrollment is partially due to the fact that humans have more treatment options for a given disease. While enrollment delays affect veterinary studies as well, the enrollment delay in human clinical trials can significantly increase both the cost and the time component of the NPV calculation relative to the veterinary program.

VETERINARY CLINICAL WORK IS LESS RISKY

Veterinary drugs are less risky because if they fail, it is with much less investment. The reason for this is that most human drugs are first tested in laboratory animal disease models, but these models do not always accurately mimic the human disease. For example, to test neuropathic pain drugs, the animal model is to physically impair a nerve (ligation) or chemically treat the animal (pyroxiden or acrylamide) in order to damage the nerve, but the symptoms that are being studied are acutely induced (Sousa 2016). Whereas in the normal disease process, for example type 2 diabetes, it takes years of gradual tissue damage for the neuropathy to be detected. For animals, the investigational drug can be evaluated early in the actual diseased patients that make up the typical caseload of veterinary clinics and research hospitals. Being able to test a drug in the actual disease state, as opposed to an artificially induced model in a different species than the intended market, decreases the risk of false success (e.g., a chemotherapy that works in a rodent model where a tumor was grafted onto the leg of a mouse, but was not predictive of when the same drug was used to treat a dog or a child with osteosarcoma).

In addition, there are differences in physiology between animals and humans that cannot always be anticipated. This is one of the reasons that two species are required to be tested before drugs can be administered to humans. For example, acetaminophen (e.g., Tylenol®) is one of the most commonly used human analgesics and is sold without a prescription because of its benign safety profile. Yet in dogs, it can cause severe liver damage at very low doses, and cats are up to ten times more sensitive to its effects than dogs (Drugs 2020). The most definitive study to date of interspecies concordance involved an International Life Sciences Institute-sponsored review of data supplied by 12 pharmaceutical companies (Olson et al. 2000). There was an overall interspecies concordance for 61% of the compounds. Rodents alone were predictive of human toxicities for 43% of the agents, while non-rodents (primarily dogs) alone were predictive for 63%.

Effectiveness studies in humans can only be started after a significant investment in toxicology and manufacturing has been made, whereas for animals, proof of concept effectiveness studies are often done prior to, or in parallel with, major investments in formal toxicology studies and improvements in manufacturing. This parallel effort can result in a decrease in timelines and an ability to demonstrate effectiveness (or an effectiveness signal) before more significant investments. While this can result in an expanded timeline for other reasons (e.g., formulation or manufacturing delays result in delays in starting a pivotal, Phase 3-type study in veterinary patients), in general this approach positively impacts the NPV calculation for veterinary programs.

VETERINARY REGULATORY RISK IS LOWER

The US public could be characterized as wanting a free magic pill that cures its problems, but with no risks or associated side effects, a hurdle that is virtually impossible to meet. The symptoms of these unrealistic societal expectations are unwarranted tort litigations, special interest agendas, the devastating opioid epidemic, and displeasure as drug prices continue to increase, just to name a few. These societal expectations have resulted in the FDA taking the stance that their primary objective is to protect patients. This mindset has two major impacts on the drug development process: first, the human side of the FDA is likely to take the most conservative position on areas of "grey" by requiring more data, which is time-consuming and increases the expenses associated with the program and therefore negatively impacts an NPV calculation. The current increase in cost of drug development noted above is a direct response of the FDA trying to respond to societal insistence on relatively few side effects. Second, if a drug developer is not sure exactly how a specific aspect of the program will be viewed in the context of the current regulatory guidelines, they must file a formal request for information. This is time-consuming and can result in either unclear or non-committal advice.

In contrast, the veterinary side of the FDA, the CVM, and its sister agency, the CVB at the USDA, are faced with different issues. Because of the macroeconomic issues being discussed in this chapter, many drugs for companion animals are used off-label (i.e., without formal approval in the target animal). Since 1994, drugs that are approved for use in humans often may be legally used by veterinarians (www.fda.gov/animal-veterinary/resources-you/ins-and-outs-extra-label-drug-use-animals-resource-veterinarians).

If we focus on the process at the CVM, this center at the FDA requires that drugs are tested to ensure the safety of the animals, but the center actively encourages development of new drugs for animals so that there are more treatment options with clear dosing guidelines for a particular indication in a particular species. This mindset has two impacts to the drug development process that differ from development for human patients: first, the CVM has a meeting with the sponsor at the beginning of the process and issues a Memorandum of Conference (MOC). The MOC is a legal notification of information exchanged including any (potential) agreements that the sponsor and the agency make specifying what steps and studies are required for the drug's approval. This allows the investor to more accurately predict a project's cost and de-risks the NPV calculation. Second, when questions about the program arise, instead of the slow and sometimes confusing process associated with human drug development, the sponsor can correspond with the Project Manager at the CVM for input into the issue at hand. However, to be clear, the veterinary regulatory process is no less regulated than the human regulatory process.

An example of the protective (human) versus proactive (animal) mindset is the difference in how the two divisions approach clinical trial design. For humans, the process is to send a study protocol to the FDA, but the FDA is not required to comment on the protocol. If it is a "first in man" study, the sponsor must wait 30 days before initiating the study. While subsequent studies can be initiated immediately, most companies give the FDA time to comment. However, the FDA may decide to make comments at any time, increasing their inherent risk. There are examples of trials that are more than 50% complete when the FDA provided comments; these can range from simple clarifications, strong suggestions for an amendment to the study design, or a full clinical hold. In any case, the practical reality is that clinical trials are launched in clinical sites without a complete assurance that the protocol will not change based on FDA (CDER/CBER) input. Altering the trial midstream almost always causes delays, which adds to the cost of the program. In sharp contrast, the CVM encourages sponsors to discuss the protocol before starting a study and for a pivotal study, to submit it for review and concurrence. They actively respond to questions or concerns about study design and there is a clear agreement reached between the CVM and sponsor prior to the study being initiated. A similar process exists for biological and vaccine products on the animal side with the CVB. The clarity provided saves time, money, and reduces risk, all of which positively impact the NPV of the program.

Perhaps the most impactful difference is in the way New Drug Applications (NDA) are reviewed. In animals, each section of the NDA can be submitted and is reviewed separately (rolling review). This practical impact allows sponsors to fix deficiencies in a package in parallel while completing other sections of the package. In contrast, in human applications all sections of the NDA are submitted and reviewed at the same time.

One important caveat to this discussion on regulatory risk is that sponsors of human drugs can apply for several programs that are intended to help sponsors receive more expedient feedback or a rolling review that is more similar to the veterinary situation, such as fast track, breakthrough status, accelerated and priority review (FDA 2020).

HUMAN MARKETS ARE MUCH LARGER

The top-selling human drug in 2018 was Humira®, with $20.45 billion in annual sales (Group 2018). The top 50 human drugs averaged $4.94 billion in annual sales (Group 2018). The largest-selling veterinary drug is the non-steroidal anti-inflammatory drug (NSAID), Rimadyl (carprofen), with annual sales of $200 million (Bautz 2016). The 200th-largest-selling human drug, Uptravi® (selexipag), has annual sales of more than $700 million, more than triple the largest-selling veterinary drug ever marketed. Table 5.1 lists human health pharmaceutical companies with associated animal health companies.

This huge discrepancy in the potential market sizes would on the surface suggest the NPV would never be in favor of the veterinary drug. However, human sales forces and direct-to-consumer advertising can be very expensive. Therefore, while the human market is larger, the relative profit for the veterinary product may be higher. For a standalone veterinary company, the calculus of a new opportunity must be made solely on the merits of the opportunity in animals and not the opportunity cost associated with the human market. Historically, for companies with both human and veterinary divisions, the human pharmaceutical division rarely has risked allowing a novel proprietary compound to be developed for animals until the patent has expired and it is considered a generic compound. The growing willingness of investors to invest in standalone veterinary companies is likely to encourage more compounds to enter into veterinary development. There are likely many compounds for which human development was discontinued but could be rescued and repurposed for veterinary use. Anivive Lifesciences Inc. is an example of a company focused on such repurposing of compounds (2020a).

TABLE 5.1

List of Human Health Companies with Associated Animal Health Subsidiary (Updated May 2020)

Human Health Company	Animal Health Subsidiary	Standalone Animal Health
Pfizer	Pfizer Animal Health	Zoetis
Merck & Co.	Merck Animal Health	
Eli Lilly	Elanco Animal Health	Elanco
Novartis	Novartis Animal Health	Acquired by Elanco
Bayer	Bayer Animal Heath	Acquired by Elanco
Boehringer Ingelheim	Boehringer Ingelheim Animal Health	
Merck & Co. (MSD AgVet) and Sanofi-Aventis (Rhône-Mérieux)	Merial	Purchased by Boehringer Ingelheim Animal Health
Sorrento Therapeutics	Ark Animal Health	

INTELLECTUAL PROPERTY AND REIMBURSEMENT DIFFERENCES

While the disparity of the market size potential is enormous, veterinary drugs have the advantage that the pressure of generic drugs is not as severe. In the United States, a new human compound is protected from competition for 20 years from the filing of the patent. After that, a generic version of the drug can be approved just by showing that blood levels of the new compound are equivalent to the originally approved compound. The confounding issue is that it often takes between 10 and 20 years to get a drug approved, so its original patent may no longer be valid or is near expiring. The Hatch-Waxman Act of 1984 was instituted to control how innovator and generic drugs are regulated in terms of exclusivity. Key components of this legislation include:

1. A compound without a patent (or an expiring patent) is given 7 years of marketing exclusivity, regardless of its patent status.
2. Part of the time required for the development of a new drug can be added back to the expiration date of the patent (patent term extension).

There also are some practical hurdles based on the FDA filing schedule and approval times for a generic product that can extend the period of market exclusivity. The bottom line is that on average, 12 years after a human drug is approved, a generic version starts to be sold and the market can evaporate for the original sponsor (Kesselheim 2017).

The veterinary situation is slightly different. While the patent laws are the same, there is not as much pressure by payors (i.e., insurance companies) to reduce drug costs because most costs are paid directly by the animal owner. Even in the setting of pet insurance, which is increasingly popular, there are not the same pressures as in the human marketplace. As a consequence, most veterinarians purchase the drug and mark up that cost when the drug is sold to the pet owner. For example, if the originator drug costs $20 wholesale, the veterinarian may purchase the drug, and mark it up by 20% and sell it to the owner for $24. The veterinarian serves in the role of a pharmacy and makes a profit of $4. Whereas if a generic drug is approved and costs $5, with a 20% markup, the veterinarian makes $1. While there have been generic veterinary drugs approved, they have not been nearly as successful as their human counterparts. This means the veterinary innovator drug company doesn't face as much market erosion (i.e., the difference in annual markets between human and veterinary medicine is greater than the difference in total markets over the lifecycle of the product).

CMC IS ESSENTIALLY THE SAME FOR HUMAN AND ANIMALS

Chemistry and Manufacturing Controls (CMC) are the procedures and protocols put in place to ensure that each batch of drug has the same purity profile and delivers the same dose of the active ingredient. Drugs that are tested in or sold to patients (human or animal) must be manufactured under these controls, referred to as Good Manufacturing Practices (GMP). Note that Figure 5.1 combined a large number of studies into a single category because for the purposes of this chapter, there are no meaningful cost or timeline differences between the human and veterinary CMC requirements.

For the NPV consideration, the differences are primarily in the timing of the risk. For animals, it is possible to test the compound and confirm its activity before investing in formal GMP manufacturing activities. As discussed above, for humans, there are toxicology and Phase 1 requirements that need GMP-produced drug product, before human studies can be initiated. This means that much more capital has to be put at risk earlier in the process for a human product, which negatively impacts the NPV calculation.

A UNIQUE DEVELOPMENT PATH IN ANIMALS (MUMS)

There is a unique offering in the development of a drug for animals, provided the indication meets strict criteria, called a Minor Use / Minor Species (MUMS) designation (2020b). Ostensibly, this compares to the orphan drug designation in humans, but with several critical differences. In humans, orphan drug designation has some benefits in the numbers of subjects required for approval which reduces cost, but the sponsor cannot sell the drug until after approval. In animals, if manufacturing and target animal safety studies support full approval, there is a lowering of the threshold for effectiveness to needing to demonstrate a "reasonable expectation of effectiveness (RXE)", rather than "substantial evidence of effectiveness". Provided the initial criteria are met and continue to be met, the sponsor company is allowed to sell the drug under a label for "conditional approval" for up to 5 years during which time they must perform the studies and submit the data for review to receive full approval. The criteria mentioned above are included in the name of the designation and the office at the CVM that oversees this program – the indication needs to be for a minor use or in a minor species, both of which are defined in the regulations (21 CFR part 516). The fact the sponsor can complete informal efficacy studies in animals prior to making the next investments in manufacturing and other studies allows for the data to support a discussion of RXE with CVM staff. This may shorten the time to return on investment and the risk of achieving the target market. The MUMS designation was created in large part because it encourages the effort toward the approval of drugs that would never be developed based on the traditional investment calculations. Further, MUMS and orphan designation both grant the sponsor company some benefit in regard to a reduction in fees and market exclusivity (7 years).

SPECIAL CASES IN ANIMALS (BIOLOGICS/PROTEINS)

Twenty-seven of the 50 largest-selling human drugs are based on recombinant DNA (i.e., biologics as opposed to small organic molecules) (Group 2018). Most of these are antibodies intended to treat inflammatory disease or cancer. In recent years, a number of companies have explored developing biologics for use in animals. However, there are several challenges. First, a human antibody will cause an adverse immune reaction in an animal, especially human antibodies in dogs (Gearing 2013, Maekawa 2017). This means that a generic antibody cannot be developed; instead the antibody has to be reengineered for the targeted species. Second, as discussed above, CMC requirements are the same between human and animal, but a reengineered antibody is a different product and will need its own manufacturing specifications and controls. Biologics are typically more costly programs to run than small organic molecules and since it will be an entirely new protein sequence, the sponsor can't leverage the human CMC data, which negatively impacts the NPV calculation. Lastly, most of the human biological drugs have achieved the market sizes described above, not so much because of patient numbers, but because of the cost of treatment. For example, the treatment regimen with an antibody against PD1 for small cell lung cancer currently cost $350,000 per year, but only 12.5% of patients are expected to respond to such treatment (Haslam and Prasad 2019). Since insurance does not cover most veterinary drugs, or often is limited in coverage of therapies for life-threatening diseases such as cancer, there are few owners in the United States that choose to pay those types of costs for their pet. The cost of antibody production is decreasing and the willingness of paying for pets is increasing in a small percentage of the population. Perhaps in time the NPV calculation for a biologic will definitively shift to positive for animals. In the meantime, most development in this area serves to support human clinical development.

WHERE IS THE VETERINARY INDUSTRY HEADED?

Prior to 1990, the pharmaceutical industry was primarily focused on making small molecule, organic compounds for treating human patients (Oxtoby 2019). In the late 1970s and early 1980s, companies such as Genentech and Amgen pioneered the efforts to make recombinant DNA-based drugs more accessible. As reliance on these drugs grew, the drug development landscape changed. The industry as a whole (regulators and investors/companies) became more comfortable with biologics, as well as the approval process being better defined and standardized. In parallel, markets have fragmented into smaller and smaller markets (Smietana 2019). This means companies are developing drugs for smaller populations of patients, but with that specification (and more and more frequently, supplemental indications for the same drug), companies are charging higher prices. The success of the smaller research and development companies has driven the trend to more clearly defining specific patient populations. In 2020, an estimated 276,480 new cases of invasive breast cancer are expected to be diagnosed in women in the United States, along with 48,530 new cases of non-invasive (in situ) breast cancer (breastcancer.org). Instead of a new drug targeting all 276,480 newly diagnosed cases, drugs are being developed to target subsets of patients, for example, subgroups HR–/HER2+ (4%), HR+/HER2+ (11%), HR–/HER2– (12%), and HR+/HER2– (73%) (AmericanBreastCancerSociety.org).

Early on, recombinant DNA companies were called "biotech" and the larger pharmaceutical companies focused on small molecules. But as the larger pharmaceutical companies became more comfortable with biologics, there has been a shift to larger companies controlling the biologics markets as well, because of their large sales forces and commercial infrastructure and frankly, their clinical and commercial success. Biotech or "specialty pharma" is increasingly becoming the research arm of the industry (Forbes.com). To the extent that the smaller biotech or specialty pharma companies are more efficient at keeping expenses low, the NPV calculation is positive for smaller opportunities. This translates to veterinary opportunities being increasingly attractive. A $50 million veterinary product can be sufficiently profitable to warrant development if the company can get to market with significantly less than the $2.5 billion a human drug costs, particularly if the veterinary company continues to sell the product for years, potentially with less competition. The willingness to invest in this space can be demonstrated by Initial Public Offerings (IPOs) of the stock of KindredBio ($50M in 2013) and Aratana Therapeutics ($35M in 2013), which sold fundamentally all their commercial assets or were acquired, respectively, in the past few years. Recent spinoffs of Zoetis (the Pfizer Animal Health arm of Pfizer) in 2014 and Elanco (the animal health subsidiary of Eli Lilly) in 2019 contributed to the changes in the investment landscape within animal health. Like many innovator companies, there are going to be successes as well as setbacks. In the 1980s, Genetic Systems and Hybridtech were two of the first companies making antibody therapeutics. They had relatively modest financial success when they were purchased, but they set the stage for the current industry of biologics/antibodies, which is expected to account for 25% of the total pharmaceutical market by 2020 (Oxtoby 2019). While the veterinary market will not approach the magnitude of success on biologics, as more veterinary programs generate positive results, investments are likely to continue to grow.

ADVICE TO THE VETERINARY ENTREPRENEUR

Because veterinary products are well suited to an NPV analysis and startup company dynamics, many scientists may have made a discovery that they feel would be beneficial to animal health and get the entrepreneurial bug. Listed below are several key steps to get started.

1. *File a provisional patent* to protect your idea before you publish it. Otherwise your publication will be considered "prior art" and will prevent a patent from being issued. The cost to file is minimal and there is a 1-year period to advance the project before the larger patent prosecution costs begin to be incurred.
2. *Incorporate your company* before you talk to investors. It will give you more negotiating power in how the company is set up following an investment. It costs very little to incorporate in Delaware. It can be done by a single person, but often University incubators or technology transfer offices can help. Many law firms also offer this service. While the value of the company is important and your ideas or data are worthwhile, do not fall into the trap of thinking you will become a millionaire overnight

by becoming an entrepreneur. On the other hand, equity is something to protect at this stage, so ideally set up the corporate structure and operating agreement with someone who has prior experience and can protect you from common mistakes.

3. *Prepare a development plan* and discuss with the appropriate regulatory agency. The knowledge gained makes it much easier to raise money because the timelines and budgets are less of an unknown risk. There are many consultants that can help put the development plan together and assist with the meeting. It is not as daunting a hurdle as it may sound.

4. *Think carefully about the market opportunity.* Is the idea a better mousetrap or a fundamental advancement in animal health that veterinarians have an interest in and will support and owners will pay for?

5. *Put your ego aside when raising money.* There is a joke in the industry that says Step 1 is to fund the company and Step 2 is to fire the founders. While a bit tongue in cheek, the reality is that stepping from University faculty to CEO is not a transition that everyone can make successfully. Investors have multiple scars from their past, often associated (fairly or not) with "founders' syndrome". Hire an experienced industry staff and take a role where you can help drive the company forward with your experience and enthusiasm for the product.

Abbreviation	Definition	Description
CMC	Chemical and Manufacturing Controls	The activities, processes, and controls required to manufacture a drug and to prove every batch is consistently and safely made.
CVB	Center for Veterinary Biologics	Division of the USDA responsible for biologics and vaccines.
CVM	Center for Veterinary Medicine	Division of the FDA responsible for new animal drugs.
FDA	Food and Drug Administration	Regulatory agency responsible for drugs (human and animal), biologics and vaccines (human only), devices (human), food, cosmetics, radiation, and tobacco within the United States.
GMP	Good Manufacturing Practices	Practices required to support that drugs are being made with the proper testing and documentation.
IND or pre-IND (or INAD or pre-INAD for animal drugs)	Investigational New Drug (or Investigational New Animal Drug)	Document with the studies needed to allow testing of an investigational drug in subjects. Often a sponsor will ask questions of the regulatory agencies in a pre-IN(A)D meeting prior to filing or requesting the IN(A)D.

MAD	Multiply Ascending Dose	Clinical study to test safety, exposing the subject to repeated doses.
MOC	Memorandum of Conference	Document outlining the discussion and agreement between all meetings between regulatory agency (e.g., CVM); the first meeting between regulatory agency and sponsor may include what studies are required to get a new drug approved. CVM sends the sponsor an MOC within 45 days of the meeting.
MUMS	Minor Use / Minor Species	Drug development pathway offered by CVM in unique populations that allows for conditional approval on a path to full approval.
NCE	New Chemical Entity	Compound that has not been previously approved as a drug.
NPV	Net Present Value	The difference between the present value of cash inflows and the present value of cash outflows over a period of time, with a discount applied.
PK/PD	Pharmacokinetic to Pharmacodynamic ratio	Assessment of where the drug concentration in the blood stream causes a measurable biologic effect.
SAD	Single Ascending Dose	Clinical study to test drug safety by escalating the dose, but exposing the subject to only a single dose.
USDA	United States Department of Agriculture	Regulatory agency responsible for biologics and vaccines (animal only), in addition to other responsibilities related to a safe food supply within the Unites States.

REFERENCES

2019. "Total U. S. Pet Industry Expenditures." *APPA*. www.americanpetproducts.org/press_industrytrends.asp.

2020. "Industry Snapshot; Who We Are and What We Do." *The Animal Health Industry*. https://ahi.org/the-animal-health-industry/.

2020a. "Anivive Lifesciences Inc." Accessed May 2, 2020. www.anivive.com.

2020b. "Title I-Minor Use and Minor Species Health." Accessed May 2, 2020. www.anivive.com.

AmericanBreastCancerSociety.org. www.cancer.org/content/dam/cancer-org/research/cancer-facts-and-statistics/breast-cancer-facts-and-figures/breast-cancer-facts-and-figures-2019-2020.pdf.

Bautz, D. 2016. "Zacks Small-Cap Research." *scr.zacks.com*. Accessed March 7, 2016. http://s1.q4cdn.com/460208960/files/March-7-2016_PARN_Bautz.pdf.

Breastcancer.Org. www.breastcancer.org/symptoms/understand_bc/statistics.

CBInsignts. 2018. "The Future of Clinical Trials: How AI & Big Tech Could Make Drug Development Cheaper, Faster, & More Effective." Accessed August 7, 2018 www.cbinsights.com/research/clinical-trials-ai-tech-disruption/.

Drugs, Plumb's Veterinary. 2020. "Acetaminophen." *Plumb's Veterinary Drugs*. www.plumbsveterinarydrugs.com/#!/monograph/OLX391xuRg/.

Duijnhoven, R. G., S. M. Straus, J. M. Raine, A. de Boer, A. W. Hoes, and M. L. De Bruin 2013. "Number of Patients Studied Prior to Approval of New Medicines: A Database Analysis." *PLoS Medicine* 10(3):e1001407. doi:10.1371/journal.pmed.1001407.

FDA, US. 2020. "Fast Track, Breakthrough Therapy, Accelerated Approval, Priority Review." Accessed May 2, 2020 www.fda.gov/patients/learn-about-drug-and-dev ice-approvals/fast-track-breakthrough-therapy-accelerated-approval-priority-review.

Forbes.com. www.forbes.com/sites/forbestechcouncil/2019/05/29/the-future-of-pharma -the-role-of-biotech-companies/#4a9d47666bb3.

Gearing, D. et. al. 2013. "A Fully Caninised Anti-NGF Monoclonal Antibody for Pain Relief in Dogs." *BMC Veterinary Research* 9:226. www.biomedcentral. com/1746-6148/9/226.

Group, the Njaroarson. 2018. "Top 200 Pharmaceutical Products by Retail Sales." https://nj ardarson.lab.arizona.edu/sites/njardarson.lab.arizona.edu/files/2018Top200Pharma ceuticalRetailSalesPosterLowResFinalV2.pdf.

Haslam, A., and V. Prasad 2019. Estimation of the Percentage of US Patients with Cancer Who Are Eligible for and Respond to Checkpoint Inhibitor Immunotherapy Drugs. 2(5):3192535. doi:10.1001/jamanetworkopen.2019.2535.

Institute, Animal Health. 2020. "Federal Approval." https://ahi.org/approval-and-regula tion-of-animal-medicines/.

Kesselheim, A. 2017. "Determinants of Market Exclusivity for Prescription Drugs in the United States." Accessed September 13, 2017 www.commonwealthfund.org/publi cations/journal-article/2017/sep/determinants-market-exclusivity-prescription-dr ugs-united.

Kleinman, M. 2012. "Pharma Shifts Focus from Small Molecules to Biologics." *PearlIRB*. Accessed April 16, 2012. www.pearlirb.com/pharma-shifts-focus-from-small-mo lecules-to-biologics/.

Lopienski, K. 2017. "Why Do Recruitment Efforts Fail to Enroll Enough Participants?" https://forteresearch.com/news/recruitment-efforts-fail-enroll-enough-patients/.

Maekawa, N. et al. 2017. "A Canine Chimeric Monoclonal Antibody Targeting PD-L1 and Its Clinical Efficacy in Canine Oral Malignant Melanoma or Undifferentiated Sarcoma. Nature." *Scientific Reports* 7(1):8951. doi:10.1038/s41598-017-09444-2.

Moore, T. J., H. Zhang, G. Anderson, and G. C. Alexander 2018. "Estimated Costs of Pivotal Trials for Novel Therapeutic Agents Approved by the US Food and Drug Administration, 2015–2016." *JAMA Internal Medicine* 178(11):1451–1457. doi:10.1001/jamainternmed.2018.3931.

Oxtoby 2019. www.chemistryworld.com/molecule-to-market/how-biologics-have-chan ged-the-rules-for-pharma/3010301.article.

Smietana, K. et al. 2019. "The Fragmentation of Biopharmaceutical Innovation." *Nature*. www.nature.com/articles/d41573-019-00046-3.

Sousa, A., G. Lages, C. Pereira, and A. Siullitel 2016. "Experimental Models for the Study of Neuropathic Pain." www.scielo.br/scielo.php?script=sci_arttext&pid=S1806-0 0132016000500027&lng=en&nrm=iso&tlng=en&ORIGINALLANG=en.

Svennebring, A., and J. Wikberg 2013. "Net Present Value Approaches for Drug Discovery." *Springerplus* 2(1):140. PMID 23586005. doi:10.1186/2193-1801-2-140.

6 How to Perform Research in Spontaneous Models of Disease

Kristen V. Khanna and Philippe Brianceau

CONTENTS

INTRODUCTION

"Spontaneous model" has become a catchphrase for a study of an investigational intervention (e.g., a drug or procedure), performed in companion animals with naturally occurring disease, that may serve basic research and inform applications in human medicine as well as meet the need for applied knowledge in animal health. The latter path may lead to the development of a new therapeutic in veterinary medicine. This type of cross-species, cross-functional, and cross-disciplinary research is often associated with topics in One Health, translational, and comparative medicine. This initiative has gained increasing interest and traction over the past decade, with real-life examples of success and advocates for its use, as shared in this book.

Each spontaneous animal model study that successfully translates and/or informs human clinical research serves as a positive example, and also invites evaluation as a unique case study. However, without someone sharing the details of each project or study, it is natural to ask, *how* did they do it? Specifically, how would an individual or research team at a University, early-stage biotech, or pharmaceutical company incorporate pets with a disease or condition of interest into a research project? How would individuals, with different backgrounds and different resources available to them, design and manage a study that involves pets and owners and practicing veterinarians? Furthermore, how could these individuals manage a project that may very well have oversight from, and potentially be inspected by, a regulatory agency in the veterinary sphere (e.g., FDA's Center for Veterinary Medicine or USDA)?

While each setting (e.g., University, biotech/pharma, private practice, etc.) and study poses its own challenges, there are certain attributes and requirements or best practices for studies that work well. There are studies for which risks can be mitigated and studies involving "spontaneous models" that may be advantageous over traditional animal models. Like all good research, studies involving animals with naturally occurring disease need to be motivated by meaningful objectives and appropriate questions.

THE OBJECTIVE

A primary purpose of addressing a research question in animals with spontaneous disease is to better understand the biological and/or clinical outcome(s) of exposure to an investigational therapy, product, procedure, or intervention; or to characterize the natural history of a disease. When evaluated in the context of translational medicine, these endpoints are often designed in a manner to answer a research question that could not easily be addressed in the human population or in conventional animal models (most commonly rodents; purpose-bred dogs, cats, rabbits, or pigs). Another, equally compelling, purpose of these studies can be to develop a product for use in veterinary medicine. University technology transfer offices and start-up companies find this latter aspect of translational research of interest, as it creates an asset that may be monetized and directed back into development programs. Overall, the purpose should revolve around answering questions and thereby making progress in both human and animal health in a way that cannot scientifically be accomplished another way.

THE RESEARCH QUESTION

While a book chapter cannot provide an answer as to which research questions should be asked, it can provide a new lens through which to see. If the research question that is best addressed in the translational setting is one that cannot be answered another way, studies designed to better understand how a drug might behave in humans with the same disease or condition as a pet may be informative. Research questions that are addressed in proof-of-concept (POC) type studies can be helpful and typically revolve around questions of dose, schedule, determining the appropriate primary (and secondary) endpoints, determining the appropriate timepoint(s) for measurements and evaluations, and often provide safety and effectiveness data in the setting of naturally occurring disease. In the "go/no-go" language of the pharmaceutical industry, there should be sufficient data in support of activity (or endpoint of interest) to maintain continued investment in the project.

If the purpose of the research is truly dual in nature – to address human and veterinary medicine – it would be a missed opportunity not to answer questions pertinent to both.

The development of a working hypothesis may be demonstrated with an example, albeit one that is more than a decade old. Anti-angiogenic drugs garnered great interest in the oncology field in the late 1990s and early 2000s. Due to their known mechanisms of action, they were believed to require extended exposure times prior to establishing an anti-cancer effect, specifically on the primary outcome measure of tumor size. As a result, drugs in this class could not be easily studied in tumor models in rodents, based on the relatively short lifespan of mice and rats. The classic model was flawed simply by the host not living long enough for the drug to potentially have a beneficial effect. Therefore, a working hypothesis that a longer duration of exposure to these drugs would result in a measurable benefit (i.e., an objective response) was pursued in pet dogs with cancer culminating in data that benefited human medicine. Notably deemed a "pre-clinical" study for human medicine, a series of studies in tumor-bearing dogs not only allowed canine patients to be on the drug a sufficient length of time to observe a benefit (either complete or partial responses in a subpopulation of dogs), but results collected from these dogs served to provide supportive data that informed clinical trials of anti-angiogenic drugs in human patients (Rusk et al. 2006a; Rusk et al. 2006b; Sahora, 2012). The translational research question asked was whether dosing the investigational drug in tumor-bearing dogs with an expected lifespan of at least 30 days would result in an anti-tumor effect. The answer was yes.

In addition to these clinical data, the pharmacokinetics in the dog study also informed subsequent human studies. Previous studies on this class of compounds in humans had selected earlier endpoints and had not allowed patients to continue receiving the drug if anti-tumor activity was not observed in the first weeks of therapy. This timeline was changed in at least one human study protocol following the results of studies in dogs.

The research questions addressed in these studies went further, beyond what may have been needed to provide evidence of safety and effectiveness for the drug to become an approved veterinary therapeutic, to addressing surrogate biomarkers of activity. The biomarkers evaluated were similarly informative for human clinical trials.

While the investigational drug evaluated in these studies did not receive FDA approval for use in human patients, it is in the same class as Avastin® (bevacizumab), which has been used by more than 2 million cancer patients (Genentech, Inc. website and data on file). These studies in dogs contributed to a body of knowledge

TABLE 6.1

Angiogenesis Inhibitors Approved for Human Use

Name	Link
Axitinib (Inlyta®)	www.cancer.gov/about-cancer/treatment/drugs/axitinib
Bevacizumab (Avastin®)	www.cancer.gov/about-cancer/treatment/drugs/bevacizumab
Cabozantinib (Cometriq®)	www.cancer.gov/about-cancer/treatment/drugs/cabozantinib-s-malate
Everolimus (Afinitor®)	www.cancer.gov/about-cancer/treatment/drugs/everolimus
Lenalidomide (Revlimid®)	www.cancer.gov/about-cancer/treatment/drugs/lenalidomide
Lenvatinib mesylate (Lenvima®)	www.cancer.gov/about-cancer/treatment/drugs/lenvatinibmesylate
Pazopanib (Votrient®)	www.cancer.gov/about-cancer/treatment/drugs/pazopanibhydrochloride
Ramucirumab (Cyramza®)	www.cancer.gov/about-cancer/treatment/drugs/ramucirumab
Regorafenib (Stivarga®)	www.cancer.gov/about-cancer/treatment/drugs/regorafenib
Sorafenib (Nexavar®)	www.cancer.gov/about-cancer/treatment/drugs/sorafenibtosylate
Sunitinib (Sutent®)	www.cancer.gov/about-cancer/treatment/drugs/sunitinibmalate
Thalidomide (Synovir, Thalomid®)	www.cancer.gov/about-cancer/treatment/drugs/thalidomide
Vandetanib (Caprelsa®)	www.cancer.gov/about-cancer/treatment/drugs/vandetanib
Ziv-aflibercept (Zaltrap®)	www.cancer.gov/about-cancer/treatment/drugs/ziv-aflibercept

about this class of therapeutic agents and how they might be successfully used. A list of currently approved angiogenesis inhibitors is found in Table 6.1.

THE RESEARCH STANDARD

Studies in dogs leading to new products in animal health have to comply with the research standards set by the US Food and Drug Administration (FDA), Center for Veterinary Medicine (CVM). This standard is not a requirement for translational medicine studies and, in fact, in many cases would lead investigators away from pursuing research in disease-bearing, client-owned animals. Knowing the difference between animal and human standards can help those working in human scientific and medical research determine which is suited best for the research goals. In most cases, a regulatory study is best reserved for an animal health partner seeking to develop an animal health product, perhaps synergistic but also independent of the translation to a human health product.

Some readers will be familiar with the research standards, Good Laboratory Practice (GLP) and Good Clinical Practice (GCP). GLP is a federal regulation, 21 Code of Federal Regulation (CFR) Part 58, that defines a process and set of expectations for conducting nonclinical laboratory studies ensuring the quality and integrity of the data generated by these studies. Apart from this brief introduction and mention of its contrast with GCP, the GLP standard of study conduct is beyond the scope of this chapter.

GCP is a research standard intended to provide guidance on how to design, conduct, monitor, record, audit, analyze, and report clinical studies, largely through strict documentation practices, ensuring the ethical conduct of a study that delivers consistent, reproduceable, and high-quality data. GCP terminology may be applied in human or veterinary medicine, although veterinary research has its own GCP standards based on the International Cooperation on Harmonisation of Technical Requirements for Registration of Veterinary Medicinal Products (VICH); internationally referred to as VICH GL-9. The FDA-CVM issues a guidance document with the same content, Guidance for Industry #85. This document is similar to the human GCP Code, but uses language that is appropriate for the research setting involving pets, owners, and veterinary hospitals or veterinary clinics.

The principles of GCP are as follows:

1. **Ethical conduct of the study is imperative**. Thus, GCP outlines practices that ensure accuracy and integrity of the data collected, and takes into consideration the welfare of animals, study personnel, and the environment.

2. **The proposed research must be described in a protocol**. To this end, the study is described through "pre-established, systematic, written procedures".

3. **Informed consent must be obtained from the pet owner before initiating any study-related procedures**. While all documentation is important to GCP, the informed consent of the owner is arguably the single most important document in any study involving client-owned animals.

4. **A reasonable safety profile in the target species should be known and is a primary ongoing consideration of the study**. By definition, the drug being assessed in an investigational study has not been proved to be safe and effective, sufficient safety data should be known prior to initiating a study of a drug in client-owned animals, such that the safety risks have been adequately identified including risks to other animals and the "human user population" (made up of veterinarians, veterinary clinic staff, owners, caregivers, and the pet's human family members). There should be a mechanism for ongoing risk assessment during the conduct of the study.

5. **Expected benefits should be believed to outweigh the risks**. The expected benefits should be greater than the known or expected risks, including a full description of known adverse events (i.e., side effects). It is understood that it is impossible for all risks to be identified at the start of a study and risk identification is the reason some studies are completed.

6. **The study may be reviewed by a qualified ethics committee**. While not legally required, it is good practice that an Institutional Animal Care and Use Committee, an *ad hoc* Animal Care and Use Committee, and/ or a more recent player, a veterinary IRB, reviews the protocol in the interest of protecting the patient and its owner.

7. **The study must engage a qualified Investigator and study staff**. A veterinarian should have credentials and the authority to support medical care and decision-making during the study. Similarly, the training of the support staff of veterinary nurses and technicians should be well documented. The Investigator may delegate certain study responsibilities to other individuals, but has the ultimate responsibility for the conduct of the study.

8. **The Investigator must ensure compliance with the protocol**. This means the right population of animals is enrolled (based on inclusion and exclusion criteria) and treated according to the protocol-mandated delivery of the drug; that study visits occur as scheduled (or deviations written accordingly); and that all data are documented according to the protocol.

9. **The records of the study must be maintained in a secure and highly professional manner**. Data capture forms (DCFs), also called case report forms (CRFs), should be completed in a timely manner (in most cases meaning contemporaneously with study activities), stored safely and protected from damage, and with the utmost integrity to protect the confidentiality of the study data (which legally belong to the study Sponsor or the University) and the study participants. While at this time there are not specific confidentiality requirements in the United States for pet patient data (such as HIPAA requirements for human personal/ medical information), the utmost care and specific institutional or corporate policies related to maintaining privacy should be in effect.

10. **The investigational product must be controlled and labeled properly at all times, as it is shipped, stored, and prescribed for investigational use**. As appropriate for the level of study, the investigational product should be manufactured to the standard of current Good Manufacturing Practice (cGMP).

11. **Quality systems should be engaged to ensure oversight and compliance with the above principles**. This may include external monitoring of data and clinical study materials, and a quality assurance review (i.e., a meta-review of processes at the site, including the quality control provided by the monitor).

Regulatory agencies expect that studies that lead to the regulatory approval of a veterinary product are conducted to GCP standards. However, despite this, and the above description of and focus on GCP study conduct, most translational studies will not require adherence to this standard. In this setting, GCP may be described as informing best practices. Many translational and POC studies are described as being "GCP-like", in that the study is engaged in the spirit of GCP, but may make exceptions to the most arduous documentation practices. However a study is completed, it is unfair and time-consuming to begin a study according to one standard and shift to a more or less stringent standard during the study, particularly a shift from non-GCP to GCP.

Just as client-owned animal studies may inform the human clinical development pathway for a drug, the GCP standard can inform best practices for study conduct. We provide two approaches for consideration by Sponsors to describe the study conduct standard in the setting of non-GCP that may be appropriate for studies of spontaneous disease in pets. First, for a study that is not conducted to a GCP standard outline, there could be explicit documentation in the study protocol in what ways the study team is allowed to deviate from GCP practices, such that investigators and support staff have a complete understanding of habits and expectations for study conduct. As an alternative, the scientific standards of a study may be defined in one or more Standard Operating Procedures (SOPs).

Just because a study is not GCP does not imply it has no regulatory value. Nor does this mean that the data cannot or should not inform development of a novel animal health product. In fact, many early stage studies, such as those that characterize dosage or early proof-of-concept studies, are essential to a regulatory package and are not conducted to GCP standard. Universities are increasingly looking for ways to commercialize technology and to license drugs for development in the veterinary market. In fact, one can argue that ethics demand progress for four-legged family members. The question becomes who will pick up the task, and the expense, of GCP study conduct.

All research in pets with naturally occurring disease should comply with a standard that takes into full consideration the ethical conduct, the need for a protocol that clearly outlines the purpose and primary endpoint of the study, the rights of the owner, the proper care and delivery of the investigational product, the handling and flow of study data, an *a priori* monitoring plan, a plan for safety reporting, an *a priori* statistical plan, and the structure for reporting the findings of the study once the data are clean and the database is locked. These would be the minimum expectations of a scientifically valid study.

THE TOOLS

The Protocol

The foundation of a well-designed and successfully implemented clinical study is a clearly written protocol that contains sufficient detail to allow all critical study procedures to be conducted in a repeatable fashion across all animals enrolled in the study and across all clinical sites involved. VICH GL-9 defines the protocol as the document that is signed and dated by the Investigator and the author (typically the study Sponsor and/or a contract research organization (CRO), if applicable) that fully describes the study objectives, design, methodology, statistical considerations, and organization of a study. The study protocol may provide background and a justification for the study, but these elements are not required.

Some Universities may not explicitly require a protocol (fitting this definition) for the conduct of translational research in pet animals, but it would be very rare that an IACUC or other ethics review board would not expect detailed information in the form of a protocol or similar format.

While studies may vary widely in their specifications and requirements, it is best to include certain elements in all protocols whether purely exploratory or pivotal in nature, and whether a study of an animal drug, a biological product, a device, or a product intended first (and perhaps only) for use in human patients.

While protocols differ in their expected level of data specificity, protocols that are as rigorous as possible given the limitations of what may be known at study outset will serve every project well. To that end, we recommend clinical study protocols contain the elements below:

- Study title
- Unique study identifier (e.g., study protocol number or study code)
- The version number and/or date and the status of the study protocol (i.e., draft, final, amended)
- Study contacts including the Investigator, representative(s) of the Sponsor, and all other participants responsible for major aspects of the study
- Identity of the site(s); it is recommended but not required that each Investigator and site be identified on his/her own individual copy of the protocol
- Objective(s) of the study
- Justification: a description of all information relevant to the objective of the study (e.g., pre-clinical or clinical data, published or otherwise available)
- Schedule of events, most often presented in table form for ease of reference by study staff
- Study design
  - The overall design of the study (e.g., a placebo-controlled clinical field effectiveness study)
  - The treatment, if any, to be applied to control group(s) and/or for control period(s)
  - The randomization method, if applicable, including the procedures to be adopted and practical arrangements to be followed to allocate animals to treatment groups and treatment groups to experimental units
  - The extent and methods of masking and other bias-reducing techniques to be used and state the provisions, including procedures and personnel, for access to treatment codes
- Animal identification method
- Specification of the animal's source (e.g., client-owned), number, species, age, sex, breed, weight, physiological status, reproductive status

- Other inclusion criteria, exclusion criteria, which should clearly define the study population
- Post-enrollment removal criteria
- Permissible and non-permissible concomitant veterinary care, medications, and therapy; specify objective criteria when concomitant medications may be used including prohibited medications (the use of which may result in an animal's removal from the study)
- Any special management of food and/or water including fasting periods, measurement of food during study, and any food(s) to be excluded so as not to compromise the objectives of the study, if applicable
- Identity of the investigational product
  - Site of manufacture
  - Lot number
  - Expiration date or date of next re-test
  - Instructions for preparation or mixing (if any)
  - Description of packaging and storage requirements
  - Dose and justification
  - Administration instructions
  - Labeling to conform with regulatory requirements (see the FDA's Code of Federal Regulations 21 CFR 511)
- Identity of control product(s) or procedures (e.g., sham surgery); if a product, include:
  - Generic or trade name
  - Dosage form
  - Dose and justification
  - Formulation (ingredients)
  - Concentration
  - Batch number
  - Expiration date
  - Administration instructions
  - Storage instructions (according to label directions if an approved drug)
- Describe the methods and precautions to be taken for the safety of study personnel handling investigational and control products
- Disposal and/or disposition of the investigational and control product(s)
- Describe the care to be given to animals removed from the study
- Describe the primary variable assessment
- Define the endpoints and measurements in the greatest specificity possible for the type of study
  - Describe what and how measurements are to be made and recorded
  - Specify the timing and frequency of study observations
  - Describe any special analyses and/or tests to be performed, including the time of sampling and the interval between sampling, storage of samples, and the analysis or testing

- Select and define any scoring system and measurements that are necessary to objectively measure the targeted response(s) of the study animal and evaluate the response
- Describe the statistical methodologies to be used to the level appropriate for the nature of the study (see below for the Statistical Plan)
- Handling of records: specify procedures for recording, processing, handling, and retaining raw data and other study documentation
- Adverse events (AEs): describe procedures for recording and reporting AEs and under what conditions medical treatment may be administered and masking codes broken, if applicable
- Changes to the study protocol: provide instructions for preparation of amendments and reporting of deviations to the study protocol
- Planned authorship of the final study report ideally should be clearly delineated
- Any study-specific procedures that apply to the conduct, monitoring, and reporting of the study
- Informed owner consent form
- All case report forms to be used during the study
- Any other relevant appendices or supplements (e.g., information to be provided to the owners of animals, instructions to study personnel)
- Citations of literature referenced in the protocol

The protocol should be approved by the Investigator and Sponsor representative and/or author with a dated signature. Once approved, the protocol is expected to be signed by each Investigator as evidence that he/she acknowledges he/she has read and understands the content of the protocol and agrees to personally conduct and supervise the study as described in the protocol. It should be stated in the protocol, or in a supplemental study document, who is responsible for maintaining original approvals for all parties to a clinical study and for assuring that a true copy of the approved protocol remains at each site during the study. All amendments to the protocol must be reviewed and approved by the same signatories as the original protocol. Once approved by the Sponsor, each amendment is expected to be signed by each Investigator.

The Data Management Plan: Tools and Electronic Data Capture (EDC)

If the end-goal of studies conducted in pets is to inform basic science or human clinical trials and product development, the data management plan is at the fore of ensuring quality information to guide decisions and hypothesis-generating work. Understanding data flow, from the clinical site (Investigator and other observers) and the owner (such as in the form of a diary, checklist, or compliance record), to the final study report, is no different in these studies than what would be demanded of a clinical trial conducted in humans. The same data management tools are used. In fact, a masked dataset from a human or pet study may be indistinguishable.

Similarly, data capture methods may be interchangeable or nearly so. Most electronic data capture (EDC) software is flexible enough to allow "generic" headings that

CLIENT SPECIFIC OUTCOME MEASURE (CSOM)						
Owner First Name:				Visit Date:		
Owner Last Name:						
CSOM Scoring/Descriptor						
Please assess below based on the last 7 days.						
Altered Activity or Attribute Related to Your Dog's Disease*	1 No Problem	2 Mildly Problematic	3 Moderately Problematic	4 Severely Problematic	5 Impossible	Not Recorded
	○	○	○	○	○	
	○	○	○	○	○	
	○	○	○	○	○	
					TOTAL (Sum):	
The activities entered at screening will be used for all CSOM scores.						

FIGURE 6.1 Electronic case report forms showing client-specific outcome measure. (Courtesy of Prelude Dynamics and Ark Animal Health, Inc.)

can be modified to be appropriate for veterinary patient data. Several companies and a few universities have developed relatively inexpensive tools for this setting. The greatest differences are common sense, such as documentation of body maps and adjustments in companion animal-specific or species-specific measurement tools, examples of which are shown in Figure 6.1 (e.g., recording a client-specific outcome measure (CSOM) for a dog).

These systems are often designed in modules that allow one to adjust the features and perform some or all of the programming oneself and thereby adjust the price point of the data capture product as well.

Data may also be captured on paper CRFs and manually entered into a database. While this method is time consuming, it is very common for pilot studies in animals when a commitment to an EDC system may be viewed as a luxury or studies are evolving on a day-to-day basis. The design of CRFs is an art, whether electronic or paper, but the principles behind them are the same for all studies, irrespective of the species of interest.

The Statistical Plan

A Statistical Analysis Plan (SAP) is most often a stand-alone document for a clinical research study, but in early-stage studies it can be described in a statistics section of the protocol. The SAP should clearly state the planned statistical analyses and ideally should be approved (by dated signature) before the initiation of the study. If part of the protocol, it is agreed to with the signature(s) of the Sponsor. If a translational study is intentionally not adequately powered to draw statistical conclusions in the final study report, but rather will provide descriptive statistics, this should be stated in the protocol. A biostatistician is a critical resource in the design and reporting of the study, which bring us to the study team.

THE PEOPLE

The IACUC/Veterinary IRB

As discussed above, the conduct of research in client-owned animals is a unique and valuable opportunity to answer research questions that might not otherwise be possible in a typical research setting, in human patients or in rodent or other animal models, and/or can be used to bring new products to market in veterinary medicine. While serving as such, some researchers are dissuaded from calling these animal "models". In fact, they are animals with the same diseases as are being studied in humans, and coming from the veterinary and pet-owning communities, these animals are patients and family members. Most of the studies contemplated could be justified based on their contribution to animal health alone. Informing human medicine could be viewed as an additional, although important, benefit.

Foremost is the ethical conduct of research in client-owned animals or pets that is facilitated by the engagement of an animal care and use committee. Universities have requirements for this type of regulatory body approval and most Sponsors of clinical research in pets have some mechanism by which they have an ethics review of the work proposed. CROs conducting studies in private veterinary practices may have an *ad hoc* committee to evaluate protocols prior to and during the course of a study, as well as to serve as the equivalent of a data safety monitoring board. The role of the IACUC has evolved in recent years as the field has evolved: the traditional purview of a laboratory animal review is no longer viewed as appropriate or sufficient for research conducted in pets. Several universities have created boards that function more like an Institutional Review Board (IRB) as are convened in the review and approval of the conduct of clinical research in human patients. These Boards consider different questions on the ethics of clinical trial conduct, keeping in mind the participant is the pet owner and the pet owner must understand the potential benefits and risks of having their pet participate in the research. Considerations are generally less focused on animal husbandry, welfare, and housing (as might be expected of a rodent study conducted in a laboratory setting) so much as whether or not the owner is sufficiently informed to be able to provide informed consent, whether or not the protocol has the appropriate controls and opportunities for receiving an investigational product or a placebo, that collection of biological samples are not too intrusive or too frequent, that pain is sufficiently managed, etc., again, similar to keeping with what would be considered for a human patient to participate in a research study. A University or medical research institute or biotech/pharma company that does not have access to this type of Board can have this need met by a CRO or by its IACUC with specific attention paid to the unique setting of working in non-rodent species.

While the regulatory agencies involved in the review and potential approval of new products for the veterinary market do not have a legal requirement for this type of review, universities or organizations that conduct research in client-owned animals will be well suited to lead the way in the ethical review of these studies.

The Research Team

The team that prepares the protocol and documentation for an IACUC/Ethics Board review is typically the same team that conducts the research. Exceptions to this may include when a University or research site has a clinical trials office or department that takes on some or all of these preparatory responsibilities and may even offer adjunct staff positions such as a Clinical Trials Clinician or Veterinary Technician (Veterinary Nurse), or a Recruitment Coordinator (an individual who manages the informed consent process with all owners). Most veterinary teaching hospitals that undertake clinical research have a Clinical Trials Office. These offices may be a resource for individuals seeking to perform clinical research in pets at the same University (e.g., at a medical school or other department). At schools that do not have this resource and no affiliation with a veterinary school, there are other ways forward. Working with a Sponsor and a CRO can support studies completed within a facility that allows pets to be treated. A partnership with a local veterinary clinic can provide the human (and physical) resources for conducting such research.

Each study is likely to involve unique roles and aspects depending on the study standard (i.e., GCP or non-GCP) to include: the treatment modality and endpoints (e.g., a radiation oncologist, an anesthesiologist, a treatment coordinator who may or may not be a veterinarian); the duration of the study; whether or not certain individuals are allowed to work on the study (e.g., residents, interns); as well as whether the study requires a masked (i.e., blinded) Investigator and additional study staff. At the research site, the team is generally made up of:

- Investigator (masked or unmasked) and potentially co-Investigators (of note, it is common terminology in human medicine to refer to a Principal Investigator (PI); whereas veterinary medicine in general does not use the term PI, but rather uses the term Investigator, or perhaps Lead Investigator)
- Site (or Study) Coordinator (possibly a veterinary nurse or technician, graduate student)
- Treatment Coordinator (unmasked)
- Medical Director (optional, often desirable if a multi-site study such that medical advice and support is consistent across sites)
- Monitor
- Quality Assurance (QA) (optional)
- Statistician
- Medical Writer

The protocol will define who will make the observations and if someone else is allowed (or designated) to record it. It will define how laboratory findings are documented and who should determine and document if they are clinically significant. It will define the role of other study team members and the role of the owner (if, for example, the owner is recording observations related to a study parameter, such as quality of life). If one is doing a study to inform a human clinical development plan, this may be explicitly defined in the study protocol and consequently may change the way certain study roles are defined.

For pivotal studies in the regulatory space (when work is completed at any clinic that will be considered part of a final study report to support a veterinary drug approval or as part of a data package to support the approval of the drug for human use), the Sponsor of the research will need to provide assurance to the regulatory agency that Quality Control and Quality Assurance standards have been met. Additional staff may include an external study monitor, who reviews the data that have been entered and, without biasing data collection, issues "queries" to ensure data accuracy and integrity in accordance to all protocol requirements. This staff may review the storage of drug, for example, to be sure it was administered at the correct dose. Whether an external party, such as provided by a CRO, or from an internal Clinical Trials Office, these individuals maintain some separation and conduct their work "at arm's length", which provides the independent review of the data. This in turn increases the confidence of Sponsors and regulatory agencies concerning data integrity.

Whether at a biotech company, a University without a veterinary school or teaching hospital, or a blended setting (where research may include a veterinary school and an associated medical school), these roles are the same. Midwestern University in Arizona provides an outstanding model with its Institute for Healthcare Innovation (www.mwuihi.com).

Human Medicine Colleagues

There are a number of different programs in the United States where veterinary clinical research is associated with human medicine colleagues. For example, the Comparative Oncology Trials Consortium (COTC) is an active network of 20 academic comparative oncology centers, centrally managed by the National Institute of Health (NIH)-NCI-Center for Cancer Research's Comparative Oncology Program. Trials conducted by the COTC are designed to impact current human Phase I and II clinical trials. Another example is The Dog Aging Project conducted by the University of Washington and Texas A&M University; this project is sponsored by a U grant (a NIH-sponsored cooperative agreement) from the National Institute on Aging. The Dog Genome Project run by teams from the Broad Institute of Harvard and MIT, the University of Massachusetts Medical School, and the International Association of Animal Behavior Consultants are collecting samples and data from thousands of dogs. A final example is the Veterinary Clinical Trials Network (VCTN) located at the Johns Hopkins University School of Medicine. This program is designed to capitalize on the entrepreneurial spirit and expertise of research and medical faculty in order to find better therapeutics and diagnostics for humankind and pets, at a lower cost and in a shorter time frame than is found historically.

Owners and Pets

Pet owners have many reasons for choosing to have their pet participate in a clinical trial. Owners are likely to want to feel they have done everything they could for their beloved family member (which admittedly goes beyond what some owners feel is enough). They may or may not have the financial resources for conventional treatments, but want to do what they can to extend the life, particularly the quality of life, of their pet. They may have a personal reason, such as a desire to contribute to the well-being of all animals, to feel they have participated in something larger than themselves, or to potentially contribute to an advancement in medical understanding of a disease that affects them (e.g., their cat has diabetes and they want to help researchers better understand the biology of diabetes or a related metabolic disease that also seriously impacted the life of their parent or friend).

The value of these contributions is individual and cannot be measured. To our knowledge there has not been a study of owners whose pets have participated in a clinical trial to evaluate their perceived value. Perhaps this is asking a question that has no answer. How can one position the meaning of an effective treatment or cure in pets to an effective treatment or cure in humans? Owners understand that dogs live condensed lives – certainly "dog years" is a commonly known concept – such that 1-year survival in a dog would be perhaps a 5-year or as much as a 7-year disease-free period in a human. Some would call this a cure. Most veterinary researchers consider this a worthy goal of medical progress.

One of the primary goals of translational research and a reason for pursuing it is to provide high-quality data or information to allow a research question to be answered and to generate the next question. Ultimately, the essential decision is whether to continue to develop a line of thinking within the research study (i.e., answering an hypothesis, or developing a product), or is the hypothesis invalid and should the study or development program come to an end? There is a small world of like-minded research scientists who are interested in making these studies happen. For researchers and for pets with medical conditions that can be used as models for human disease, every author in this book is interested in supporting these interests and facilitating veterinary clinical research.

REFERENCES

Rusk, A., McKeegan, E., Haviv, F., Majest, S., Henkin, J. and Khanna, C. (2006a). Pre-clinical evaluation of antiangiogenic thrombospondin-1 peptide mimetics, ABT-526 and ABT-510, in companion dogs with naturally occurring cancers. *Clin Cancer Res* 12(24):7444–55.

Rusk, A., Cozzi, E., Stebbins, M., Vail, D., Graham, J., Valli, V., Henkin, J., Sharpee, R. and Khanna, C. (2006b). Cooperative activity of cytotoxic chemotherapy with antiangiogenic thrombospondin-I peptides, ABT-526 in pet dogs with relapsed lymphoma. *Clin Cancer Res* 12(24):7456–64.

Sahora, A.I., Rusk, A.W., Henkin, J., McKeegan, E.M., Shi, Y. and Khanna, C. (2012). Prospective study of thrombospondin-1 mimetic peptides, ABT-510 and ABT-898, in dogs with soft tissue sarcoma. *J Vet Intern Med* 26(5):1169–76.

7 The Use of Animals in Research

Victoria K. Baxter

CONTENTS

LABORATORY ANIMAL RESEARCH: IS IT NECESSARY?

New developments in medicine are allowing humans to live longer and have healthier lives, and using pets as subjects in preclinical trials provides owners and veterinarians a first-hand view of these advancements. However, the clinical trial stage usually comes very late in the process of developing procedures, diagnostics, and therapies. Before a new chemotherapeutic regimen may be used to treat a patient with lymphoma or a new anti-inflammatory drug may be tried on a patient with a herniated intervertebral disc, experiments examining the safety and efficacy of these products must first be assessed. While evaluating new products in pets with spontaneously occurring disease can play a role, this process is almost always achieved in some part by using laboratory or purpose-bred research animals.

Laboratory animals represent a vital and indispensable component of the medical advancement process for products and procedures intended for both humans and animals, and nearly every single medical advancement that has been developed in the last 100 years has at least in some part been possible because of research animals (Institute of Medicine 1991). Most clinical conditions involve complex physiological processes, and full evaluation of therapies targeted to treat these conditions requires a whole living organism to understand the influence different cells, tissues, and organ system have on each other. The United States (US) Food and Drug Administration (FDA) and Health Canada require that a new potential therapy is proven to be both safe and effective before it will grant approval for marketing (United States Food & Drug Administration 2017, Health Canada 1997). However, robust preclinical evaluation of a new product or therapy involves a combination of both *in vitro* and *in vivo* studies.

For most drugs and biologics, the development process begins with *in vitro* studies. Once a clinical condition has been selected, the first step in the drug development process is usually identification of the target, which usually consists of proteins, DNA, or RNA (United States Food & Drug Administration 2018). After a compound has been identified as a promising candidate against the chosen target, experiments evaluating the compound's absorption, distribution, and excretion, mechanism of action, ideal route of administration, interaction with other drugs, and potential adverse effects or toxicities are conducted prior to initiation of clinical trials in humans. While much of this information can be determined through in silico or *in vitro* experiments, including mechanism of action, drug interactions, and toxicity, understanding other aspects requires a complete animal system. Determining a drug's biodistribution and ideal route of administration necessitates examination of the interplay of multiple organ systems; for example, a drug that is given orally, metabolized by the liver, and excreted in the urine involves the circulatory, digestive, and urinary systems. Emerging *in vitro* technologies such as "organ-on-a-chip" recreate key aspects of organ physiology, including tissue barriers and interfaces (such as blood vessel networks within and between tissues), tissue-level organization of different cell types, and multi-organ interactions (Zhang et al. 2018). While these alternative systems to conventional preclinical assessment represent a promising complement to animal testing, for the foreseeable future, full understanding of potential therapies requires a whole-body system that can only by achieved using live organisms, whether human or animal.

Many aspects of product development or examination of a disease process require a whole animal system. Most diseases, including microbial infections, cancer, and degenerative diseases, are complex and involve a combination of genetic and environmental factors. Pathogenesis studies, which evaluate the biological mechanisms that lead to the development or outcome of a disease, often involve aspects of the body, such as the immune system, that are difficult to replicate outside of a full organism. Before moving into the ultimate end user, whether that user is a human or animal patient, the pharmacokinetics and initial safety profile of a new or repurposed drug or therapy must be established. And critical evaluation of the pathological changes induced by a disease and toxicological changes induced by a putative diagnostic, therapy, or drug should involve a comprehensive examination of all organs and tissues in a body to assess any unforeseen or off-target effects. Understanding these more basic intricacies of a disease, diagnostic, or therapy is necessary to set a solid foundation for more translational studies and, ultimately in many cases, clinical trials. While it is these clinicals trials that will produce an end product that can be utilized by both humans and animals, ethical principles more often than not dictate that these necessary basic and translational studies be conducted using laboratory animals rather than the end user when possible.

In cases where human efficacy trials may not be feasible or ethical, a new drug or biologic designed to reduce or prevent life-threatening consequences induced by biological, chemical, or radiological agents may bypass the human clinical trial phase following successful preclinical trials in animals. Known as the Animal Efficacy Rule or simply the "Animal Rule", this law was authorized by the FDA in the United States in 2002 following the September 11th terrorist attacks and designed to counter potential acts of bioterrorism (United States Food & Drug

Administration 2019a). Under the Animal Rule, the FDA may approve a new product following animal studies without human clinical trials if the mechanism by which the product works is established and well-understood, and preclinical studies demonstrate a response predictive for humans in multiple animal species. Only a handful of products have been approved by the FDA using the Animal Rule, but include treatments for plague (caused by infection with the bacterium *Yersinia pestis*) and the Ebola virus.

In some cases, using purpose-bred research animals is not necessary, and the efficacy of new products may be tested in patients (both human and animal) without the prerequisite safety testing. A prime example of this situation is a new medical device that is made up of materials that have already been established to be biocompatible with the intended tissues in which the device will be implanted (United States Food & Drug Administration 2019b). In contrast, a medical device that is completely or partially composed of materials whose biocompatibility has not been established must first undergo safety testing in animals. Determining the ideal research subject population for evaluating a disease, procedure, drug, or product should take all of these aspects and considerations into account.

REGULATIONS THAT GOVERN ANIMAL RESEARCH

Using laboratory animals in research studies is not an entitlement, but instead a privilege that involves cooperation between government agencies, research institutions, and individual investigators. Responsible animal studies require careful study design involving consideration of the 3 Rs: Reduction, Replacement, and Refinement, which were first proposed by William Russell and Rex Burch in their seminal 1959 publication *The Principles of Humane Experimental Technique* (Russell and Burch 1959). Depending on the jurisdiction, regulations cover a wide variety of ethical issues involving animals used in research, including husbandry standards, facility inspections, record keeping, veterinary care, control of animal pain and distress, animal use protocol development and critical review, and determination of investigator competency with animal techniques (Vasbinder and Locke 2016). Expanding globalization also exposes the relatively new challenge of international harmonization, where scientific community members from multiple countries must work together to ensure that animal welfare standards and policies of animal care and use programs in different jurisdictions are upheld. While some countries have well-developed legal regimes for research animals dating back to the 1800s, regulations in other regions are still being established as scientific efforts evolve in those countries (Figure 7.1).

Legislation protecting animals used in research was first enacted in Britain in 1876, and Europe has long been at the forefront of establishing and revising minimal standards of laboratory animal care (Gluck, DiPasquale, and Orlans 2002). In 1986, the Council of Europe published the European Convention for the Protection of Vertebrate Animals used for Experimental and other Scientific Purposes, and the European Economic Community (now the European Union) published Directive 86/609/EEC, which together provided guidelines and

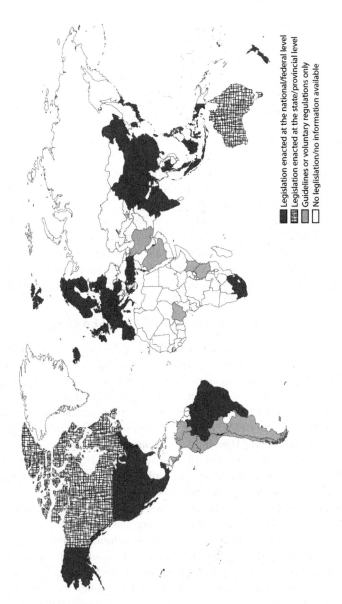

FIGURE 7.1 Animal research legislation by country.

technical details for carrying out experiments involving animals (Olsson et al. 2016). Scientific advances over the next few decades prompted a revision of the Directive to expand coverage to animals used in education and basic research, increased the focus on the 3Rs and animal welfare, and established consistent regulations among Member States of the European Union. The resulting Directive 2010/63/EU, implemented starting in 2010, provides minimal standards for housing and care of laboratory animals, restricts the use of certain animal species, and provides the framework for evaluating and authorizing research projects involving animals (European Union 2010). While the extent and implementation of animal protection standards vary among countries, transposition of Directive 2010/63/EU into national legislation has produced a strong level of harmonization among Member States, ensuring that minimal standards of animal welfare are met across most of Europe.

In North America, both the United States and Canada employ a strong emphasis on the 3Rs when approaching animal research oversight (Griffin and Locke 2016). However, while the United States has enacted two federal laws regarding animal research, Canada has no national direct legislation of animal welfare and instead relies on social contracts, emphasizing guidance and policy. While the Constitution Act 1982 forbids the Canadian government from enacting legislation if the provinces have already taken action in the matter, the federal government has taken action in three key areas involving animals in research: 1) protecting all animals in Canada from cruelty, abuse, and neglect, 2) setting regulations for testing, inspection, and quarantine activities of live animals imported into Canada, and 3) requiring research grants awarded by the government be contingent on a research institution holding a Canadian Council on Animal Care Certificate of GAP – Good Animal Practice. In contrast, the United States has enacted the Animal Welfare Act, enforced by the US Department of Agriculture, and the Health Research Extension Act, an amendment to the US Public Health Services Act that applies to any research supported by the Public Health Service, which includes the National Institutes of Health, the main federal financier of biomedical research in the United States (United States Department of Agriculture 2017; National Institutes of Health Office of Laboratory Animal Welfare 2015). While not laws, both Canada and the United States have additional published documents providing guidance on animal care and use in research: the Canadian Council on Animal Care *Guide to the Care and Use of Experimental Animals* and the US *Guide for the Care and Use of Laboratory Animals* (Canadian Council on Animal Care 1993; National Institutes of Health Office of Laboratory Animal Welfare 2010). In both countries, most of the responsibility is placed on local animal care committees (Canada) and institutional animal care and use committees (US), with individual institutions responsible for reviewing proposed experiments involving animals, guaranteeing personnel training and competency, providing appropriate animal husbandry and facilities as outlined in each respective *Guide*, and ensuring adequate veterinary care is provided. Failure to meet acceptable standards of animal welfare can result in recension of federal funds in both countries, with additional sanctions possible in the United States under the Animal Welfare Act and other federal laws.

Regulations governing the use of animals in research in Asia and Oceania vary greatly depending on the country. Countries with strong, well-established scientific communities have enacted national and provincial laws that promote principles similar to those in Western countries, including Japan (Act on Humane Treatment and Management of Animals), South Korea (Animal Protection Act and

Laboratory Animal Act), and New Zealand (Animal Welfare Act 1999) (Ogden et al. 2016). The minimal standards for research animal welfare in Australia is equitable to those of the European Union (EU) and United States, though the current framework lacks a central regulatory authority, with animal welfare legislative responsibility (except for fisheries) resting on each of the six states and two territories that make up the country (Timoshanko, Marston, and Lidbury 2016). Similar to Canada, compliance with regulatory guidelines outlined in the Australian Code for the Care and Use of Animals for Scientific Purposes and other federal regulations is required for federal funding, and every jurisdiction requires research institutions to establish an animal ethics committee that reviews proposed animal use protocols. Other countries rapidly expanding their focus on biomedical research in recent decades, including China, India, Singapore, Thailand, Indonesia, and Malaysia, have enacted national legislature and regulations with varying degrees of coverage and stringency (Ogden et al. 2016; Retnam et al. 2016).

Regulations involving laboratory animals in countries in Latin America, Africa, and the Middle East are developing but overall are lacking compared to those in Europe and North America. In Latin America, only Brazil, Mexico, and Uruguay have enacted legislation overseeing the care and use of animals in research, though other countries have anti-animal cruelty statutes that may include research animals (Rivera et al. 2016). In Africa and the Middle East, only Turkey, Israel, Qatar, and South Africa have formal legislation providing oversight and compliance regarding animal research, though countries such as Kenya and Tanzania have general animal welfare guidelines and require government-issued licenses to perform animal experimentation (Mohr et al. 2016). Development and implementation of regulations involving laboratory animals in these regions are often impeded by factors including political instability, civil unrest, economic challenges, lack of infrastructure, and culture differences.

In countries where formal guidelines regarding the humane care and use of research animals do not exist, individual institutions and members of the scientific community often recognize and follow guidelines implemented by the European Union and United States. Voluntary accreditation organizations, such as AAALAC International, promote international harmonization and provide opportunities for individual institutions to comply with internationally accepted minimum standards, regardless of the national regulatory framework (Guillén, Gettayacamin, and Swearengen 2016). And professional organizations that promote the humane care and use of research animals, including the Federation of European Laboratory Animal Science Associations, American Association for Laboratory Animal Science, Institute for Laboratory Animal Research, Universities Federation for Animal Welfare, and World Organization for Animal Health, provide and disseminate information, research, training, and collegiality among members of the laboratory animal science and welfare communities. Because it is becoming better recognized and acknowledged that good animal welfare produces good research data, establishing and revising the regulations that govern animal research will only result in better translational research outcomes.

USING PURPOSE-BRED LABORATORY ANIMALS VERSUS PETS FOR RESEARCH

Whether using pets or purpose-bred laboratory animals for preclinical research studies, each presents advantages and disadvantages (Table 7.1 and 7.2). Using pets in preclinical studies offers many advantages that allow easy translation to human studies. Most pets possess an intact immune system similar to humans and comparable physiologic parameters, such as heart rate, body temperature, and respiratory rate, making it easier to translate study outcomes to humans than in smaller model organisms more commonly used in laboratory settings, such as mice and rats. Tertiary care animal hospitals and veterinary schools usually possess and use the same equipment used in human hospitals, such as MR scanners and anesthesia monitoring equipment. Because diseases seen in pets are spontaneous and not experimentally induced, study outcomes are more likely to mimic those seen in human clinical trials. Additionally, because pets are kept in privately owned homes by pet owners, the effect of environmental factors and

TABLE 7.1

Advantages of Using Pets Versus Purpose-Bred Laboratory Animals for Research Studies

Pets	Purpose-Bred Research Animals
Comparable physiologic parameters (i.e. heart rate, body temperature, respiratory rate) to humans	Can be less expensive
Possess an intact immune system similar to human patients	Ability to control most, if not all, environmental factors, such as food intake, housing, temperature, and humidity
Clinical setting often uses the same equipment (i.e. imaging equipment, anesthetic equipment) as in human hospitals/clinics	Easier to achieve adequate sample size required to appropriately power studies
Spontaneously developed disease more likely to mimic disease seen in humans, such as tumors developing resistance to treatment	Many model species (mice, rats) have shorter life spans with accelerated growth rates
Allow for a more genetically diverse study population	Ability to evaluate a comprehensive study from start to finish and collect tissue samples following euthanasia
Ability to assess the effect of a "normal" home environment on study outcomes	Often able to specifically define genetic background to evaluate the genetic influence on a disease process or treatment
Owners are often intimately familiar with their pets and can monitor for subtle changes to behavior, feed intake, etc.	Able to employ genetic and experimental technologies not feasible for pet subjects
	Able to address complications immediately without communication with a pet owner

TABLE 7.2

Disadvantages of Using Pets Versus Purpose-Bred Laboratory Animals for Research Studies

Pets	Purpose-Bred Research Animals
Require a significant amount of pet owner and referring veterinarian communication	Expensive to conduct studies on larger species or for models of spontaneous disease (due to long-term housing requirements and low morbidity rates)
Require owner consent and often IACUC and IRB approval as well	Large amount of regulatory oversight required, including IACUC approval
Significantly more expensive than smaller model species (i.e. rodents)	Diseases are often experimentally induced and therefore do not always mimic natural disease seen in humans
More expensive to house during in-depth or invasive treatments or analyses (i.e. require a 24-hour pet hospital with a fully staffed ICU)	Controlled housing limits the effects environmental factors may play in a disease or treatment outcome
Insufficient owner compliance or loss of patient(s) to follow-up can occur	Specialized equipment often required for smaller model species
Co-morbidities can confound study outcomes	Study participants are often genetically homogenous or immune-modulated and therefore may not reflect the outcomes that would be seen in human populations
Pending the disease being evaluated, a control group may not be possible; standard of care should always be discussed and offered	Negative public perception to inducing a disease state in an otherwise healthy animal or euthanizing an animal specifically for a study

co-morbidities, which humans more often than not also possess, on a disease or treatment outcome are able to be evaluated.

However, animals that are purpose-bred for research offer many advantages for studying diseases over pets with spontaneously occurring disease. Arguably the greatest benefit of using laboratory animals in research is the high level of control that can be exerted over most aspects of a study. Laboratory animals can be kept in very controlled conditions, where food, water, housing, temperature, humidity, and light are closely monitored and managed. Implementing these controls can reduce factors that could potentially confound experimental results or disrupt the study outcome. Laboratory animals are also closely monitored by individuals who are experts in their care, from the husbandry technician to the veterinarian, allowing for earlier identification of clinical disease signs, drug side effects, or other study-related phenotypes that an untrained pet owner may not appreciate or recognize as important. Studies of complete animal cohorts, including both experimental and control groups, can often be conducted at the same time when using laboratory animals, whereas pets used in clinical trials must be enrolled individually as they are identified. Additionally, laboratory animals can be closely monitored for the entirety of a study, whether the study lasts an hour or the full life of the animal, with little chance of loss to follow-up, a major risk when using privately owned pets. And finally, when properly justified, a laboratory animal can be euthanized at the end of the study for full post-mortem evaluation of disease or drug/treatment effects and collection of critical tissues, allowing for the most in-depth understanding of all possible aspects of a study.

Research developments over the past few decades have provided additional advantages for using laboratory animals for studies. Technological advancements, particularly genetic modification of full organisms, allow investigators to create animal models of human or animal disease to examine how specific mutations contribute to the pathogenesis of a disease or effect a potential drug treatment. Engineered endonuclease technology, particularly CRISPR-Cas9, which allows for precise and efficient targeted genome editing, has resulted in an explosion of genetically modified animal models over the last 5 years, from fruit flies to zebrafish to mice to dogs to nonhuman primates (Lee, Sung, and Baek 2018). Targeted genome editing allows a disease to be studied or treatments identified and evaluated in multiple animals in a much more time-efficient manner than can be done by identifying sporadic cases in the pet population. Inducing disease in laboratory animals is also a commonly employed method in animal research, whether through inducing diabetes through streptozotocin administration in mice or performing a partial hepatectomy in dogs to study liver regeneration. These controlled experimental methods using laboratory animals allow the investigator to evaluate the clinical condition as early or as late in the process as desired, whereas in spontaneously occurring conditions in pets, the disease can only be studied after it is diagnosed, usually well into the course of disease.

Using pets with spontaneously occurring diseases in research does provide some advantages over purpose-bred laboratory animals. Because of Russell and Burch's concept of the Three Rs, most initial experiments using laboratory animals are performed on lower order organisms, such as fruit flies or mice, before progressing to higher order mammals and humans. As a result, the vast majority of drugs and therapies that perform well against a disease in laboratory animal models do not successfully translate to higher order animals or humans due to inherent differences in anatomy, physiology, or immunology (Mak, Evaniew, and Ghert 2014). Evaluating disease that is naturally occurring in the end user (the pet) presents the best possible model for evaluating potential treatments for that disease in that species. Co-morbidities, prior pathogen infection, and genetic heterogeneity, which are often discouraged in controlled experiments using laboratory animals but are almost always found in pet populations, can help find ideal therapies that have a greater chance of working across multiple animals that have a disease. Additionally, using laboratory animals for research, even for research that will ultimately end up benefiting animals, is controversial. Public perception of animal research is much more positive when the experiment being performed or treatment being evaluated directly impacts the animal on which it is being conducted.

While there are advantages and disadvantages to each, when used together, purpose-bred laboratory animals and pets with spontaneously occurring disease can provide a comprehensive view of a disease or potential treatment. Laboratory animal studies can be used as a complement to clinical trials in privately owned animals; for example, healthy purpose-bred research dogs may be used to determine normal canine values for a new functional MRI technique or in pharmacokinetic and safety studies for a putative chemotherapeutic drug for treating gliomas before that imaging technique or that drug is evaluated as a potential diagnostic or treatment for pet dogs with that particular brain tumor. Additionally, studies performed in laboratory animals and privately owned pets can work synergistically towards the goal of bringing therapies to clinical trials in humans. Investigators and veterinarians benefit from working together to determine the optimal course of action in producing a new diagnostic, procedure, or therapy for the end user, whether that user is an animal or a human.

REFERENCES

Canadian Council on Animal Care. 1993. *Guide to the Care and Use of Experimental Animals*, 2nd ed. Ottawa (Ontario): Canadian Council on Animal Care.

European Union. 2010. *Directive 2010/63/EU of the European Parliament and of the Council of 22 September 2010 on the Protection of Animals Used for Scientific Purposes Text with EEA Relevance.*

Gluck, John P, Tony DiPasquale, and F Barbara Orlans. 2002. *Applied Ethics in Animal Research: Philosophy, Regulation, and Laboratory Applications*. Ebook. Purdue University Press E-Books.

Griffin, Gilly, and Paul Locke. 2016. "Comparison of the Canadian and US Laws, Regulations, Policies, and Systems of Oversight for Animals in Research." *ILAR Journal* 57(3): 271–84.

Guillén, Javier, Montip Gettayacamin, and James R Swearengen. 2016. "Challenges and Opportunities in Implementation: The AAALAC International Perspective." *ILAR Journal* 57(3): 368–77.

Health Canada. 1997. *Guidance for Industry: General Considerations for Clinical Trials, ICH Topic E8*. Ottawa (Ontario): Health Canada – Publications.

Institute of Medicine. 1991. *Science, Medicine, and Animals*. Washington (DC): National Academies Press.

Lee, Jong Geol, Young Hoon Sung, and In-Jeoung Baek. 2018. "Generation of Genetically-Engineered Animals Using Engineered Endonucleases." *Archives of Pharmacology Research* 41: 885–97.

Mak, Isabella W. Y., Nathan Evaniew, and Michelle Ghert. 2014. "Lost in Translation: Animal Models and Clinical Trials in Cancer Treatment." *American Journal of Translational Research* 6(2): 114–8.

Mohr, Bert J, Francis A Fakoya, Jann Hau, Ouajdi Souilem, and Lida Anestidou. 2016. "The Governance of Animal Care and Use for Scientific Purposes in Africa and the Middle East." *ILAR Journal* 57(3): 333–46.

National Institutes of Health Office of Laboratory Animal Welfare. 2010. *Guide for the Care and Use of Laboratory Animals*, 8th ed. Washington (DC): National Academies Press.

National Institutes of Health Office of Laboratory Animal Welfare. 2015. *Public Health Service Policy on Humane Care and Use of Laboratory Animals Office.*

Ogden, Bryan E, Wanyong Pang William, Takashi Agui, and Byeong Han Lee. 2016. "Laboratory Animal Laws, Regulations, Guidelines and Standards in China Mainland, Japan, and Korea." *ILAR Journal* 57(3): 301–11.

Olsson, I, S Anna, Sandra Pinto da Silva, David Townend, and Peter Sandøe. 2016. "Protecting Animals and Enabling Research in the European Union: An Overview of Development and Implementation of Directive 2010/63/EU." *ILAR Journal* 57(3): 347–57.

Retnam, Leslie, Pradon Chatikavanij, Pattamarat Kunjara, Yasmina A Paramastri, Yong Meng Goh, Fuzina Nor Hussein, Abdul Rahim Mutalib, and Suresh Poosala. 2016. "Laws, Regulations, Guidelines and Standards for Animal Care and Use for Scientific Purposes in the Countries of Singapore, Thailand, Indonesia, Malaysia, and India." *ILAR Journal* 57(3): 312–23.

Rivera, E, R Hernandez, A S Carissimi, and C Pekow. 2016. "Laboratory Animal Legislation in Latin America." *ILAR Journal* 57(3): 293–300.

Russell, W M S, and R L Burch. 1959. *The Principles of Humane Experimental Technique.* London: Methuen.

Timoshanko, Aaron C, Helen Marston, and Brett A Lidbury. 2016. "Australian Regulation of Animal Use in Science and Education: A Critical Appraisal." *ILAR Journal* 57(3): 324–32.

United States Department of Agriculture. 2017. *Animal Welfare Act and Animal Welfare Regulations.*

United States Food & Drug Administration. 2017. "The FDA's Drug Review Process: Ensuring Drugs Are Safe and Effective." Last modified November 24, 2017. www.fda.gov/drugs/drug-information-consumers/fdas-drug-review-process-ensuring-drugs-are-safe-and-effective.

United States Food & Drug Administration. 2018. "The Drug Development Process." Last modified January 4, 2018. www.fda.gov/patients/drug-development-process/step-1-discovery-and-development.

United States Food & Drug Administration. 2019a. "Animal Rule Information." Last modified May 21, 2019. www.fda.gov/emergency-preparedness-and-response/mcm-regulatory-science/animal-rule-information.

United States Food & Drug Administration. 2019b. "Why Are Animals Used for Testing Medical Products?" Last modified June 18, 2019. www.fda.gov/about-fda/fda-basics/why-are-animals-used-testing-medical-products.

Vasbinder, Mary Ann, and Paul Locke. 2016. "Introduction: Global Laws, Regulations, and Standards for Animals in Research." *ILAR Journal* 57(3): 261–5.

Zhang, Boyang, Anastasia Korolj, Benjamin Fook Lun Lai, and Milica Radisic. 2018. "Advances in Organ-On-a-Chip Engineering." *Nature Reviews Materials* 3(8): 257–78.

8 DNA Methods in Veterinary Medicine

Alan F. Scott

CONTENTS

INTRODUCTION

All animals share a common evolutionary ancestor and have a similar repertoire of genes in their genomes, often performing the same or similar functions. This fact enables animal models to be so successful in biology, in general, and medicine, in particular. In genetics, animal models are especially invaluable as they often allow information learned from one species to be directly transferred to another. The "genetics revolution" of recent decades is having a growing impact on human health and will increasingly impact the health of captive animals, particularly our pets. In this chapter I will briefly summarize the main DNA methods that are in use today and their application to other species.

Both mitochondrial (mtDNA) and genomic DNA (gDNA) are present in most cells; the most prominent exception being mammalian red blood cells which lack nuclei, and therefore, lack DNA. Although scientists had studied DNA for many years, it was not until the 1970s, with the advent of DNA cloning (inserting foreign DNA into viruses or bacteria where they can be cultured as pure molecules and purified for study) that the field quickly changed. Plasmid and bacteriophage cloning, in particular, provided a method for easily creating large amounts of otherwise rare DNA sequences. This vast increase in the molarity made DNA hybridization and sequencing techniques feasible. Subsequently, in the early 1980s, Kary Mullis invented the polymerase chain reaction (PCR) which allowed for segments of DNA to be amplified without cloning. Today, PCR and other amplification methods (such as whole genome amplification or WGA) are the cornerstones of the key technologies of genotyping and sequencing which have grown into multi-billion dollar industries that increasingly impact all aspects of biology and medicine. The discovery of short tandem repeats by Alec Jeffreys (Jeffreys et al., 1985) whose length varied between individuals, coupled with the advent of PCR led to the first use of DNA variants to study inheritance in pedigrees and for use in the identification of individuals for forensic and other applications. Although the early DNA sequencing methods were slow and expensive, when investigators applied sequencing mainly to identify the genes causing human disease, they noticed that there was a surprising amount of variability in genomes, much of it outside of the coding regions. As the human genome project progressed and technology improved to the point that more genomes could be efficiently sequenced, data repositories of variants were built and made available. These variants could then be used for linkage studies in pedigrees, for identifying mutations causing disease and, potentially, for studies to find variants that "mark" regions of the genome with loci that are involved in the genetics of complex traits such as risk for late-onset diabetes, cleft lip, heart disease and hundreds more. The key to unlocking all of this potential was first to find and catalog these thousands of variable sites scattered across the genome, mostly single-nucleotide polymorphisms (SNPs), especially those with fairly high allele frequencies, and second to develop efficient methods to score these in thousands of samples. Two companies, Illumina and Affymetrix, were instrumental in commercializing SNP genotyping in the 2000s and array-based genotyping is used by companies such as 23andMe and Ancestry.com for humans, while veterinary testing companies such as Embark and Wisdom use arrays designed for dogs.

Genotyping is performed by hybridizing DNA from an individual to a chip which has short DNA molecules (oligos) bound to it. These oligomers are synthetic fragments of DNA which match sequences adjacent to known variable positions in that species. In order to increase the number of targets that can anneal (the process by which single DNA strands find complementary DNA sequences and pair by hydrogen bonding) to the oligos on an array, the genomic DNA originally added to the array is first amplified using WGA to increase the molarity by thousands of fold. This increase in molarity drives the kinetics of binding so that the gDNA templates and allele-specific primers on the arrays will hybridize relatively quickly. Once the WGA DNA is bound to the oligomers on the array, chemically modified nucleotides are added by another polymerase reaction. Each of the two alleles at a position on the array has a different fluorescent tag. Those tags are then used to distinguish the alleles. Software determines if a given array position is homozygous or heterozygous. A final report lists the genotype at each of the positions interrogated. For humans, arrays with up to 5M SNPs are available and versions with different or specialized content continue to be developed. Similarly, agricultural and veterinary arrays are also produced based on sequence data for different species. Because of the cost of design and manufacturing commercial SNP arrays are seldom worthwhile for non-commercial species, although the decreasing cost of whole genome sequencing can produce similar data for a similar price. Also, there is often enough similarity between species that at least some arrays can be used with related animals (e.g., the human methylation array, a variety of the SNP array that measures the relative amount of methylated cytosines at particular genomic locations, provides data from great apes; pers. comm.). The widespread availability of relatively inexpensive arrays has led to the growth of a large commercial market that continues to grow and is having consequences on human health, forensics, ancestry studies, population genetics, etc. It should be noted that the sites used for these arrays were obtained by sequencing the genomes of representative individuals. In humans the first genotyping arrays had a European bias because the initial human sequencing data was derived from that ethnicity. There are many current efforts underway to increase the diversity of the ethnic groups represented in the human databases. A lack of ethnic diversity can have unintended consequences. In the case of ancestry testing, SNPs are compared to "reference" populations of a given ethnicity. Discrepancies between reports from different genotyping companies are largely based on which individuals were picked, for example, as the "Irish" reference. While ancestry, or in the case of dog breeds "purity", is of interest, the real value of genotyping is that it can, and has, been used to compare individuals with specific phenotypes or disorders to healthy controls as a way to identify genes segregating in populations that may underlie those conditions. Studies using these techniques are called genome-wide association studies (GWAS).

Genome-wide association studies have been used in human genetics for several years to identify blocks of DNA with shared alleles, referred to as haplotypes, that are statistically associated with the risk for developing particular diseases. These haplotype blocks are shorter in larger and more outbred populations but are often much larger in more inbred populations because a relatively small founder population will have less heterogeneity and, therefore, a reduced opportunity for recombination events to break haplotypes at each generation. In humans, many of the first disease hunting GWAS studies were undertaken in populations that were genetically closed (e.g., Amish) or were relatively isolated (e.g., Iceland, Finland, etc.). Because such groups had gone through genetic bottlenecks it was reasoned that individuals with similar complex phenotypes might be more genetically similar to each other than individuals with those phenotypes in outbred populations. Haplotypes are also larger in newer populations where there has not been sufficient time for recombination. In humans, Europeans have larger haplotype blocks than Africans. Also, haplotypes are more alike in closely related family members. Within dog breeds, shared haplotypes are about as similar as those among human cousins (E. Karlsson, pers. comm.). These differences in haplotypes are used by commercial companies that genotype pets to identify their breed. Similarly, when we breed plants and animals for particular traits we lose heterogeneity. This can have both positive and negative consequences that can now be understood with DNA-based testing.

Using GWAS arrays (Figure 8.1) and DNA from cohorts with different disease phenotypes, it has been possible to find statistically significant associations for thousands of human phenotypes (see GWAS catalog, www.ebi.ac.uk/gwas/, with

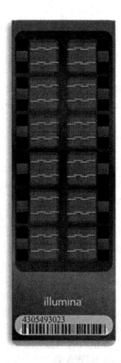

FIGURE 8.1   The Illumina Canine Genotyping array (CanFam2.0) can analyze 12 samples at a time, interrogating about 170,000 SNPs across the dog genome. The SNPs on the chip were designed to maximize information from multiple breeds and can be used in association studies for susceptibility to inherited disorders as well as distinguishing breed admixture. This array is used by commercial test providers such as Mars Wisdom Health™ to provide reports of breed identification and admixture and identifies particular variants known to cause or be associated with over 150 inherited disorders. The array was used by Dreger et al. (2019) to study coat color and other morphometric traits in over 11,000 dogs from 212 breeds. Although many breeds have been "closed" for over 100 years they found that rare variants persisted in most of them.

approximately 140,000 associations as of 2019). The usefulness of associated SNPs for particular common traits continues to grow and can be used to produce polygenic risk scores (PRS) which are increasingly being used in personalized medicine. A recent example is a study of obesity by Khera et al. (Khera et al., 2019) that looked at genotypes from over 300,000 individuals mostly from the UK whose medical records are known through the National Health Service and genotypes from the UK Biobank study. By algorithmically analyzing 2.1M SNPs across the genome they were able to find significant correlations with BMI. It is likely that polygenic risk scores will become an increasingly important part of human health. This can be seen in the commercial market that has developed for genetic testing and an increasingly large number of people have been genotyped using commercial arrays (23andMe, Ancestry.com, National Geographic, etc.). Some of these companies allow users to participate in crowd-sourced research by answering questions online related to their health, etc. To date, this data has been used to identify particular genes associated with traits and will certainly be used for PRS assessments in the future. Pharmaceutical companies can also use the data from large GWAS studies and a method called Mendelian randomization to find traits that might benefit from drug interventions as opposed to those that are likely benign (e.g., HDL levels). For non-human, non-laboratory species much less genotyping has been published, but identification of agriculturally important traits using these informatic techniques is gaining importance.

The success of GWAS studies requires that there is genetic and phenotypic variation in a species and that the two can be correlated. However, if the phenotype is "new" or too rare to collect a sufficient number of cases, then GWAS studies may not be fruitful. In species with long haplotypes, such as dogs (because of their fairly recent domestication), there may not be enough time for recombination to "break" the haplotypes to narrow the region of the suspected gene. Also, a particular phenotype may be caused by any of several different genes. In these instances, DNA sequencing is a better tool.

The limitations of genotyping and the lower costs of sequencing are now resulting in an increasing number of ambitious projects, sponsored by both governments and the commercial sector, to sequence very large numbers of humans. As of 2019, well over a million human genomes are likely to have been sequenced and the rate of sequencing is increasing as costs decrease. The increasing interest by diagnostic and pharmaceutical companies, as well as health care providers, in mining sequence data is an additional driver of the market. A consequence of these studies is that we have an increasingly good understanding of what the 20,000 or so genes do in humans and can infer what they likely do in other species. The OMIM database (OMIM.org) culls the literature for human diseases, while the mouse genome database (MGD.org) records data for that species. OMIA (Online Mendelian Inheritance in Animals) largely collects reports from the veterinary literature. As public and private efforts to link human sequence to electronic medical records increases it is hoped that medical care supported by genetics will better predict disease risk for which interventions can be specifically targeted. Ideally, a similar approach could be realized in veterinary medicine.

As of 2019, most DNA testing is carried out by the sequencing by synthesis (SBS) method that was developed in the 1970s and is still the basis of most commercial sequencers. SBS takes individual DNA molecules and copies them, adding labeled nucleotides into the "synthesized" strand. For most commercial sequencers this is done using fluorescent nucleotides that are imaged after each cycle of synthesis. As of 2020, the leading commercial manufacturer of high-throughput fluorescent sequencers is Illumina, Inc. In their latest sequencer, DNA is captured into nanowells by hybridization of short pieces of DNA of known sequences called adaptors which have been ligated to the DNA to be sequenced to short complementary oligomers on the flow cell. Once captured, the library DNAs are denatured into single-stranded molecules, amplified by PCR to make clusters of ~1,000–10,000 copies, denatured again and then sequenced in a series of cycles which are imaged sequentially over ~1–2 days. As many as 25 individual whole genomes can run at a time on a flow cell, with an average read depth at any position of 30-fold. This depth provides about 15 reads from each of the maternal and paternal chromosomes and, typically, will find about 99.9+ percent of all variants in human samples. Figure 8.2 illustrates an example of reads from the same region of a genome aligned and shown using the Integrated Genome Viewer (IGV; Thorvaldsdottir et al., 2013). Bases that differ from reference are shown as shaded vertical bars. A consensus view is shown at the top which also graphs the read depth. Initially, most sequencing of humans was done using a method which captured and enriched for the coding regions of the genome, which make about 1–2% of the genome. This approach is called whole exome sequencing (WES). The motivation for exome or other targeted capture methods was the cost of WGS, the difficulty of interpreting non-coding sequence and the fact that most Mendelian disorders are caused by mutations in coding sequence. As throughput and costs have come down, however, whole genome sequencing (WGS) is becoming the dominant method of clinical sequencing, due to its speed and ease of library preparation. Targeted and exome sequencing is likely to continue in use, especially for identifying somatic mutations in tumors where greater read depth is needed because only a fraction of cells in the tumor may have the mutation of interest.

There is an increasing interest in the genomics and genetics communities to look at long-range effects on the genome that involve structural variants (SVs) such as insertions of transposable elements, duplications, inversions or deletions of large blocks of DNA at a scale finer than can be carried out using traditional microscopy. Being able to characterize large blocks of DNA is also paramount for *de novo* genome assembly. One method to accomplish this is to use linked-read sequencing—a technique where a few large DNA molecules are captured in oil droplets, randomly nicked and copied using DNA polymerase and specialized oligomers so that each newly synthesized DNA fragment from a long DNA template in the droplet also includes a unique molecular identifier (UMI) tag. These tagged fragments are then sequenced using the methods described above (SBS). After sequencing, the UMI tag can be used to group all related reads together and the short individual reads can be assembled into longer scaffolds. This method is used for *de novo* assembly of genomes from different species (e.g., Hawaiian monk seal; Mohr et al., 2017) and scimitar oryx (Humble et al., 2019) and can also be used to identify structural variants and haplotype blocks from the parents. Haplotypes are particularly useful for certain gene regions such as the major histocompatibility complex (MHC) loci that are routinely tested to determine tissue matches for transplant surgery. Figure 8.3 shows an example of a region sequenced using linked reads and for which variants have been sorted into two haplotype blocks.

Alternatives to SBS are becoming available. In one technology now marketed by MGI Genomics as a less expensive alternative, patient DNA is sequentially hybridized to short labeled DNAs with all possible combinations of bases found in the genome. This method has been refined for human sequencing and may be on par with SBS sequencing for most applications, although it does have limitations, especially for animals without a reference sequence.

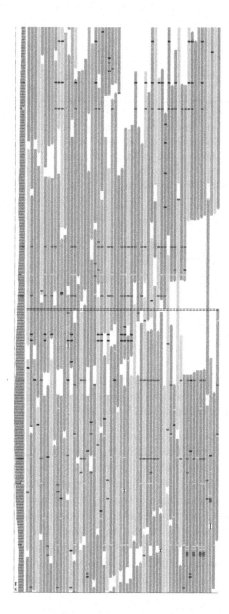

FIGURE 8.2 Typical sequence data is shown aligned in the lower panel. Each horizontal line is a read aligned to a reference and the vertical lines correspond to positions that are heterozygous.

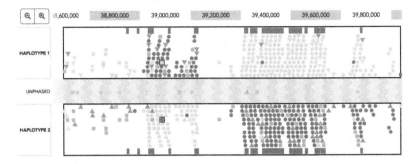

FIGURE 8.3 In this example, linked read sequencing (Mohr et al., 2017) was used to assign variants to parental haplotypes. The total region shown here is about 1.2 Mb. Along with assigning SNPs to haplotypes, this technique can also identify structural variants such as insertions or deletions only occurring on one chromosome. The symbols indicate haplotype-specific differences (SNPs and indels).

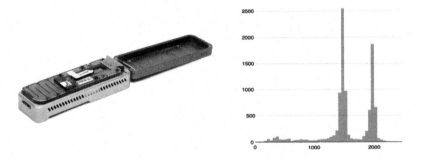

FIGURE 8.4 (a) An Oxford Nanopore MinION flow cell (see www.nanoporetech.com for details). (b) Histogram of total reads vs. fragment length for two different PCR products run together on a Oxford Nanopore ver 9.4 flow cell.

Perhaps the most radical new approach is the use of nanopores to sequence DNA directly (Figure 8.4). This fast, relatively inexpensive method looks at large, intact molecules of DNA in their native (unamplified) state and can detect large insertions, translocations as well as modified (e.g., methylated) DNA bases. The current disadvantages are that it has a lower single molecule accuracy than SBS and can be confounded by short insertions or deletions (indels) or by homopolymeric regions (e.g., six or more bases of a single type). The only current (as of January 2020) manufacturer of this technology is Oxford Nanopore, which offers multiple device formats from small flow cells that can be run in the field or office using a laptop or cell phone to larger units that can sequence hundreds of gigabases (Gb) at a time.

When nanopore sequencing is used with high molecular weight DNA it can produce reads well over 100 kb. Because of the long reads, this method is an excellent complement to the short-read, but more accurate, SBS sequencing and is being used more often in assembling large genomes (Miga et al., 2019;

Lind et al., 2019) and detecting structural variants, as in tomato cultivars (Sedlazeck et al., 2018).

Another long-read method was pioneered by PacBio, Inc. (www.pacb.com; Eid, 2009) in which DNA molecules (~10–50 kb) are ligated into circles which are captured, one each, into nanowells, and sequenced by incorporating fluorescent bases. The method can now do multiple rounds of reads around the circle to produce a consensus sequence of very high quality (Wenger et al., 2019). The costs and throughput are still higher than traditional SBS short-read sequencing but are likely to improve with more widespread adoption or if the library prep method can be optimized to use less input DNA; a limitation in some studies.

An orthogonal method to identify larger scale variation that complements sequencing is optical mapping. In this approach, long DNA molecules are isolated, tagged by incorporating fluorescent nucleotides at specific DNA sequences and then electrophoresed as single DNA molecules through nanochannels where the patterns of marked sites are imaged. The single molecule images are then reassembled into maps which can be aligned to a reference sequence for the species. This method, and variants of it, are being used to aid *de novo* gene assembly and to look at changes in genomes that can occur in cancer and certain inherited diseases. A commercial supplier of optical mapping technology is Bionano Genomics (www.bionanogenomics.com) and optical maps have been used as an adjunct to the assembly of many genomes (e.g., Miga et al., 2019; Kronenberg et al., 2018) or characterizing regions with repetitive sequences that are hard to assemble with most DNA sequencing methods (e.g., Demaerel et al., 2019) (Figure 8.5). As with other long DNA methods, optical mapping also requires

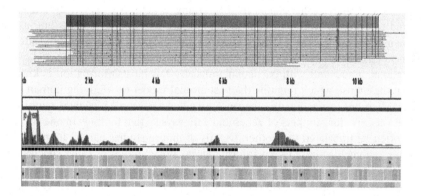

FIGURE 8.5 A comparison of optical maps (top panel) with sequence reads. Each horizontal line represents the image of an individual molecule image labeled at a specific nucleotide sequence (vertical bars). The software takes the molecular images and makes a best fit alignment which can then be "matched" against an actual sequence. In this case, the optical maps are likely from the telomeric end of a chromosome. In the corresponding DNA sequence, there are "peaks" of highly similar sequence motifs that are expected at telomeres.

long DNA (ideally greater than 300 kb) which is best obtained from nucleated cells ($\sim$1–2 $\times$ 10^6).

Lastly, another approach to genome assembly is the use of Hi-C, so named because it uses high-throughput sequencing on chromatin. Hi-C is a form of chromatin confirmation techniques. It uses the way that DNA is wound around chromatin to gain information about that DNA. In this method, chromatin is isolated with the bound DNA. Formaldehyde is added, which causes the different pieces of DNA that are close to each other to link together. More links will occur with nearby sequences than distant ones. After the formaldehyde step, the DNA is digested with one or more restriction enzymes, which leaves the linked DNA pieces stuck together. Those linked fragments are then ligated together to form chimeric molecules whose ends originate at different positions along the chromosome (Dudchenko et al., 2018). After standard paired-end Illumina sequencing the number of near to distant joins can be determined by comparing the reads to scaffolds generated by other methods described above. Hi-C has been used to assemble genomes for dozens of animals (e.g., Humble et al., 2019; see also, DNAzoo.org).

APPLICATIONS IN VETERINARY MEDICINE

GENETIC TRAIT TESTING

The largest source of new human Mendelian disorders (i.e., disorders that are inherited within pedigrees) are from consanguineous marriages, usually of cousins. This has been known for a long time and is likely the reason for various cultural prohibitions of incest. Interestingly, Darwin was aware of the risks of this when he married his cousin in 1839. Many, if not most, captive animals are inbred in order to "fix" particular traits that are of value to humans but, as in humans, this can lead to increased risks for particular disorders. With the advent of inexpensive testing there is an increasing understanding of the genes, and often mutations, associated with particular traits. By far, most information is known about the mouse which remains the best animal model for studying human disease. Mice are useful for this, because as noted above, all placental mammals share very similar numbers of genes and pathways so that findings in one species can often be translated to another. Details of mouse studies can be found at the mouse genome database (www.informatics.jax.org). Studies of other species are available at OMIA (omia.org). OMIM, the human genetic disorder database, has some 640 entries with model organism data, about 50 of which include examples from dogs.

Dog genomes seem especially amenable to tolerating change and producing a wide range of phenotypes, the demand for which has encouraged breeders to exaggerate traits perhaps beyond what is in the best interest of those animals (e.g., https://dogbehaviorscience.wordpress.com/2012/09/29/100-years-of-breed-impr ovement/).

As costs drop for genotyping, and especially WGS, it would be extremely valuable if breeders would analyze the genomes of individual animals that have long, healthy lives, behave as expected for the breed but still retain desirable characteristics for the breed. A breed-specific genome project is certainly within the scope of current technology and could be performed in 2020 at a reasonable cost. The availability of a healthy reference for each breed would be a way to more easily identify deleterious mutations that appear on that genetic background. Because breeds typically are inbred to the same extent as human cousins, creating a reference genome should be fairly easy. Dogs are a particularly interesting case because humans may very well have selected characteristics during domestication so that, to some extent, they can understand our motivations better than we can interpret theirs. A reference genome of "exceptional" individuals from different species would complement longitudinal studies such as the UK Biobank which has genotyped and plans to sequence 500,000 older adults whose medical records are tracked and who can be used to identify genetic risks as we age. A similar study in the United States, called AllofUs (allofus.nih.gov) is beginning in 2020, but will likely take years to provide the insights that animal genomes might be able to do in just a few years.

SELECTED OBSERVATIONS ABOUT DOG GENES FROM DNA-BASED STUDIES

The first dog genome was reported by Kirkness et al. (Kirkness et al., 2003) of a Poodle named Shadow. By today's standards the genome was low depth (~1.5X) but it identified approximately the same number of genes as in humans and mice. Two years later, a more complete genome of a Boxer was published (Lindblad-Toh et al., 2005). That study found that the genome was about 2.4 Gb and showed that haplotype blocks were approximately 50X longer than in humans which would make genetic mapping easier for simple Mendelian traits. In 2016 Hayward et al. (Hayward et al., 2016) used the canine array to do a genome-wide association study of 4,200 dogs. They identified chromosomal regions associated with a number of disorders such as hip dysplasia, idiopathic epilepsy and mast cell tumors. They also looked at traits such as body size, fur length and shedding. Other examples include Baker et al. (2017) who used the canine SNP array in an association study to evaluate risk for anterior cruciate ligament rupture and found about 170 loci that underlie risk in the Labrador Retriever. Batcher et al. (2019) found a strong association between a retrogene for FGFR4 and disc herniation with a relative risk varying from 5.5 to 15.1 in different breeds. Using whole genome sequencing, Bauer et al. (in press; Bauer et al., 2019) identified *de novo* mutations in the collagen gene, COL5A1 (OMIM 120215), that cause a canine equivalent of Ehlers-Danlos syndromes, type 1 which is characterized by hyperextensible skin, hypermobility of the limbs and tissue fragility. In a separate paper Bauer et al.

(2018) showed that a splicing defect in the gene for muskelin, MKLN1, causes lethal acrodermatitis in dogs. While MKLN1 mutations have not yet been identified in humans this study makes human geneticists aware that this is a candidate gene for similar phenotypes in humans. In 2018 Deane-Coe et al. (2018) used the canine array and testing of some 6,000 dogs to identify a ~100 kb duplication near the ALX4 gene that is associated with blue eyes in Siberian Huskies. ALX4 is expressed in the retinal pigment epithelium and the authors propose that the duplication affects expression of the gene. Donner et al (2018), in one of the largest genetic epidemiology studies of its kind thus far, studied the frequency of 152 disease variants in over 100,000 dogs from mixed breeds and purebreds. They found, as expected, that mixed breeds were more likely to carry *recessive* mutations that are deleterious in purebred animals. Hitti et al. (2019) found that a mutation in the NECAP1 gene caused a progressive retinal atrophy in the Giant Schnauzer, mutations of which have been reported to cause early infantile epileptic encephalopathy in humans. Letko et al. (2019) reported a missense variant in SCN8a causing spinocerebellar ataxia in Alpine Dachsbrackes, a phenotype similarly seen in some humans with mutations in this gene. Mansour el al. (2018) showed that a frameshift mutation in the DVL2 gene was strongly associated with a Robinow-like syndrome in Bulldogs and related breeds with screw tails. In humans Robinow syndrome, which is characterized by dysmorphic facial features, frontal bossing, hypertelorism, a broad nose and short limbs has been reported to be caused by mutations in either DVL1 or DVL3. Parker et al. (2017) reported that the American Hairless Terrier has a deleted SGK3 (Serum/Glucocorticoid-regulated kinase 3) gene. Mutations in a mouse model have defective hair growth with short, thin hair. Raffan et al. (2016) observed that a deletion in the POMC gene was associated with Labrador Retrievers that were prone to obesity. The Arg236Gly polymorphism in POMC in humans has been associated with increased susceptibility to obesity (Challis et al., 2002) and several human variants have been identified in children with early-onset obesity along with adrenal insufficiency and red hair. vonHoldt et al. (2017) observed structural variants in a region of canine chromosome 6 associated with hypersociability and Tandon et al. (2019) found that the presence of a canine transposable element in the canine WBSCR17 gene is a strong predictor of dog social behavior with respect to humans. In humans, WBSCR17, a GalNAC transferase, lies in what is referred to as the Williams-Beuren syndrome (WBS) chromosome region with approximately 28 genes. WBS is a contiguous gene deletion syndrome that is caused by hemizygous deletion of DNA from this region of chromosome 7q11.23. The severity and features of the human disorder can vary widely and can include intellectual disability and aortic stenosis and "elfin." A characteristic of patients with deletions in the WBSCR is that they have a notably friendly personality and has led to the speculation that changes in WBSCR genes may be involved in the domestication of both dogs and foxes (Wilkins et al., 2014).

CANCER TESTING

Two of the major applications of DNA methods to human cancers are analysis of DNA from tumors to identify particular mutations associated with specific treatment plans or to improve prognosis. For example, if deep sequencing of a melanoma or melanoma-derived tumor identifies a mutation at codon 600 from valine to glutamic acid in BRAF1, then treatments such as Vemurafenib can be very successful. Second, monitoring DNA methylation profiles in tumors, especially brain tumors, is proving to be an especially helpful tool for tumor staging. This method uses a variant of the GWAS arrays, except that the genomic positions interrogated are known to have variable methylation. How these tools and others can be transferred to non-human animals will require large studies, the results of which are likely to be informative to human health as well.

PATHOGEN TESTING

Traditional testing for pathogens can be time-consuming and require specialized laboratories. Human medicine is beginning to move towards DNA-based testing that can be completed more quickly and with higher precision. The current limitations of DNA sequencing are related to speed, cost and sensitivity. Nanopore sequencing may partially solve these issues by providing a relatively low cost and rapid technology, that despite having a much higher error rate than traditional sequencing can overcome that limitation by creating consensus sequences from many individually erroneous reads. An interesting application of nanopore sequencing is that it can be used in the field to monitor infectious disease (e.g., cholera; Acharya et al., 2019) and Ebola (Quick et al., 2016), where sequences from the pathogen of interest are amplified by PCR and samples loaded and run on a nanopore flow cell. For cholera and other prokaryotes the regions applied are usually the 16s rRNA genes whose sequences vary between species and can serve as a reliable taxonomic biomarker (Cheng et al., 2018). The relative speed (as little as a few hours), cost and portability of nanopore sequencing is likely to see it become used in ERs and clinics in the near term. In veterinary medicine nanopore sequencing has been demonstrated as a tool to diagnose distemper virus (Peserico et al., 2019) and to monitor antibiotic resistance in a veterinary hospital (Kamathewatta, et al., 2019). As the technology continues to improve in both read accuracy and ease of use it is likely that nanopore sequencing will find many applications in veterinary medicine, environmental monitoring and biohazard identification, among others.

PHARMACOLOGICAL TESTING

In humans, allelic differences in various drug metabolism genes can play a major role in selecting the correct medication and its dose. Increasingly, DNA-based testing of specific drug-metabolism genes will be accomplished clinically either through rapid DNA tests under development or by having genetic profiles of individuals in online health records. This latter approach, not unlike having a blood type on file, is often referred to as sequence-once and read-many times. The strategy is already being implemented in some countries and US healthcare systems. Veterinarians may be able to use similar techniques to provide appropriate dosing of drugs for the animals in their clinics, once similar profiles are created for different species.

In summary, the delineation of an increasingly large number of genetic diseases in dogs and genetic associations with morphological, behavioral and other traits will increase the value of genetic testing (e.g., Mealey et al., 2019) and, as DNA-based therapies are developed they are likely to be available for our pets before they find widespread use in human medicine (e.g., Nghiem and Kornegay, 2019). As observed by Ostrander et al. (2017) gene editing using CRISPR-Cas9 or other technologies is expected to become more widespread in coming years. The authors cite an example of a 2015 study where the MSTN (myostatin) gene of Beagles was edited to produce a phenotype similar to that seen in Whippets where it causes increased muscle mass.

Table 8.1 summarizes the technologies currently available and which applications they are best suited for.

LIMITATIONS

Genetics is an unusual discipline because it touches on so many aspects of life both for ourselves and the animals whose lives we interact with. Unfortunately, it can be misused, over-interpreted and, consequently, its promise can be negated by unscrupulous individuals and companies that make claims based on complete fabrications or a poor understanding of the science. Unlike with human testing which is scrutinized by governments, health managers and legal and ethical communities, there are fewer safeguards for veterinary testing. Hopefully, responsible test providers will emerge that can be trusted to provide accurate and well-reasoned information so that pets and pet owners will benefit from genetic testing (see Shaffer et al., 2019).

CONCLUSION

In the next few years, DNA-based testing is likely to become a part of routine veterinary care. In order to achieve this, however, we will need to improve our understanding of animal genomes and the significance of genetic variation in particular species and breeds. In humans with suspected genetic disorders, we can currently make a diagnosis about one-third of the time. We can expect this rate to be even lower in animals at this moment. Currently, we don't know if this is a limitation of technology or interpretation of the data. Over time both will improve and as they do, we can expect that our efforts to improve the lives of ourselves and our pets and livestock will improve as well.

TABLE 8.1

Choosing the Right Technology

1. Breed/individual identification and common variants affecting phenotype: Genotyping arrays
   a. As arrays have a fixed content determined by the manufacturer, newly described rare variants are unlikely to be assayable.
2. Identifying a rare variant or new mutation in an animal: Exome or whole genome sequencing
   a. Exomes are less expensive to screen than whole genomes but the cost of creating "bait" panels is high and these products will not be available for most non-human species.
   b. Whole genome sequencing (both exons and non-coding DNA) can be performed on any species; interpreting variants is difficult for genomes of non-model/atypical veterinary species.
3. Panel sequencing: Targeting specific genes
   a. Panels are used primarily to focus on specific genes implicated in cancers or for phenotypes with one or a few likely causative genes (e.g., cystic fibrosis in humans).
   b. The target genes are usually amplified by PCR and sequenced. For inherited disease genes where two alleles are expected, the inexpensive Sanger sequencing is generally performed. For tumors where the mutation may be "diluted" with normal cells, deep sequencing (often several hundred-fold read depth) is used. In humans, identification of the causative mutation in tumors can be used to target therapy. A variation of this method can be used to identify mutations in circulating cancer cells in blood which can be used to follow the success of treatment, track remission or suggest when to change treatment strategies.
4. Methylation arrays:
   a. Human methylation arrays are now beginning to be used for epigenetic studies with special interest on cancers that often are characterized by abnormally methylated DNAs. Methylation arrays are not available for non-human species, although the human array can be used to provide less complete data for closely related primates.
   b. Lower throughput and custom assays can be developed for veterinary species but generally the data to decide which genes undergo epigenetic modifications is based on specialized whole genome sequencing that can assay the percent methylation at specific bases. Nanopore sequencing would be an alternative to a specialized array for many species.
5. Pathogen identification:
   a. Identifying bacterial, viral and parasitic diseases can be achieved using whole genome sequencing. Although more expensive than traditional methods, new sequencing methods, such as nanopore sequencing, may allow rapid sample testing including tests in the field.

ACKNOWLEDGEMENTS

I thank Roxann Ashworth for her suggestions and corrections.

REFERENCES

Acharya, K, S Khanal, K Pantha, N Amatya, RJ Davenport, and D Werner. "A Comparative Assessment of Conventional and Molecular Methods, Including Minion Nanopore Sequencing, for Surveying Water Quality." *Scientific Reports* 9(1) (2019): 15726.

Baker, LA, B Kirkpatrick, GJM Rosa, D Gianola, B Valente, JP Sumner, W Baltzer, Z Hao, EE Binversie, N Volstad, A Piazza, SJ Sample, and P Muir. "Genome-Wide Association Analysis in Dogs Implicates 99 Loci as Risk Variants for Anterior Cruciate Ligament Rupture." *PLoS One* 12(4) (2017).

Batcher, K, P Dickinson, M Giuffrida, B Sturges, K Vernau, M Knipe, SH Rasouliha, C Drögemüller, T Leeb, K Maciejczyk, CA Jenkins, C Mellersh, and D Bannasch. "Phenotypic Effects of Fgf4 Retrogenes on Intervertebral Disc Disease in Dogs." *Genes (Basel)* 10(6) (2019).

Bauer, A, JF Bateman, SR Lamandé, E Hanssen, SGM Kirejczyk, M Yee, A Ramiche, V Jagannathan, M Welle, T Leeb, and FL Bateman. "Identification of Two Independent Col5a1 Variants in Dogs With Ehlers-Danlos Syndrome." *Genes (Basel)* 10(10) (2019).

Bauer, A, V Jagannathan, S Högler, B Richter, NA McEwan, A Thomas, E Cadieu, C André, MK Hytönen, H Lohi, MM Welle, P Roosje, C Mellersh, ML Casal, and T Leeb. "Mkln1 Splicing Defect in Dogs With Lethal Acrodermatitis." *PLoS Genetics* 14(3) (2018): e1007264.

Challis, BG, LE Pritchard, JW Creemers, J Delplanque, JM Keogh, J Luan, NJ Wareham, GS Yeo, S Bhattacharyya, P Froguel, A White, IS Farooqi, and S O'Rahilly. "A Missense Mutation Disrupting a Dibasic Prohormone Processing Site in Pro-Opiomelanocortin (Pomc) Increases Susceptibility to Early-Onset Obesity Through a Novel Molecular Mechanism." *Human Molecular Genetics* 11(17) (2002): 1997–2004.

Cheng, J, H Hu, Y Kang, W Chen, W Fang, K Wang, Q Zhang, A Fu, S Zhou, C Cheng, Q Cao, F Wang, S Lee, and Z Zhou. "Identification of Pathogens in Culture-Negative Infective Endocarditis Cases by Metagenomic Analysis." *Annals of Clinical Microbiology & Antimicrobials* 17(1) (2018): 43.

Deane-Coe, PE, ET Chu, A Slavney, AR Boyko, and AJ Sams. "Direct-to-Consumer DNA Testing of 6,000 Dogs Reveals 98.6-Kb Duplication Associated With Blue Eyes and Heterochromia in Siberian Huskies." *PLoS Genetics* 14(10) (2018): e1007648.

Demaerel, W, Y Mostovoy, F Yilmaz, L Vervoort, S Pastor, MS Hestand, A Swillen, E Vergaelen, EA Geiger, CR Coughlin, SK Chow, D McDonald-McGinn, B Morrow, PY Kwok, M Xiao, BS Emanuel, TH Shaikh, and JR Vermeesch. "The 22q11 Low Copy Repeats Are Characterized by Unprecedented Size and Structural Variability." *Genome Research* 29(9) (2019): 1389–401.

Donner, J, H Anderson, S Davison, AM Hughes, J Bouirmane, J Lindqvist, KM Lytle, B Ganesan, C Ottka, P Ruotanen, M Kaukonen, OP Forman, N Fretwell, CA Cole, and H Lohi. "Frequency and Distribution of 152 Genetic Disease Variants in Over 100,000 Mixed Breed and Purebred Dogs." *PLoS Genetics* 14(4) (2018): e1007361.

Dreger, DL, Blair N Hooser, Angela M Hughes, Balasubramanian Ganesan, Jonas Donner, Heidi Anderson, Lauren Holtvoigt, Kari J Ekenstedt. "True Colors: Commercially-Acquired Morphological Genotypes Reveal Hidden Allele Variation among Dog Breeds, Informing Both Trait Ancestry and Breed Potential." *PLOS One* 14(10) (2019): e0223995. https://doi.org/10.1371/journal.pone.0223995.

Dudchenko, Olga, Muhammad S Shamim, Sanjit Batra, Neva C Durand, Nathaniel T Musial, Ragib Mostofa, Melanie Pham, Brian Glenn St Hilaire, Weijie Yao, Elena Stamenova, Marie Hoeger, Sarah K Nyquist, Valeriya Korchina, Kelcie Pletch, Joseph P Flanagan, Ania Tomaszewicz, Denise McAloose, Cynthia Pérez Estrada, Ben J Novak, Arina D Omer, and Erez Lieberman Aiden. "The Juicebox Assembly Tools Module Facilitates De Novo Assembly of Mammalian Genomes with Chromosome-Length Scaffolds for Under $1000." *bioRxiv*. 2018 doi: https://doi.org/10.1101/254797

Eid, John "Real-Time DNA Sequencing From Single Polymerase Molecules." *Science* 323(5910) (2009): 133.

Hayward, JJ, MG Castelhano, KC Oliveira, E Corey, C Balkman, TL Baxter, ML Casal, SA Center, M Fang, SJ Garrison, SE Kalla, P Korniliev, MI Kotlikoff, NS Moise, LM Shannon, KW Simpson, NB Sutter, RJ Todhunter, and AR Boyko. "Complex Disease and Phenotype Mapping in the Domestic Dog." *Nature Communications* 7 (2016): 10460.

Hitti, Rebekkah J, James AC Oliver, Ellen C Schofield, Anina Bauer, Maria Kaukonen, Oliver P Forman, Tosso Leeb, Hannes Lohi, Louise M Burmeister, David Sargan, and Cathryn S Mellersh. "Whole Genome Sequencing of Giant Schnauzer Dogs With Progressive Retinal Atrophy Establishes Necap1 as a Novel Candidate Gene for Retinal Degeneration." *GenGes* 10(5) (2019): 385.

Humble, Emily, Pavel Dobrynin, Helen Senn, Justin Chuven, Alan F Scott, David W Mohr, Olga Dudchenko, Arina D Omer, Zane Colaric, Erez Lieberman Aiden, David Wildt, Shireen Oliaji, Gaik Tamazian, Budhan Pukazhenthi, Rob Ogden, and Klaus-Peter Koepfli. "Chromosomal-Level Genome Assembly of the Scimitar-Horned Oryx: Insights Into Diversity and Demography of a Species Extinct in the Wild." (2019).

Jeffreys, Alec J, Victoria Wilson, and Swee Lay Thein. "Hypervariable'Minisatellite'regi ons in Human DNA." *Nature* 314 (6006) (1985): 67.

Kamathewatta, KI, RN Bushell, ND Young, MA Stevenson, H Billman-Jacobe, GF Browning, and MS Marenda. "Exploration of Antibiotic Resistance Risks in a Veterinary Teaching Hospital with Oxford Nanopore Long Read Sequencing." *PLoS One* 14(5) (2019): e0217600.

Khera, AV, M Chaffin, KH Wade, S Zahid, J Brancale, R Xia, M Distefano, O Senol-Cosar, ME Haas, A Bick, KG Aragam, ES Lander, GD Smith, H Mason-Suares, M Fornage, M Lebo, NJ Timpson, LM Kaplan, and S Kathiresan. "Polygenic Prediction of Weight and Obesity Trajectories From Birth to Adulthood." *Cell* 177(3) (2019): 587–596.e9.

Kirkness, EF, V Bafna, AL Halpern, S Levy, K Remington, DB Rusch, AL Delcher, M Pop, W Wang, CM Fraser, and JC Venter. "The Dog Genome: Survey Sequencing and Comparative Analysis." *Science* 301(5641) (2003): 1898.

Kronenberg, Zev N, Ian T Fiddes, David Gordon, Shwetha Murali, Stuart Cantsilieris et al. "High-Resolution Comparative Analysis of Great Ape Genomes." *Science* 360(6393) (2018): eaar6343.

Letko, A, E Dietschi, M Nieburg, V Jagannathan, C Gurtner, A Oevermann, and C Drögemüller. "A Missense Variant in Scn8a in Alpine Dachsbracke Dogs Affected by Spinocerebellar Ataxia." *Genes (Basel)* 10(5) (2019).

Lind, AL, YYY Lai, Y Mostovoy, AK Holloway, A Iannucci, ACY Mak, M Fondi, V Orlandini, WL Eckalbar, M Milan, M Rovatsos, IG Kichigin, AI Makunin, M Johnson Pokorná, M Altmanová, VA Trifonov, E Schijlen, L Kratochvíl, R Fani, P Velenský, I Rehák, T Patarnello, TS Jessop, JW Hicks, OA Ryder, JR Mendelson, C Ciofi, PY Kwok, KS Pollard, and BG Bruneau. "Genome of the Komodo Dragon Reveals Adaptations in the Cardiovascular and Chemosensory Systems of Monitor Lizards." *Nature Ecology & Evolution* 3(8) (2019): 1241.

Lindblad-Toh, K, CM Wade, TS Mikkelsen, EK Karlsson, DB Jaffe et al. "Genome Sequence, Comparative Analysis and Haplotype Structure of the Domestic Dog." *Nature* 438(7069) (2005): 803.

Mansour, TA, K Lucot, SE Konopelski, PJ Dickinson, BK Sturges, KL Vernau, S Choi, JA Stern, SM Thomasy, S Döring, FJM Verstraete, EG Johnson, D York, RB Rebhun, HH Ho, CT Brown, and DL Bannasch. "Whole Genome Variant Association Across

100 Dogs Identifies a Frame Shift Mutation in Dishevelled 2 Which Contributes to Robinow-Like Syndrome in Bulldogs and Related Screw Tail Dog Breeds." *PLoS Genetics* 14(12) (2018): e1007850.

Mealey, KL, SE Martinez, NF Villarino, and MH Court. "Personalized Medicine: Going to the Dogs?" *Human Genetics* 138(5) (2019): 467.

Miga, Karen H, Sergey Koren, Arang Rhie, Mitchell R Vollger, Ariel Gershman et al. "Telomere-to-telomere Assembly of a Complete Human X Chromosome." (2019).

Mohr, DW, A Naguib, NI Weisenfeld, V Kumar, P Shah, DM Church, D Jaffe, and AF Scott. "Improved *De Novo* Genome Assembly: Linked-Read Sequencing Combined With Optical Mapping Produce a High Quality Mammalian Genome at Relatively Low Cos." *bioRxiv* (2017).

Nghiem, PP, and JN Kornegay. "Gene Therapies in Canine Models for Duchenne Muscular Dystrophy." *Human Genetics* 138(5) (2019): 483–89.

Ostrander, EA, RK Wayne, AH Freedman, and BW Davis. "Demographic History, Selection and Functional Diversity of the Canine Genome." *Nature Reviews. Genetics* 18(12) (2017): 705–20.

Parker, HG, A Harris, DL Dreger, BW Davis, and EA Ostrander. "The Bald and the Beautiful: Hairlessness in Domestic Dog Breeds." *Philosophical Transactions of the Royal Society of London. Series B: Biological Sciences* 372(1713) (2017).

Peserico, A, M Marcacci, D Malatesta, M Di Domenico, A Pratelli, I Mangone, N D'Alterio, F Pizzurro, F Cirone, G Zaccaria, C Cammà, and A Lorusso. "Diagnosis and Characterization of Canine Distemper Virus Through Sequencing by Minion Nanopore Technology." *Scientific Reports* 9(1) (2019): 1714.

Quick, J, NJ Loman, S Duraffour, JT Simpson, E Severi et al. "Real-Time, Portable Genome Sequencing for Ebola Surveillance." *Nature* 530(7589) (2016): 228.

Raffan, E, RJ Dennis, CJ O'Donovan, JM Becker, RA Scott, SP Smith, DJ Withers, CJ Wood, E Conci, DN Clements, KM Summers, AJ German, CS Mellersh, ML Arendt, VP Iyemere, E Withers, J Söder, S Wernersson, G Andersson, K Lindblad-Toh, GS Yeo, and S O'Rahilly. "A Deletion in the Canine Pomc Gene Is Associated With Weight and Appetite in Obesity-Prone Labrador Retriever Dogs." *Cell Metabolism* 23(5) (2016): 893–900.

Sedlazeck, Fritz J, Zachary Lemmon, Sebastian Soyk, William J Salerno, Zachary Lippman, and Michael C Schatz. "Svcollector: Optimized Sample Selection for Validating and Long-Read Resequencing of Structural Variants." (2018).

Shaffer, LG, K Sundin, A Geretschlaeger, J Segert, JE Swinburne, R Royal, R Loechel, CJ Ramirez, and BC Ballif. "Standards and Guidelines for Canine Clinical Genetic Testing Laboratories." *Human Genetics* 138(5) (2019): 493–99.

Tandon, D, K Ressler, D Petticord, A Papa, J Jiranek, R Wilkinson, RY Kartzinel, EA Ostrander, N Burney, C Borden, MAR Udell, and BM VonHoldt. "Homozygosity for Mobile Element Insertions Associated With Wbscr17 Could Predict Success in Assistance Dog Training Programs." *Genes (Basel)* 10(6) (2019).

Thorvaldsdottir, H, JT Robinson, and JP Mesirov. "Integrative Genomics Viewer (Igv): High-Performance Genomics Data Visualization and Exploration." *Briefings in Bioinformatics* 14(2) (2013): 178–92.

vonHoldt, Bridgett M, Emily Shuldiner, Ilana Janowitz Koch, Rebecca Y Kartzinel, Andrew Hogan, Lauren Brubaker, Shelby Wanser, Daniel Stahler, Clive DL Wynne, Elaine A Ostrander, Janet S Sinsheimer, and Monique AR Udell. "Structural Variants in Genes Associated With Human Williams-Beuren Syndrome Underlie Stereotypical Hypersociability in Domestic Dogs." *Science Advances* 3(7) (2017): e1700398.

Wenger, Aaron M, Paul Peluso, William J Rowell, Pi-Chuan Chang, Richard J Hall, Gregory T Concepcion, Jana Ebler, Arkarachai Fungtammasan, Alexey Kolesnikov, Nathan D Olson, Armin Töpfer, Michael Alonge, Medhat Mahmoud, Yufeng Qian, Chen-Shan Chin, Adam M Phillippy, Michael C Schatz, Gene Myers, Mark A DePristo, Jue Ruan, Tobias Marschall, Fritz J Sedlazeck, Justin M Zook, Heng Li, Sergey Koren, Andrew Carroll, David R Rank, and Michael W Hunkapiller. "Highly-Accurate Long-Read Sequencing Improves Variant Detection and Assembly of a Human Genome." *Nature Biotechnology* 37(10) (2019): 1155–62.

Wilkins, AS, RW Wrangham, and WT Fitch. "The "Domestication Syndrome" in Mammals: A Unified Explanation Based on Neural Crest Cell Behavior and Genetics." *Genetics* 197(3) (2014): 795–808.

9 The Importance of Collecting Tissue from Pets (Alive and Deceased)

Rebecca A. Krimins

CONTENTS

INTRODUCTION

Performing clinical trials in veterinary patients typically begins with a significant amount of data collection and testing that must be performed long in advance of a pet becoming a participant in a trial. Quite often *ex vivo* testing of specific tissue is necessary. For example, if the scientific team is researching allergic dermatitis, specimens of tissue from dogs or cats with that condition may be necessary. For a team that is studying bladder stones, a sampling of stones from different patients may need to be evaluated. For a team that is evaluating if a certain molecule will bind to prostate tissue, biopsies of prostate tissue may be necessary and so forth for the many different types of disease entities that are considered in medicine.

Historically, trying to obtain the necessary tissue specimen in a condition (i.e. fresh tissue, frozen tissue, formalin-fixed tissue, etc.) and time frame (i.e. immediate, 2 hours post collection, within 1 day of collection, etc.) that are necessary for the research team, has not always been possible and is often not easily accomplished. There are many different types of pet owners, some who want to help, some who do not want to help, and most who simply are not aware that their pets' tissues may be of help to the scientific community. In addition, there has long been a component of veterinary clinical trials (this stems from human clinical trials) where pet owners are concerned that their pet may be 'experimented' on and thus, do not feel comfortable contributing to research science. However, this author has found that once a pet owner/family member is educated on the process and the goals of the research study, the pet owner/family member understands and wants to be a part of the process as well.

This chapter is to offer researchers suggested tools and methods necessary in order to effectively collect tissue samples from a living or deceased pet.

BIOPSY AND DISCARDED TISSUE SPECIMENS VS NECROPSY SAMPLES

Obtaining tissue from biopsy samples and/or discarded tissue specimens requires a different process than collecting post-mortem samples. Collecting tissue samples from live veterinary patients is best accomplished through communications with local referring veterinarians who perform procedures on a daily basis. Nowhere in this chapter is it recommended to collect tissue from a veterinary patient that is not undergoing a scheduled procedure; rather, this chapter focuses on the use of collecting tissue samples that are scheduled to be removed by the local veterinarian for an associated or unassociated procedure (i.e. ovariohysterectomy, castration, cystotomy, splenectomy, amputation, etc.). When a tissue is biopsied or a surgery is performed, often a sample is submitted to a histopathology lab. If a surgery is performed and no tissue samples are being submitted to a lab, then the tissue specimens are discarded in a specific receptacle used for the collection of discarded tissue. Referring veterinarians can assist with tissue collection in several ways. One of these ways is by requesting that the tissue sample be returned to their office *after* it has been processed and analyzed (in other words, the original sample can be returned after receiving information in regards to the original goal). Another way referring veterinarians can aid tissue collection is by requesting the veterinarian collect a tissue sample that he/she would have otherwise discarded. Once veterinarians are aware of what is needed, many veterinarians become team players and will assist with tissue collection.

COMMUNICATION

Communication is key and the researcher can use various methods to educate the recipient (veterinarian, pet owner, front office staff, etc.) on the goal of the research. Methods include building websites, printing brochures, making PowerPoint lectures, and delivering those lectures to target audiences, scheduling in-person meetings, and more. It is important to explain the research to the organization and what all is required; these explanations should involve all persons who have any connection to the procedure being performed on the pet (i.e. receptionists at veterinary hospitals, cleaning staff, instrument washers, veterinary technicians, veterinary technician assistants, veterinarians, office administrators, etc.) Once folks hear the research goal, the vast majority quickly get onboard and are willing to work towards the common goal(s). For the office leaders who need to know what is going on (i.e. hospital owners, office managers, etc.), schedule an appointment to discuss the work. In addition, there are additional people and teams that can be invaluable to helping assist in tissue sample collections, for example social workers, hospice workers, and advocacy groups. Get on social media and involve social media programs with links to websites about the research/clinical trial. Testimonials from pet owners can be especially beneficial to advocating for clinical trial work. It is important to tell pet owners, family members, and the public what is needed in a manner that they want to hear it. This often means being professional yet stripping the scientific jargon that researchers are accustomed to having to use in a scientific journal. If the research team has a local artist or graduate art program, ask a student to draw up animations as educational pieces. If a necropsy is part of the procedure that will need to be performed as part of the trial, explain that a necropsy is a type of post-mortem surgical procedure performed on a pet after death.

CONSENT FORMS

It is imperative to have a consent form and explain to members (these may be members of the research team and/or referring veterinarians and/or others) that a consent form is necessary for tissue collection. Some veterinary employees and/or pet owners may get stressed if the consent form comes into a play when a pet has not yet died. Explain that just because a consent form is being discussed it has no impact on when the pet will die. In human medicine, there are human subjects that have been on programs (signed a consent) for years; all this means is that arrangements have been made for what will happen with tissue samples after death.

We live in an age where nobody picks up the phone anymore, and everyone just wants to email. Be wary of emailing this information at all times; if the information is being delivered or discussed during a sensitive time, a phone call or in person meeting may be the best way to communicate. Always remember that the clinical trial experts are helping veterinarians, veterinary staff, pet owners, and family members manage an extremely difficult experience. Most of these people will be grateful for this assistance. Do not be surprised if pet owners request being part of the research program in the future after having participated in the tissue submission process.

Geography is also very important. These cases and tissue collection often only work for the geographic area in which the research is located (i.e. local area). If a pet family is not local to an area, it may be helpful to have a list of expanded veterinary offices to which this pet family can be sent.

GEOGRAPHY

Always let the family members and pet owners know that someone will learn from their pet's tissue and never say 'we don't need your pet's tissue', 'we don't have time for this now', or 'we are not going to do this now'. That does not mean that the research team has to be available 24/7 in order to pick up tissue specimens, rather that this is a sensitive topic and if the team is not going to accept tissue, this needs to be communicated in a delicate manner. Sometimes it is not possible to get a tissue sample (i.e. the researcher is going on a long-needed vacation, or the researcher is in another country attending a conference, etc.) and if this is the case, one can respectfully say 'unfortunately, we simply do not have the resources right now to pick up these tissue samples but we absolutely appreciate you and your family'.

DETAILED COMMENTS

Some additional comments about tissue collection. Never rush a family with decision making. Try to pick up tissue as soon as possible. Even if the research team is unable to use the tissue, someone should go and pick it up. Publicize the research. Pet owners are some of the most resilient people this author has met and most owners want to do something good. Once a research team is able to get a single pet owner to say 'I want to do this', then typically the rest of the family will be on board.

A recent publication by Ableman et al. describes a program that was implemented in 2012 in the state of New York in order to improve methods for performing chronic wasting disease surveillance in cervids. This program, called the Taxidermy Partnership Program, has proven to be a success and initially started with letters outlining the program that were sent to all state taxidermists in an attempt to solicit participants to aid in sampling tissues. Participants were paid for their time and effort in submitting samples. All supplies sent to participants contain a kit with pre-labeled tissue containers, tools for obtaining the tissue, written instructions, payment paperwork, and a New York State Wildlife Health Cooperator patch. These authors found that taxidermists were an untapped source of valuable tissue samples and that the taxidermists could be successfully trained with minimal agency effort and expense (Ableman et al. 2019). There are numerous other programs that supply free kits to aid in specimen collecting. For example, the Dog Aging Project, out of the University of Washington, recently received a 15-million-dollar grant from the National Institute on Aging and is currently enrolling 10,000 dogs that will be followed for 10 years (Kaeberlein, Creevy, and Promislow 2016). This author believes similar programs can be created to collect specimens in pets by working with state shelters, rescue organizations, and humane societies that often see high volumes of animals undergoing daily surgical procedures.

In addition to the availability and use of tissue from companion animals, numerous other sources for tissues/samples are available through private and commercial entities, some of which are highlighted below.

TISSUE BANKING

https://vhc.missouri.edu/small-animal-hospital/oncology/tissue-collect
ion-bank

Canine and Feline Genomics studies
https://familydogproject.elte.hu/canine-tissue-bank/
Canine Brain and Tissue Bank, collects and stores biological samples from pet dogs
http://ccogc.net
Canine Comparative Oncology and Genomics Consortium

COMMERCIAL

www.kerafast.com/productgroup/535/dog-mixed-breed-tissue-samples
Tissue samples from various organs of mixed-breed dogs. Available in histological tissue section on glass slide (HS) or paraffin-embedded tissue block (PETB) formats.
https://bioivt.com/search?string=dog
BioIVT provides animal tissue from any commercially available animal research model. Custom preparations from tissue types such as brain, kidney, lung, intestine, heart, and skin are readily available. Animal tissues are collected at facilities located in the United States, using BioIVT Standard Operating Procedures.
www.amsbio.com/Tissues.aspx
AMSBIO supplies a comprehensive range of tissues available in frozen and formalin-fixed, paraffin embedded (FFPE) in all formats.
www.biocompare.com/pfu/124211/soids/112498-269767/Blood_and_Tissue_Products/Canine_Tissue
Dog (mixed breed) tissue samples

ACKNOWLEDGEMENTS

Many of the concepts discussed in this chapter were based on comments and recommendations provided by Jody Hooper, MD, the Director of the Rapid Autopsy Program, at Johns Hopkins University (Hooper 2018).

REFERENCES

Ableman, A., K. Hynes, K. Schuler, and A. Martin. 2019. "Partnering with Taxidermists for Improved Chronic Wasting Disease Surveillance." *Animals (Basel)* 9(12). doi: 10.3390/ani9121113.
Hooper, J., and E. Duregon 2018. "Performance of Rapid Research Autopsy." In J. Hooper and A. Williamson, eds: *Autopsy in the 21st Century*, 167–185. Springer, Cham.
Kaeberlein, M., K. E. Creevy, and D. E. Promislow. 2016. "The Dog Aging Project: Translational Geroscience in Companion Animals." *Mammalian Genome* 27(7–8):279–288. doi: 10.1007/s00335-016-9638-7.

10 The FDA New Animal Drug Approval Process

Jacob Michael Froehlich, Alice Ignaszewski, and Anna O'Brien

CONTENTS

INTRODUCTION

Scientific study of disease in animals often leads to improvements in existing therapies or the discovery of novel treatments. This research has the potential to positively impact large populations of both humans and animals. In order to reach these patients and translate discovery to the bed-, cage-, or stall-side, these products are often commercialized and marketed. Likewise, veterinarians rely on these commercially marketed products to diagnose, cure, treat, or otherwise improve the quality of life for their animal patients. In the United States, the legal marketing of new animal drugs requires the demonstration of safety, effectiveness, quality manufacturing, and appropriate labeling, culminating in an approval from the US Food and Drug Administration. After reading this chapter, researchers should gain a basic understanding of the approval process for a new animal drug and the ways in which researchers can contribute to or navigate that approval process.

US FOOD AND DRUG ADMINISTRATION'S CENTER FOR VETERINARY MEDICINE

Many animal products are regulated by the United States federal government. However, the laws, regulations, and government agency which govern an individual product depend on that product's classification. Under current federal law, most products administered or applied to animals are regulated as either an animal drug, an animal device, food for animals, a veterinary biologic, or a pesticide. Animal drugs, animal devices, and food for animals are regulated by the US Food and Drug Administration's Center for Veterinary Medicine (FDA-CVM). Veterinary biologics are regulated by the Animal and Plant Health Inspection Service (APHIS)'s Center for Veterinary Biologics (CVB) of the US Department of Agriculture (USDA), while pesticides are regulated by the US Environmental Protection Agency (EPA).

The FDA-CVM regulates animal drugs, animal devices, and food for animals under the Federal Food, Drug, and Cosmetic Act (hereinafter, "the Act"). Originally passed in 1938, the Act has been amended by Congress on multiple occasions, leading to a modern regulatory structure which functions to protect both human and animal health. Under the auspices of the Act, the FDA-CVM:

- Ensures new animal drugs are safe and effective
- Monitors the safety and effectiveness of approved new animal drugs on the market
- Ensures that food products made from treated animals are safe for people to consume
- Ensures food for animals – including animal feed, pet treats, and pet food – is safe, made under sanitary conditions, and properly labeled
- Provides regulatory oversight over animal devices
- Ensures additives for use in food for animals are safe and effective
- Conducts research that helps the FDA-CVM ensure the safety of new animal drugs, food for animals, and food products made from animals
- Incentivizes the development of legally available new animal drugs for minor species and for minor uses in major species

The FDA-CVM is organized into six Offices that all work toward achieving the core mission of protecting human and animal health. The six Offices are the Office of the Director, Office of Management, Office of Surveillance and

Compliance, Office of New Animal Drug Evaluation, Office of Research, and the Office of Minor Use and Minor Species Animal Drug Development. The Office of New Animal Drug Evaluation (ONADE) is responsible for approval of new animal drugs.

While the word "drug" may mean many things in everyday language, this term is specifically defined under the Act. In this context, the term "drug" means, in part, "articles intended for use in the diagnosis, cure, mitigation, treatment, or prevention of disease in man or other animals" or "articles (other than food) intended to affect the structure or any function of the body of man or other animals."* While people generally think of drugs as being traditional small molecule drugs such as non-steroidal anti-inflammatory drugs (NSAIDs) and antimicrobials; purified proteins such as monoclonal antibodies and recombinant cytokines; and cells, tissues, and their derivatives (see *New Animal Drugs: Animal Cell-Based Products* below) can also be drugs.

Similarly, the Act defines the term "new animal drug" as "any drug intended for use for animals other than man" that is not generally recognized as safe and effective "for use under the conditions prescribed, recommended, or suggested in the labeling."† Here, the word "new" does not necessarily mean novel to science or medicine, but that the product is not commonly recognized as safe and effective within the literature and scientific community. While new animal drugs and human drugs are both covered by the same Act, they are reviewed by different Centers within the FDA and fall under different regulations. However, both human and animal drugs are held to similar standards.

Under the Act, "device" is defined, in part, as "an instrument, apparatus, implement, machine, contrivance, implant, *in vitro* reagent, or other similar or related article" that is "intended for use in the diagnosis, cure, mitigation, treatment, or prevention of disease in man or other animals" or "intended to affect the structure or any function of the body of man or other animals" *but* "does not achieve its primary intended purposes through chemical action" or "being metabolized." While the FDA-CVM does have regulatory oversight over animal devices and can take appropriate regulatory action if an animal device is misbranded or adulterated, the Act does not require pre-market approval for animal devices.

OVERVIEW OF THE PHASED REVIEW PROCESS

To begin the new animal drug approval process, a sponsor generally opens an Investigational New Animal Drug (INAD) file under which data can be submitted. The term "sponsor" is used to refer to an individual or organization involved in the development and approval of a new animal drug. The sponsor is the point of contact with the FDA-CVM during the approval process and is responsible for compliance with applicable provisions of the Act and regulations. Once the INAD file is open, the FDA-CVM typically reviews the data that are intended to support

---

* Section 201(g) of the Act
† Section 201(v) of the Act

TABLE 10.1

Technical Sections of (J)INAD Files by Product Type

PRODUCT TYPE

New animal drug	Generic new animal drug
Target animal safety (TAS)	Bioequivalence (BE)
Effectiveness (EFF)	Patent certification and marketing
Human food safety (HFS)*	exclusivity
Chemistry, manufacturing,	Chemistry, manufacturing, and
and controls (CMC)	controls (CMC)
Environmental impact (NV)	Environmental impact (NV)
Labeling	Labeling
All other information (AOI)	Human food safety (HFS)*

* The human food safety (HFS) technical section is not completed if the target animal species is a non-food animal.

approval of the new animal drug under a phased review process. This means that the different types of data intended to support approval (e.g., target animal safety, effectiveness, chemistry, manufacturing, and controls, etc.) can be submitted independently as components of the INAD file called technical sections. As submissions to technical sections are received, the FDA-CVM will review the data and provide feedback on the acceptability of the information. Once all necessary data within a technical section are deemed acceptable, a technical section complete letter is issued by the FDA-CVM. The technical sections supporting approval are listed in Table 10.1. Trade secrets and commercial or financial information submitted to the FDA-CVM are not available for public disclosure.

A sponsor may work on the technical sections in any order, or even simultaneously, and may start or stop when needed until all technical sections are completed under the INAD file; there is no set order to the phased review process. It is the responsibility of the sponsor to ensure studies supporting approval are conducted in accordance with applicable standards, e.g., Good Laboratory Practices (GLPs),* Good Clinical Practices (GCPs),† and/or other appropriate regulations. Generally, for studies used in support of an approval, it is important that the product being tested is the same formulation intended for marketing.

The final stage of the approval process is the filing of an administrative New Animal Drug Application (NADA). The administrative NADA is submitted after all technical section complete letters supporting approval have been received by the sponsor and represents a formal request for approval from the FDA-CVM for the sponsor's new animal drug. After the FDA-CVM determines that all required information is included under the administrative NADA, the FDA-CVM will

---

* 21 CFR Part 58
† GFI #85 (VICH GL9): Good Clinical Practice

send a letter to the sponsor indicating that the drug is approved, and they can now legally market their new animal drug.

NEW ANIMAL DRUGS: SMALL MOLECULES, PURIFIED PROTEINS, AND RECOMBINANT TECHNOLOGIES

A sponsor will generally begin discussions with the FDA-CVM after proof-of-concept work has been completed, and the sponsor has developed an idea for the drug's proposed indication(s) (i.e., what the drug is intended to do), the dosage form (e.g., injectable solution, tablet), and the dosage regimen (e.g., single or multiple doses). The FDA-CVM's review considers many factors, including:

- Safety, which includes safety in the target animal, human food safety for new animal drugs used in food animals, and human user safety for individuals administering the new animal drug
- Effectiveness
- Quality manufacturing
- Labeling
- Impact on the environment

These factors are reflected in the technical sections, of which there are typically seven. The technical sections, in no particular order, are as follows and will each be discussed in greater detail below: target animal safety; effectiveness; human food safety (if required); chemistry, manufacturing, and controls; environmental impact; labeling; and all other information. Sponsors are encouraged to submit protocols to the FDA-CVM for review prior to conducting their studies. While submission of study protocols is not required, protocol review by the FDA-CVM may be helpful to ensuring that the study design satisfies scientific and regulatory requirements.

TARGET ANIMAL SAFETY (TAS)*

The TAS technical section includes data, scientific literature, and/or other information that demonstrates the drug is safe for use under the conditions prescribed, recommended, or suggested in the proposed labeling in the intended class of animal. The purpose of the studies conducted for this technical section is to evaluate possible toxic effects of the new animal drug in a controlled setting with the intent of extrapolating those findings to the target population at large.

The specific studies and information needed to assess target animal safety is highly dependent on the characteristics of the particular new animal drug. However, one of the most common studies that is conducted for this technical section is called a margin of safety study. A margin of safety study is essentially an overdose study, evaluating dose levels above the proposed labeled dose (e.g.,

---

* 21 CFR Part 514.1(b)(8)(i)

1X, 3X, and 5X) for three times the labeled duration in comparison to a nontreated control group.* End points generally include physical examinations; daily health observations; repeated blood and urine collections for hematology, clinical chemistry, and urinalysis; and necropsies with histopathology at the study's termination. Injection site and application site safety may also be evaluated in this study if the product is administered via injection or topically, respectively.

Additional safety studies may be appropriate for a particular drug, depending on the conditions of use and the drug's characteristics. For example, if the product is intended for use in reproducing animals, male and female reproductive safety studies are typically conducted. The TAS technical section also contains any relevant studies or references regarding the safety of humans that administer or may come into direct contact with the new animal drug (user safety).

EFFECTIVENESS (EFF)†

A sponsor is required to demonstrate by substantial evidence that the new animal drug has the effect it purports or is represented to have under the proposed conditions of use suggested in the labeling. To demonstrate substantial evidence of effectiveness, sponsors generally conduct one or more adequate and well-controlled study evaluating the new animal drug under the proposed conditions of use. The data from these studies demonstrate that the new animal drug is effective for the labeled indication(s).

The number and types of studies required to demonstrate substantial evidence of effectiveness is dependent on the new animal drug's indication and may include both laboratory studies and field studies conducted under the proposed conditions of use. The field studies are also used to gather in-use safety data. Effectiveness studies typically compare an investigational drug treated group to an untreated (negative) control or to a positive control treated with an approved drug for the same indication. Variations in study design are utilized where appropriate based on the indication and pharmacokinetic profile of the new animal drug.

CHEMISTRY, MANUFACTURING, AND CONTROLS (CMC)‡

An FDA-approved new animal drug must meet certain manufacturing standards to ensure consistent quality of the product. For example, the new animal drug must be manufactured in accordance with current Good Manufacturing Practices (cGMPs) and confirm the identity, strength, quality, and purity of the final formulation of the new animal drug prior to approval. This provides assurance to the end users that each tablet, injection, or topical product purchased remains physically and chemically the same (with the same safety and effectiveness profile), as the product evaluated prior to approval.

---

* GFI #185 (VICH GL43): Target Animal Safety for Veterinary Pharmaceutical Products
† 21 CFR Parts 514.1(b)(2) and (b)(3)
‡ 21 CFR Part 514.1

A full description of the methods used in and the facilities and controls used for the manufacture, processing, and packaging of the new animal drug is provided in the CMC technical section. Manufacturing procedures, analytical specifications, method validation data, and stability data to support expiry periods and storage conditions are provided as well, along with demonstrated cGMP compliance. Manufacturing facilities are also inspected as part of the requirements for this technical section; this ensures that the sponsor is utilizing facilities with the correct equipment and methods to consistently produce a high-quality, safe, and effective drug.

HUMAN FOOD SAFETY (HFS)

New animal drugs approved for use in food-producing species (e.g., beef and dairy cattle, swine, goats, sheep, chickens, turkeys, some species of fish) are evaluated for human food safety to ensure that food derived from treated animals is safe for human consumption. The HFS technical section includes scientific data or information necessary to demonstrate that residues of the new animal drug in the edible tissues of treated animals are safe.* Edible tissues are defined as muscle, liver, kidney, fat, skin with fat in natural proportions, whole eggs, whole milk, and honey.† Drugs for use in companion animals (e.g., dogs, cats, horses) are considered non-food-producing animals and do not have to address human food safety.

For drugs used in food-producing animals, the HFS technical section is comprised of three parts: toxicology; residue chemistry, which includes the analytical method for detecting residues; and microbial food safety. Toxicology generally evaluates a series of studies such as testing for systemic toxicity, developmental and reproductive toxicity, genotoxicity, and when applicable, carcinogenicity, effects on human intestinal flora, neurotoxicity, and immunotoxicity. Information from these studies is used to establish the acceptable daily intake (ADI), which most often will be set on the basis of the drug's toxicological, microbiological, or pharmacological properties. This value, usually expressed in micrograms or milligrams of the total drug residues per kilogram of body weight per day, represents the daily intake of drug residue in animal tissue that may be consumed during the entire life of a human without adverse effects or harm to the health of the consumer. This ADI, together with food consumption values for edible tissues, is then used to determine safe concentrations. The safe concentration is the amount of total residue of a new animal drug that can be consumed from each edible tissue every day for up to the lifetime of a human without exposing the human to residues in excess of the ADI. Safe concentrations, expressed as parts per million (ppm) or parts per billion (ppb), are used for tolerance determinations.

Information from residue chemistry studies is used to assess the quantity and nature of residues in tissues derived from animals treated with new animal drugs.

---

* Section 512(b)(1) of the Act
† 21 CFR Part 556.3

The metabolites humans may be exposed to when consuming meat from a treated animal are evaluated during toxicological studies using laboratory animals. A target tissue and a marker residue* are selected from the information provided about the drug metabolism in the target animal. A tolerance for the marker residue is determined using the safe concentration and by examining total residue and marker residue depletion data. The tolerance is the maximum concentration of a marker residue, or other residue indicated for monitoring, that can legally remain in a specific edible tissue of a treated animal.†

Marker residue depletion data are also collected to demonstrate the depletion of the marker residue post-treatment to below the tolerance and to provide data for calculating a withdrawal period and, if the drug is used in dairy animals, a milk discard time. A withdrawal period or milk discard time is the interval between the time of the last administration of a new animal drug and the time when the animal can be safely slaughtered for food or its milk can be safely consumed. Along with providing information about the quantity and nature of residues, the sponsor must provide a practicable analytical method for measuring tissue residues. The analytical method is used to ensure that tissue residues don't exceed the legal tolerance after the withdrawal period or milk discard time have been completed. If the new animal drug has antimicrobial activity, the FDA-CVM evaluates if use of the drug will promote emergence or selection of antimicrobial-resistant bacteria of public health concern, such as *Salmonella* spp., *Escherichia coli*, and *Campylobacter* spp., in or on treated food-producing animals.

As mentioned above, a battery of genotoxicity studies is typically conducted and, if a drug is determined to be genotoxic or is a known potential carcinogen, additional testing may be conducted to assess carcinogenicity. Drugs that are determined to be carcinogenic are then subject to the Delaney Clause, a provision in the Act. Under the Delaney Clause, a NADA cannot be approved if "such drug induces cancer when ingested by man or animal or, after tests which are appropriate for the evaluation of the safety of such drug, induces cancer in man or animal."‡ The diethylstilbestrol (DES) proviso exception to the Delaney Clause allows a carcinogenic animal drug to be approved if: (1) the drug will not adversely affect the animals treated with the drug and (2) no residue of such drug will be found in any edible portion of the treated animal after slaughter or in any food yielded by or derived from the living animal section.§ The regulations define the requirement of no residue as the residue of carcinogenic concern in edible tissues that will not exceed concentrations that represent no significant increase in the risk of cancer to humans.¶

---

* 21 CFR Part 556.3
† 21 CFR Part 556.3
‡ Section 512(d)(1)(I) of the Act
§ Section 512(d)(1)(I)(i)–(ii) of the Act
¶ 21 CFR Part 500.80 Subpart E

Environmental Impact (NV)

The National Environmental Policy Act of 1969 (NEPA) requires the FDA-CVM to evaluate all major agency actions to determine if the action will have a significant impact on the human environment. To implement NEPA, the FDA-CVM requires[*] sponsors to submit either an environmental assessment (EA) or a claim of categorical exclusion from preparation of an EA for their environmental impact technical section.

A categorical exclusion is a class of actions that the FDA-CVM has determined from past experience do not individually or cumulatively have a significant effect on the human environment. Therefore, these actions do not normally require the preparation of an EA or an environmental impact statement. Actions that meet the criteria of categorical exclusion are specified in the regulations[†] and include drugs intended for use in non-food animals, drugs intended for use under prescription or veterinarian's order (i.e., veterinary feed directive) for therapeutic use in terrestrial species, and actions that do not increase the use of a drug. If extraordinary circumstances indicate that a specific proposed action normally categorically excluded may significantly affect the quality of the human environment, then an EA or an environmental impact statement is prepared.[‡]

If a claim of categorical exclusion is not applicable, or not accepted due to extraordinary circumstances, the sponsor will prepare an EA. An EA is a concise public document that evaluates the potential for the drug to result in significant environmental impacts. Typically, EAs will describe the potential environmental fate and exposure of the drug and its potential effects on non-target organisms (e.g., earthworms, soil microorganisms, plants, dung fauna, fish, aquatic invertebrates, algae). The EA may include relevant scientific literature and/or sponsor-generated studies. An EA adequate for approval is one that contains sufficient information for the FDA-CVM to determine whether the proposed action may significantly affect the quality of the human environment. If the EA indicates that no significant impacts to the environment will occur, the FDA-CVM will prepare a Finding of No Significant Impact (FONSI). If significant environmental impacts are expected, the FDA-CVM will prepare an environmental impact statement.

Labeling

A drug label provides the information necessary for the safe and effective use of the drug, which includes the indication(s), dosage, appropriate animal classes, warnings, and precautions, along with storage and disposal requirements. Depending on the drug, there may be numerous labeling components, including but not limited to the package insert, the immediate container label, any outer packaging such as the box or carton, and shipper labeling for multiple containers. The information on the drug labeling comes from studies submitted by the

---

[*] 21 CFR Part 25
[†] 21 CFR Part 25.33
[‡] 21 CFR Part 25.21

sponsor in the above-mentioned technical sections, as well as information known about the drug or drug class. This language is typically drafted during the evaluation of each technical section and the sponsor submits relevant portions of the labeling with each section.

Labeling language must not be false or misleading* and is intended to provide clear instructions for the drug's use in a proper, safe, and effective manner. The proprietary (trade) name is also reviewed by the FDA-CVM and is evaluated in a similar manner, identifying names that may be promotional, false, or misleading. In addition, the FDA-CVM ensures that a proprietary name for a specific new animal drug is not too similar in spelling, or sounds too similar in speech, to the proprietary name of another drug. This review guards against inadvertent medication errors that could threaten both human and animal health.

ALL OTHER INFORMATION (AOI)

As the name suggests, the AOI technical section is the opportunity for the sponsor to submit other information not included in any of the other technical sections that is relevant to the safety and effectiveness evaluation of the drug. Information submitted may include, but is not limited to, both favorable and unfavorable published scientific literature on the drug product, adverse event reporting and/or foreign experience/marketing if the drug is approved in other countries, and other studies that have been completed by the sponsor but not submitted in any other technical section.

NEW ANIMAL DRUGS: ANIMAL CELL-BASED PRODUCTS

Animal cell-based products are defined as products which meet the definition of a new animal drug *and* contain, consist of, or are derived "from cells that are intended for implantation, transplantation, infusion, or transfer into an animal recipient."† Because these products meet the definition of a new animal drug, they are regulated by the FDA-CVM. This broad category of products includes, amongst others, stem, progenitor, and precursor cells such as multipotent stromal cells (MSCs) and hematopoietic stem cells (HSCs), differentiated cells such as dermal fibroblasts, reprogrammed differentiated cells (e.g., induced pluripotent stem cells, iPSCs), and tissue derivatives such as platelet-rich plasma (PRP), autologous conditioned serum (ACS), and amnion-based products. While the FDA-CVM recognizes that each cell or tissue product possesses unique characteristics, the term "animal cell-based product" will be used for the remainder of this section, unless a specific example is warranted.

The FDA-CVM categorizes animal cell-based products as autologous, allogeneic, or xenogeneic products, based on the relationship between the donor and recipient animals. Autologous animal cell-based products are further

---

* Section 502(a) of the Act
† GFI #218: Cell-Based Products for Animal Use

subcategorized as Type I and Type II products. Type II autologous animal cell-based products are those products that are minimally manipulated (e.g., centrifugation of whole blood to produce packed erythrocytes for autotransfusion), used for a homologous purpose (e.g., autologous cartilage-derived cells used to repair a chondral defect), used in non-food animal species (e.g., an equine patient), and produced without the addition of another article,[*] drug, or device. Type I autologous animal cell-based products are those autologous products that do not meet *each* of the aforementioned criteria. For example, an animal cell-based product that is formulated with culture-expanded cells is a Type I product because the cells are more than minimally manipulated, even if the product meets all of the other criteria for a Type II product. Similarly, an animal cell-based product that is not intended to perform the same basic function in the recipient as in the donor is a Type I product because it is intended for a non-homologous use (e.g., autologous cartilage-derived cells used to treat a neurological condition). Under the new animal drug provisions of the Act, all animal cell-based products, regardless of their donor–recipient relationship, require premarket review and an approved NADA to be legally marketed in the United States (as described above in *New Animal Drugs: Small Molecules, Purified Proteins, and Recombinant Technologies*).[†]

Early and frequent communication with the FDA-CVM during the development of an animal cell-based product is critical to ensuring an efficient review process. Due to the ever-evolving scientific knowledge related to these products, the FDA-CVM often works with sponsors of animal cell-based products during the research or pre-investigational development (PID) phase, prior to opening an INAD file. PID refers to the early stages of product development for an animal cell-based product which typically occur before the precise constituents, formulation, manufacturing process, or indication for that product have been determined. Under PID, the FDA-CVM and sponsors discuss the evolving science and challenges related to the product, exchange information which may facilitate the development of the product, and begin to define the pathway to approval. Once a specific product is developed and the sponsor is ready to enter into binding discussions with the FDA-CVM, an INAD file is opened and the approval process begins. Sponsors are strongly encouraged to contact the FDA-CVM early in the development process to determine what information should be submitted and the appropriate file type to utilize. Information submitted to the FDA-CVM both early in development under PID and during the approval process under the INAD file is confidential.

---

[*] Water, crystalloids, or sterilizing, preserving, or storage agents are generally permissible and do not preclude classification of a product as a Type II animal cell-based product, unless the addition of the agent raises new safety concerns with respect to the product.

[†] The FDA-CVM recognizes that Type II autologous animal cell-based products pose a lower risk to human and animal safety than other categories of animal cell-based products when used in non-food-producing animals and are, therefore, a lower enforcement priority. However, persons marketing such products should be aware that the agency may take enforcement action against them at any time when the agency concludes it is necessary to further the purposes of the FD&C Act.

Unique Considerations for Animal Cell-Based Products

The FDA-CVM uses a risk-based approach to the premarket evaluation of new animal drugs. Therefore, the development plan for approval of an animal cell-based product is dependent on the attributes and characteristics specific to an individual animal cell-based product and the unique safety, effectiveness, and manufacturing considerations associated with that product. In addition to the principles discussed above (see *New Animal Drugs: Small Molecules, Purified Proteins, and Recombinant Technologies*), unique considerations for animal cell-based products may include, in part:

- Characterization of the product
- Demonstrated control of the manufacturing process
- Comparability between product batches
- Potential for disease transmission
- Safety considerations related to the cell or tissue components of the product
- Species-specific considerations related to the cell or tissue components of the product

Characterization of an animal cell-based product is important to understanding the attributes and characteristics of that specific product, as it provides the basis for understanding both the functionality and variability of the product. Animal cell-based products are biologically complex, and methods for identifying critical quality attributes are often not well established. Characterization of an animal cell-based product may involve measuring various macromolecules, describing physical properties, and assaying functional ability of the constituent cells, tissues, and biological derivatives. Because each specific product is unique, the methodology used to characterize the animal cell-based product may differ based on the product itself, processing and manufacturing involved in the generation of the final product, and intended functionality of the constituent cells or tissues.

Demonstrating control of the manufacturing process is also an important consideration, as changes in the source tissue, manufacturing process, storage conditions, or even end user instructions may impact the biological activity of the product. Characterizing and establishing the manufacturing process for an animal cell-based product early in development allows regulatory considerations impacting safety, effectiveness, and quality of the product to be identified and addressed before safety and effectiveness studies are conducted. Reaching fundamental agreement between the FDA-CVM and the sponsor on these considerations may prevent unnecessary studies from being conducted or necessary studies from being repeated.

Another unique scientific challenge for animal cell-based products is demonstrating comparability of the product from batch to batch (i.e., each batch of the product has consistent safety, effectiveness, and quality). The unique genetic background of individual donor animals and intangible variations in the manufacturing process such as the inherent variability associated with cell culture components may contribute to variability in individual batches of the final product. Likewise, the biological characteristics of the product may be adversely affected, and this in turn may impact the safety and effectiveness profile of individual batches, leading to unpredictable clinical outcomes. Additionally, critical quality attributes of the product that affect safety and effectiveness outcomes are often challenging to identify. Similarly, *in vitro* methods to assess the comparability of animal cell-based products across batches are not yet well defined, and it is often difficult to associate clinical outcomes with the end points of laboratory assays. Due to the interconnected nature of safety, effectiveness, and quality, it is critical to assess the variability between product batches to ensure that each new batch continues to be safe and effective, no matter when that batch is manufactured.

The potential for disease transmission is another unique consideration for animal cell-based products. Because these products are sourced from the cells and tissues of donor animals, they present a risk for transmission of disease agents from these donor animals to the recipients of the product. The potential for transmission of a disease agent is dependent on the characteristics of the donor population, as well as the manufacturing process. Strategies to mitigate the risk of disease agent transmission may include appropriate donor screening and demonstrated control over the manufacturing process. For donor screening, considerations may include medical and vaccination history, geographic location and travel history, housing and animal management, and disease agent testing. To control for disease transmission in the manufacturing process, in-process and end-product testing including disease agent and sterility testing are typically utilized and can provide assurance of control over the process.

Safety considerations for an animal cell-based product may also differ in some respects from those of small molecule drugs or purified, recombinant proteins. Unique safety considerations for animal cell-based products may include, in part, immunogenicity, biodistribution, cell survival, tumorigenicity, and ectopic tissue formation. The specific safety considerations of each animal cell-based product are dependent on the biologic properties of that product. For example, for a live cell product with significant differentiation potential, tumorigenicity and ectopic tissue formation evaluations may be potential safety considerations. Similarly, a product containing allogeneic or xenogeneic tissues may pose immunogenicity considerations.

Species-specific considerations may affect the safety, effectiveness, or quality of an animal cell-based product. Examples of these considerations include product use in association with common co-morbidities in the target animal population, sensitivities resulting in increased immunogenic responses, anatomical, or physiological characteristics that may affect how the cells or tissues function once administered, and challenges related to administering cells or tissues. Additionally, cells and tissues from certain species may pose challenges to *in vitro* manipulation or other processes during manufacturing, and these challenges may in turn affect safety, effectiveness, or quality of the final product.

Whether for a species-specific consideration or any of the other considerations discussed above, the FDA-CVM utilizes a risk-based approach to the regulation of animal cell-based products. This approach is informed by the individual risks associated with the specific constituents of the product, the donor animals from which those constituents are derived, the manufacturing process, and the intended population of recipient animals. Together, these risks are critical to determining the safety, effectiveness, and quality of each individual product.

The scientific understanding of animal cell-based products is rapidly evolving due to intense scientific study and interest from the research community, veterinarians, and animal owners. As these innovative technologies and their therapeutic applications are further developed, the FDA-CVM encourages sponsors to discuss the development plan and unique considerations for their products with the FDA-CVM as early as possible in product development. To promote the development of these products and to enhance communication between the FDA-CVM and sponsors, the FDA-CVM has developed a pilot Veterinary Innovation Program (VIP). This program, discussed at the end of this chapter in *Navigating the New Animal Drug Approval Process: A Roadmap for Researchers*, underscores not only the importance of communication between the FDA-CVM and sponsors of animal cell-based products, but also the FDA-CVM's commitment to facilitating advancements in development of innovative animal products, including those products manufactured from animal cells and tissues.

GENERIC NEW ANIMAL DRUGS

In 1988, the Generic Animal Drug and Patent Term Restoration Act (GADPTRA) was signed into law, amending the Act. GADPTRA allows for the approval of a generic copy of a new animal drug previously found safe and effective by the FDA-CVM. A generic new animal drug is required to contain the same active ingredient, in the same concentration, dosage form, and route of administration as the new animal drug being copied.* Additionally, the generic new animal drug must be bioequivalent to, and have labeling that is the same as, the new animal drug.† The patent term restoration provision of GADPTRA allows for extension of new animal drug patents based on the time required for drug approval. It also establishes periods of exclusive marketing for a newly approved new animal drug or for an already approved new animal drug in which a new species or claim has been added to the drug label.

The approval process for a generic new animal drug is similar to the approval process detailed above (see *Overview of the Phased Review Process*). Instead of opening an INAD file, the sponsor will open a Generic Investigational New Animal Drug (JINAD) file under which data can be submitted. When a sponsor opens a JINAD file to initiate the phased review process, the appropriate new animal drug that is being copied, referred to as the Reference Listed New Animal Drug (RLNAD), is identified, along with its approved indications. In contrast to the seven technical sections that make up the INAD file, there are six technical sections that make up the JINAD file. The technical sections under a JINAD are: bioequivalence (BE); patent certification and marketing exclusivity; chemistry,

---

* Section 512(n)(1) of the Act
† Section 512(n)(1) of the Act

manufacturing, and controls (CMC); environmental impact (NV); labeling; and human food safety (HFS) (if applicable). The information required to support the completion of the CMC, NV, and HFS technical sections is the same for both new animal drugs and generic new animal drugs (see *New Animal Drugs: Small Molecules, Purified Proteins, and Recombinant Technologies* above). Upon completion of the required technical sections for a generic new animal drug, the sponsor will request approval by filing an administrative Abbreviated New Animal Drug Application (ANADA). It should be noted that the TAS and EFF technical sections are not components of an administrative ANADA, as a generic new animal drug is a copy of a new animal drug that has already been demonstrated to be safe and effective. Instead, the BE technical section acts as a link to the TAS and EFF technical sections and is the reason why the application for approval of a generic new animal drug is considered "abbreviated."

BIOEQUIVALENCE (BE)[*,†,‡]

The bioavailability of a generic new animal drug and the RLNAD must be the same, meaning that the extent and rate of absorption of the active pharmaceutical ingredient(s) (API) or its metabolite(s) are equal.[§,¶] To demonstrate BE, an *in vivo* blood level bioequivalence study is generally conducted. The absorbed drug concentration of the API(s) or its metabolite(s) in the blood of animals after administration of either the generic (test) or reference drug is measured at multiple time-points. It is important that the drug concentration of the API(s) or its metabolite(s) be measured for a long enough duration to capture the absorption, distribution, and elimination phases of the drug concentration versus time profile. The extent of absorption is estimated by the area under the blood concentration versus time curve (AUC), and the rate of absorption is estimated by the maximum observed drug concentration (C_{max}) and the corresponding time to reach this maximum concentration (T_{max}). When the confidence intervals of these two pivotal parameters fall within 0.80 and 1.25, the two products are determined to be bioequivalent.

In vivo blood level BE studies are conducted using the target animal species as described on the RLNAD labeling. The typical study design of an *in vivo* blood level BE study is a two-period, two-sequence, crossover study.

Period	Sequence A	Sequence B
1	Test	Reference
2	Reference	Test

---

[*] GFI #35: Bioequivalence Guidance
[†] GFI #224 (VICH GL52): Bioequivalence: Blood Level Bioequivalence Study
[‡] 21 CFR Part 58
[§] 21 CFR Part 314.3
[¶] Section 512(n)(1)(E) of the Act

A pre-determined number of animals is randomly assigned to either sequence A or sequence B and dosed accordingly. Generally, the highest dose approved for the RLNAD is used. After the dose is administered, blood samples are collected to capture the concentration versus time curve. Each period is separated by a washout period, which is a pre-specified amount of time to allow for the treatment administered in period 1 to be cleared from the body prior to the subject receiving the treatment in period 2.

There are circumstances in which a drug may not be systemically absorbed, and, in these cases, alternative BE study designs can be considered. A pharmacologic end-point study design is used to evaluate a drug-induced physiologic change related to the labeled indications. A clinical end-point study design may be used if the concentration of drug in the blood is not measurable and there are no appropriate pharmacologic effects that can be monitored. Prior to conducting any type of BE study, a sponsor may meet with the FDA-CVM to discuss the development plan of the proposed generic new animal drug. Additionally, the sponsor is encouraged to submit a study protocol for the FDA-CVM to review.

Certain generic new animal drugs may qualify for a waiver from the requirement to demonstrate *in vivo* bioequivalence (biowaiver).* The products eligible for a biowaiver are typically highly soluble, which means the factors that would normally impact the bioavailability of the API (e.g., dissolution of a tablet in the stomach), are removed. Examples of product categories that may be eligible for a biowaiver are parenteral solutions, oral solutions or other solubilized forms, topically applied solutions intended for local therapeutic effects, and inhalant volatile anesthetic solutions.† In general, the generic new animal drug contains the same active and inactive ingredients in the same concentrations, are of the same dosage form, and have the same physico-chemical characteristics, which includes being within or equal to the pH range of the RLNAD, in order to be eligible for a biowaiver.

The final component of the BE technical section is AOI. AOI for a generic new animal drug is part of the BE technical section rather than its own technical section since the AOI pertains solely to the Agency's determination of BE.‡

PATENT CERTIFICATION AND MARKETING EXCLUSIVITY§,¶

As part of the generic new animal drug approval process, a patent certification is required for all patents claiming the drug substance, drug product, or method of use (indication) for the RLNAD. For each patent, the patent number must be provided along with a certification that, in the sponsor's opinion and to the best of their knowledge, one of the following applies:

---

* Section 512(n)(1)(E) of the Act
† GFI #35: Bioequivalence Guidance
‡ 21 CFR 314.94(a)(7)
§ Section 512(n)(1)(H) of the Act
¶ Section 512(c)(2)(F) of the Act

1. The patent information has not been submitted to the FDA (Paragraph I Certification)
2. The patent has expired (Paragraph II Certification)
3. The patent remains enforceable until a specific date on which the patent will expire (Paragraph III Certification)
4. That the patent is invalid, unenforceable, or will not be infringed by the manufacture, use, or sale of the generic new animal drug product (Paragraph IV Certification)

If there are no listed patents for the RLNAD, a No Relevant Patent statement is provided, stating that no patent exists for the RLNAD claiming the drug substance, drug product, or method of use. For situations in which a patent claims a method of use for the RLNAD that the labeling of the proposed generic new animal drug does not include, a statement must be submitted explaining that the method of use patent does not claim any of the proposed indications for the generic new animal drug.[*]

As mentioned above, GADPTRA establishes periods of marketing exclusivity for reference products. A marketing exclusivity is the period of time during which the FDA-CVM will not approve a generic copy of the approved RLNAD. The Act provides for 5 years of marketing exclusivity for a new animal drug product that has not been previously approved in any NADA, or 3 years of marketing exclusivity for a new approved use of a NADA (e.g., adding a new parasite to the label of an anthelminthic).[†‡] Patent information and exclusivity periods of NADAs are made available to the public through a publication known as the Green Book.[§]

LABELING[¶]

All proposed generic new animal drugs will be labeled for the same species and claim(s) as the RLNAD, unless there are species or claims covered by patent or exclusivity protection. Additionally, the generic new animal drug labeling will be the same as the RLNAD labeling, meaning that the organization and content of the labeling are the same. Exceptions to the "same as" rule include items specific to the generic new animal drug, such as proprietary name, logo, company name and address, and changes resulting from an approved suitability petition (see below), or differences in the manufacturers distributing or producing the product.

SUITABILITY PETITIONS[**]

There are certain differences between a proposed generic new animal drug and an RLNAD that may be allowed through a suitability petition (SP). By submitting an

---

[*] Section 512(n)(1)(I) of the Act
[†] Section 512(c)(2)(F)(i) of the Act
[‡] Section 512(c)(2)(F)(ii) of the Act
[§] https://animaldrugsatfda.fda.gov/adafda/views/#/search
[¶] Section 512(n)(1)(F) of the Act
[**] Section 512(n)(3) of the Act

SP, permission is requested to submit an ANADA for a generic new animal drug that differs from the RLNAD in one of the active ingredients in a combination product, its route of administration, dosage form, strength, or in its use with other animal drugs in animal feed. If the differences between the proposed generic new animal drug and RLNAD are such that safety and effectiveness studies are not required, the SP is approved. The sponsor can file an ANADA after the SP is approved. Ideally, the sponsor would seek SP approval prior to opening a JINAD file.

ALTERNATIVE APPROVAL PATHWAYS: CONDITIONAL APPROVAL AND INDEX LISTING*

Under the Act, seven animal species are defined as "major species": dogs, cats, horses, cattle, pigs, chickens, and turkeys. All other species are considered "minor species." Under this dichotomy, ferrets are considered a minor species, as are goats, scarlet macaws, leopard geckos, red-eyed tree frogs, bettas, and, yes, even honeybees! Similarly, the Act defines a "minor use" as the use of a new animal drug in a major species for a condition which occurs either infrequently or in a limited geographical area and in a small number of animals per year. Examples of a minor use in a major species could be a rare cardiac disorder which occurs in fewer than the published "small number of animals" for dogs (currently 70,000) or an uncommon metabolic disorder in horses (the current small number is 50,000). These definitions are important to the new animal drug approval process, as the Minor Use and Minor Species Animal Health Act of 2004 (which amended the Act itself) established incentives for sponsors to pursue drug approvals for uncommon conditions in major species (similar to the Orphan Drug Act of 1983 which created financial incentives for development of a drug or biologic to treat rare or neglected tropical diseases in humans) and species with small populations. These incentives are available through the Office of Minor Use and Minor Species Animal Drug Development (OMUMS) within the FDA-CVM.

In addition to the NADA and ANADA pathways described in the preceding sections, new animal drugs can be legally marketed in the United States using the conditional approval and index listing pathways. To receive a conditional approval for a new animal drug, several requirements must be met. First, the new animal drug must be intended for use in a minor species or for a Minor Use in a Major Species (MUMS). Second, all technical sections with the exception of the EFF technical section must be complete prior to conditional approval. In place of the EFF technical section, the sponsor must show a "reasonable expectation of effectiveness" prior to conditional approval. For example, the FDA-CVM conditionally approved an anti-neoplastic drug for the treatment of lymphoma in dogs after the sponsor demonstrated positive results in two pilot studies. A conditional approval is effective for a 1-year period and is renewable for up to four additional 1-year terms, provided, amongst other things, that the sponsor demonstrates progress toward establishing effectiveness and ultimate full approval under an NADA.

---

* Section 571 of the Act

In 2018, Congress passed amendments to the Act, allowing for expanded conditional approval for new animal drugs that do not meet MUMS criteria.* Under these amendments, a new animal drug may be conditionally approved if that new animal drug meets two criteria. First, the new animal drug must either be intended to treat a serious or life-threatening disease or condition or address an unmet animal or human health need. Second, demonstrating effectiveness for the new animal drug would require a complex or particularly difficult study or studies. Sponsors who wish to pursue expanded conditional approval are encouraged to contact the FDA-CVM early in the development process for their new animal drug.

Index listing is the fourth pathway for legally marketing a new animal drug in the United States. The Index of Legally Marketed Unapproved New Animal Drugs for Minor Species (the Index) is limited to non-food-producing minor species (or some early life stages of food-producing species) that are too rare or varied for a sponsor to reasonably conduct adequately designed and well-controlled safety and effectiveness studies.† For example, a new animal drug intended to treat an infrequent neoplastic disease in a rare parrot species or a viral infection during the larval stage of an ornamental fish species may fit this pathway. Prior to listing in the index, the sponsor proposes a Qualified Expert Panel. OMUMS verifies that members of this panel are qualified and do not have any conflict of interest. OMUMS then reviews the risk–benefit analysis summarized in a final report from the panel as part of the sponsor's request for addition to the Index.

While not a pathway for legal marketing and approval, new animal drug designation is an incentive established by the MUMS Act for sponsors of MUMS drugs. Similar to the orphan drug status for human pharmaceuticals, this designation program provides incentives to sponsors. Grants are available for sponsors of designated new animal drugs to defray costs associated with conducting safety and effectiveness studies. Additionally, designation provides exclusive marketing rights for a period of 7 years following an approval or conditional approval.‡ Exclusive marketing rights for designated new animal drugs means that the sponsor will face no competition from another sponsor marketing the same drug in the same dosage form for the same intended use for 7 years (as opposed to the 3- and 5-year periods of marketing exclusivity described above in *Generic New Animal Drugs*). As a condition of this status, sponsors of these new animal drugs must demonstrate progress toward approval or conditional approval by making annual updates to the FDA-CVM once a designation status has been granted. OMUMS maintains a public list of approved or conditionally approved drugs with current designations.§ The FDA-CVM is committed not only to ensuring that marketed new animal drugs are safe and effective, but also to working with sponsors to bring new animal drugs to market, even for those species few in number or disease conditions rare in occurrence.

---

* Draft GFI #261: Eligibility Criteria for Expanded Conditional Approval for New Animal Drugs
† www.fda.gov/animal-veterinary/minor-useminor-species/index-legally-marketed-unapproved-new-animal-drugs-minor-species
‡ Section 573(c) of the Act
§ www.fda.gov/animal-veterinary/minor-useminor-species/designations-list

FDA-CVM'S POST-APPROVAL ROLE

Once a new animal drug is approved and marketed, the FDA-CVM begins post-approval monitoring to assure the continued safety and effectiveness of the marketed new animal drug. The Office of Surveillance and Compliance (OSC) is responsible for monitoring adverse drug experiences (ADEs) and changes in or lack of effectiveness for the approved new animal drug. In addition, the OSC reviews all product labeling and promotional materials, working with the sponsor and the ONADE to revise these documents as new information becomes available (e.g., if a new safety risk becomes apparent post-marketing, the label may be revised to warn veterinarians and owners of this risk). Sponsors are required to provide the FDA-CVM with regular pharmacovigilance reports and reports identifying the quantity of drug marketed in the United States.* The responsibilities of the OSC extend beyond post-approval marketing to include monitoring animal food, enforcing industry compliance with the Act, and monitoring the conduct of clinical investigators and sponsors of clinical investigations to make sure Good Laboratory Practices (GLPs) are maintained, just to name a few. The work conducted by the OSC is vital to helping the FDA-CVM protect human and animal health.

NAVIGATING THE NEW ANIMAL DRUG APPROVAL PROCESS: A ROADMAP FOR RESEARCHERS

The new animal drug approval process is based on scientific data submitted by a sponsor to support each technical section and meet regulatory requirements as discussed previously in this chapter. The planning, conducting, analyzing, and submitting of the required data and supportive information involves a significant resource investment, primarily time and money. For this reason, a large majority of approved new animal drugs are developed, owned, and marketed by large national and international pharmaceutical companies; however, smaller research groups such as academics and start-up laboratories can successfully complete the approval process as well.

Additionally, researchers can assist start-up laboratories and pharmaceutical companies with the new animal drug approval process by conducting early discovery and proof-of-concept research in accordance with new animal drug approval standards (e.g., Good Laboratory Practices, GLPs), such that this research can be readily leveraged if approval is sought for a product conceived from that research. Early quality, GLP- or GCP-conforming research can even expedite the approval process by answering essential regulatory questions, especially for animal cell-based products. For example, investigations of the biodistribution and survival of a particular cell type conducted by a researcher under GLP regulations might be used to inform the requirements for target animal safety studies for a product derived from those cells, once the approval process begins.

---

* 21 CFR 514.80

While the scope of what is required for a new animal drug approval may seem complex, the rigorous standards by which the law and regulations require a sponsor to demonstrate the safety and effectiveness of a new animal drug function to protect animals and humans alike and ensure consumer confidence in these drugs. To begin, sponsors are encouraged to visit the FDA-CVM's website. This website contains helpful information and numerous Guidance for Industry (GFI) documents which represent the agency's current thinking on various aspects of the approval process (see *References* at the end of this chapter). Sponsors new to working with the FDA-CVM are strongly encouraged to communicate with the FDA-CVM early in their product development program (e.g., at the proof-of-concept stage). The FDA-CVM is committed to open dialogue with sponsors at any point in the development of a new animal drug, from the initial experiments at the benchtop to large, multi-site field studies. The agency meets with sponsors to answer their questions and give feedback on all aspects of product development, study design, and data submissions.

For certain emerging technologies including animal cell-based products, the FDA-CVM has established a pilot Veterinary Innovation Program (VIP). The goal of the VIP is to facilitate advancements in development of innovative animal products by providing greater certainty in the regulatory process, encouraging development and research, and supporting an efficient and predictable pathway to approval. The VIP offers sponsors multiple opportunities for intensive interaction and helpful dialogue. For example, sponsors of products accepted into the VIP can take advantage of pre-review and post-review feedback prior to or following the review of each major technical section. The VIP also offers the option of stopping and restarting the review clock, allowing sponsors to address data gaps within a technical section without losing their places in the review queue. Both of these benefits may reduce the number of review cycles and reduce the overall time to approval. Sponsors of animal cell-based products are highly encouraged to explore these benefits and others described on the VIP website.*

In addition to the costs incurred by the sponsor during the drug development phase, the Animal Drug User Fee Act (ADUFA) and Animal Generic Drug User Fee Act (AGDUFA) allow the FDA-CVM to collect user fees for certain animal drug applications, products, establishments, and sponsors. However, in some specific situations, sponsors may be granted a fee waiver. Under ADUFA, sponsors may qualify for a significant barrier to innovation (BI), fees exceed costs (FEC), free choice feeds (FT), Minor Use in a Minor Species (MUMS), or small business (SB) waiver. AGDUFA provides for a MUMS waiver. As each sponsor's situation and product are different, sponsors are encouraged to talk with the FDA-CVM prior to opening an investigational file to explore the available waiver options.

By working together, researchers and the FDA-CVM can ensure that safe and effective, quality manufactured, and properly labeled new animal drugs are readily available to pet owners, livestock producers, and veterinarians. Achieving

---

* www.fda.gov/animal-veterinary/animals-intentional-genomic-alterations/vip-veterinary-innov ation-program

FDA-CVM approval for a new animal drug not only fulfills the legal responsibilities of a sponsor, but also provides animal owners, producers, and veterinarians with confidence in that approved drug. Whether a new animal drug is composed of a small molecule or living cells, or is intended for use in dogs or the rarest of endangered species, a new animal drug approval is the culmination of a sponsor's demonstration to experts in a variety of fields and disciplines that their drug is safe for the use on its label and that use is supported by sound science. Ultimately, the new animal drug approval process allows the FDA-CVM to fulfill its mission to protect human and animal health by partnering with sponsors, whether large corporations or researchers, who also have the best interests of humans, animals, and the public health at the forefront of their efforts.

Quick Acronym/Definition Guide

ACRONYM	MEANING
ACS	Autologous conditioned serum
ADE	Adverse drug experience
ADI	Acceptable daily intake
ADUFA	Animal Drug User Fee Act
AGDUFA	Animal Generic Drug User Fee Act
ANADA	Abbreviated New Animal Drug Application
AOI	All other information
APHIS	Animal and Plant Health Inspection Service
API	Active pharmaceutical ingredient
AUC	Area under the curve
BE	Bioequivalence
BI	Barrier to innovation
cGMP	Current Good Manufacturing Practices
C_{max}	Maximum observed drug concentration
CMC	Chemistry, manufacturing, and controls
CVB	Center for Veterinary Biologics
DES	Diethylstilbestrol
EA	Environmental assessment
EFF	Effectiveness
EPA	Environmental Protection Agency
FEC	Fees exceed costs
FDA	Food and Drug Administration
FDA-CVM	Food and Drug Administration Center for Veterinary Medicine
FONSI	Finding of No Significant Impact
FT	Free choice feeds
GADPTRA	Generic Animal Drug and Patent Term Restoration Act
GCP	Good Clinical Practice
GFI	Guidance for Industry
GLP	Good Laboratory Practice
HFS	Human food safety

(Continued)

Quick Acronym/Definition Guide

ACRONYM	MEANING
HSC	Hematopoietic stem cell
INAD	Investigational New Animal Drug
iPSC	Induced pluripotent stem cell
JINAD	Generic Investigational New Animal Drug
MSC	Mesenchymal/multipotent stem/stromal cell
MUMS	Minor use in a major species, minor species
NADA	New Animal Drug Application
NEPA	National Environmental Policy Act
NSAID	Non-steroidal anti-inflammatory drug
NV	Environmental impact
OMUMS	Office of Minor Use and Minor Species Animal Drug Development
ONADE	Office of New Animal Drug Evaluation
OSC	Office of Surveillance and Compliance
PID	Pre-investigational development
ppb	Parts per billion
ppm	Parts per million
PRP	Platelet-rich plasma
RLNAD	Referenced Listed New Animal Drug
SB	Small business
SP	Suitability petition
TAS	Target animal safety
T_{max}	Time to maximum concentration
USDA	United States Department of Agriculture
VIP	Veterinary Innovation Program

REFERENCES

Animal Drugs @ FDA. https://animaldrugsatfda.fda.gov/adafda/views/#/search.

Animal Drug User Fee Act (ADUFA) Website. www.fda.gov/industry/fda-user-fee-programs/animal-drug-user-fee-act-adufa.

Animal Generic Drug User Fee Act Website. www.fda.gov/industry/fda-user-fee-programs/animal-generic-drug-user-fee-act-agdufa.

Center for Veterinary Medicine Main Website. www.fda.gov/animal-veterinary.

Center for Veterinary Medicine Policies and Procedures Website. www.fda.gov/animal-veterinary/guidance-regulations/policies-procedures-manual.

Draft GFI #261: Eligibility Criteria for Expanded Conditional Approval for New Animal Drugs. www.fda.gov/media/130706/download.

Electronic Code of Federal Regulations (eCFR). www.ecfr.gov/cgi-bin/ECFR?page=browse.

Federal Food, Drug, and Cosmetic Act. https://legcounsel.house.gov/Comps/Federal%20Food,%20Drug,%20And%20Cosmetic%20Act.pdf.

From an Idea to the Marketplace: The Journey of an Animal Drug through the Approval Process. www.fda.gov/animal-veterinary/animal-health-literacy/idea-marketplace-journey-animal-drug-through-approval-process.

GFI #35: Bioequivalence Guidance. www.fda.gov/media/70115/download.

GFI #132: Administrative Applications and the Phased Review Process. www.fda.gov/media/70029/download.

GFI #185 (VICH GL43): Target Animal Safety for Veterinary Pharmaceutical Products. www.fda.gov/media/70438/download.

GFI #218: Cell-Based Products for Animal Use. www.fda.gov/media/88925/download.

GFI #224 (VICH GL52): Bioequivalence: Blood Level Bioequivalence Study. www.fda.gov/media/89840/download.

Index of FDA-CVM Guidance for Industry (GFI) Documents. www.fda.gov/animal-veterinary/guidance-regulations/guidance-industry.

Veterinary Innovation Program (VIP) Website. www.fda.gov/animal-veterinary/animals-intentional-genomic-alterations/vip-veterinary-innovation-program.

11 Clinical Trials, Patient Recruitment and Advertising

Krista K. Vermillion

CONTENTS

Coming together is a beginning, staying together is progress and working
together is *success*.

– Henry Ford

INTRODUCTION

Once study designs have been composed and contracts have been signed, investigators can find themselves geared up and ready to go with one last question,
"Where are the patients?" There is a vast amount of text that researchers can
find regarding recruitment in human clinical trials, but very little, if any, has
been published about recruitment in the animal population. Although the patient
populations differ quite a bit, *the recruitment population is the same* – humans.
With that in mind, our approach to recruitment in a veterinary trial can be based
on foundations built in human trials.

Before any trial begins, the investigator will need to come up with a plan
regarding where, when and how he/she will be recruiting participants. This chapter will walk you through the basics of what is needed to construct a recruitment
timeline, build a recruitment plan and create recruitment materials depending on
who you are approaching and your budget.

Let's get this study started!

TIMELINES

The trouble is, you think you have time.

– Buddha

Depending on how you obtained your funding, you might have already been required
to create a recruitment timeline for funders or sponsors. If not, you will still need to
spend some time mapping out a timeline in order to determine how many patients
need to be enrolled in your study weekly/monthly/quarterly/yearly. Whether or not
you are setting up a single site or a multi-site trial, a timeline is imperative. If multi-
site, then the ultimate responsibility falls to the national Principal Investigator to set
up a timeline that matches the needs of trial recruitment from site to site. It's the
same for single site trials as well. Although the study team might be smaller, there
is still a budget to adhere to, which will always drive your timelines.

I prefer a backwards approach. What is your ultimate stop? Is it 50 patients in 2
years? If so, start your timeline there; for example, let's say you're starting your trial
in January 2020. I would start planning my timeline in terms of what is needed to
bring your trial to a successful last patient enrollment in January 2022. Always give
yourself a slow period at the beginning of the timeline. This gives study teams time
to get into their own groove, learn who should be consenting (we'll talk about this
later), learn what works in approach and learn the protocol front to back. If you look
at 24 months of participants, it would be easy to determine a recruitment rate of
approximately two patients a month, with a month or two being a higher enrolling
month. But a realistic study team would automatically assume that your recruitment

rate will be lower in the first three months of your trial's enrolling period – planning for one patient a month in that time period at most. This lag will mean that you will have to enroll at least two, if not three, per month for the rest of the enrolling period. While this is a fairly simple concept, it is not uncommon for the timing of enrollment to be overlooked. You should also be holistically realistic in your timeline planning. Enrollments almost always lag from November–December because of holidays and June–August can become slow because of vacations for both study staff and possible participants. With all of this in mind, in planning a 24-month enrollment period for 50 patients, it would be smart to set your enrollment bar at three per month knowing that it will take time to create a groove in your staff and also knowing that you will have slower enrollment periods.

To prepare a professional looking timeline, there are many free programs and templates online to start with. I recommend going this route and creating an aesthetically pleasing timeline to take your study from the back of a napkin to reality. Visuals are a good way to get your study team started and to wrap their minds around the task at hand. Have fun with your timelines and if possible, bring in study team members to collaborate in their creation. Your timeline is an operational document that you will reference almost as much as your protocol or Manual of Operations.

CREATE A PLAN

The next solid step in recruitment is to create a recruitment plan. Some funding opportunities that the National Institutes of Health (NIH) presently offers require a recruitment plan as part of a grant package and also as an operational document requirement after an investigator receives funding. A recruitment plan not only helps an investigator to map out his/her approach to recruiting participants for the trial, it will also help identify barriers that might be faced along the journey to last patient in. Or, in some cases, the barriers that seem to block any patient recruitment at all. Later on in this chapter, we will break down the creation of a recruitment plan. The recruitment plan model that we will discuss in this chapter is adaptable to different types of funding, i.e., different types of advertising budgets and regulatory requirements. It is possible to recruit patients with little to no budget at all, but if an investigator has the opportunity to work advertising into their budget while working with a funder, more is better.

ADVERTISING YOUR TRIAL

Communication *works* for those who work at it.

– **John Powell**

Whether engaging in human or animal research, every investigator is faced with the daunting prospect of finding patients for their trials. Not every screened patient will meet inclusion/exclusion criteria and sometimes, an investigator will over-estimate the number of potential participants he/she sees in day-to-day practice, leaving them dazed and confused when participants don't come pouring in for their new trial. Experienced researchers value the need for advertising money and often, the more experienced researchers are also able to get a larger budget to fund these efforts. Don't get discouraged if you don't fall into the big budget category, however, because there are many different ways to recruit for a clinical trial that are free or of minimal cost.

First, get organized and take the time to consider your target audience. For veterinary trials, this audience will most likely be divided into two groups: Other veterinarians in your area and pet owners in your area. The way that you will approach them will differ across the board. This chapter section will discuss free advertising for vets and pet owners and paid advertising for vets and pet owners. No matter who your audience, it is important to think specifically, not broadly. Focus on what might work for your particular disease, animal and area.

Let's first take a look at some relatively inexpensive or free ways to spread the word about your trial.

Institutional Websites

If you are practicing research at a large academic institution, they most likely already have a website platform that will support information about your trial. Some institutions might offer help in the content for this page, while others might leave this up to the investigator to provide. When creating content for a website, a good rule of thumb is to follow most Institutional Review Boards (IRB) consent rule of keeping language to a 6th or 7th grade level. A trap more than one investigator has fallen into is writing website content (or social media content or flyer content) at a provider level, not a layman's level. Don't do that! No matter what avenue you take, the animal's owner is who you will eventually need to sign a consent form, and no one likes to be approached with information that doesn't make sense to them. Website content should be easy to understand with clear and concise ways to sign up for the trial and easy to find contact information. Don't make folks search for ways to reach you. Contact information should be available in several different places on a website and, very importantly, *updated* as personnel, numbers and emails change.

Email Blasts

Email blasts are also a free way to spread the word about your trial. Many academic research institutions offer this service and will work with an investigator to create an institutional blurb about their trial.

Flyers and Face to Face

Let's go old school for a moment. A recruitment flyer or pamphlet can take you a long way in finding participants for your trial. For any trial, be it human or animal, the best avenue will be to create two flyers – one for providers and one for pet owners. Their look and verbiage will be different although the message will be the same.

For a provider's flyer, it is a good idea to spend time explaining the history of the disease you are studying, the financial impact that this disease can have and also the opportunity to do translational research on animals for this particular disease, explaining why. A brief description of what a pet's family can expect and compensation should be included in the flyer. Also, just like the website, good contact information that is always updated should conclude the text for a flyer. For a pet owner flyer, reasoning for the trial should be included with a brief history of the disease and a focus on cost to a family and impact to the pet. Procedures and interventions that the family can expect should be briefly discussed as well. Benefits to the pet and pet family should be highlighted, for instance, if a pet gets costly imaging included in their participation, this should be outlined in the text of the flyer. A patient forward flyer should be interesting to the eye and conclude with good contact information as well. Often, across campuses and in providers' offices, you will see study flyers with tear off contact tabs running along the bottom of the flyer. This isn't a bad idea, but in this digital age, most interested parties can just take a picture of the flyer and keep contact information that way.

A study pamphlet should be considered for a more complicated trial so that more information can be poured into possible participants or their care providers. It's not a good idea to try to squeeze too much information onto a simple flyer. Too much text can make a flyer hard to read and can shut down a possible participant's interest. *Of note, it is assumed that patient facing documents will need approval from IRBs. Below, you will see two flyer examples* (Table 11.1 and Table 11.2).

SOCIAL MEDIA

Social media platforms can provide an excellent resource for recruitment into research trials. The idea of using social media for recruitment into a trial is a rather new concept and many times thought of as being a free platform for advertising

---

TABLE 11.1

Example of Pamphlet/Flyer Components Used to Advertise to Providers (i.e., Veterinarians)

A Double Blind, Randomized Interventional Trial Investigating Hemangiosarcoma in Elderly Dogs Aged 8 and Up

History	Our Research
Provide a detailed history of the disease here. Mention its impact on canine health, the instances per year and the overall costs that the disease is responsible for...	Explain what your research is about – list your inclusion/exclusion criteria and your research question. Detail is good here.
Procedures	**Contact Us**
Outline the procedures and visits that participation in this trial will entail.	Email Phone number Fax Website

TABLE 11.2

Example of a Pamphlet/Flyer Designed for Pet Owners*

A Research Study to Find Out More About Cancer in Older Pets

What Are We Trying to Find Out?	How Can You Help?
History	Highlight how the pet owner is helping your
Write a brief history regarding the	team and other pets. Make sure to drum up the
disease you're studying here.	positives – participation is simple, can be
	advantageous to you and your pet and it could
	help save pets' lives.
Procedures	**Compensation**
In this section, briefly list the procedures	If the owner is compensated, be sure to mention
the pet owner can expect.	that a study team member will discuss this with
	the pet owner.
Our Research	**Contact Us**
This is a good place to list a simple	Email
version of your inclusion/exclusion	Phone number
criteria and your research question.	Fax
	Website

* The pet owner pamphlet/flyer should be friendly and inviting. Including an illustration(s) and/or photograph(s) of a pet(s) is highly recommended.

a trial. The truth is, the most effective advertising on Facebook is actually paid for, but there are other ways to use social media to an investigator's advantage. This chapter will not delve into the ethics involved in social media recruitment, although every researcher should investigate negative aspects of social media and make the best decisions for his/her patient population based on these findings.

Social media provides an accessible way to engage an audience and find out exactly what is being said about a disease or about the research being conducted about this disease. Platforms, such as Facebook (www.facebook.com), can be cost-effective, efficient and successful in engaging a diverse range of individuals (Ryan, 2013, 35–39). When considering using social media, go back to your target. Who are you trying to engage? One thing to avoid at all costs is creating a social media page without the personnel to man it. A group or page with four members looks worse than having no group at all. For veterinary trials, it might be a good idea to reach out to the pet groups that have already been created in your area. It's easy to contact the administrator of these groups and ask if you can plug your research on their group's feed. This is an ideal place to post that flyer! If you do create your own page, make sure that there is someone on your study team to post interesting content and metrics that are relevant to your trial. For instance, you can post first participant enrolled, milestones reached and interesting articles about the particular disease cohort that is being studied. This type of engagement can go a long way and the only cost is man power.

There are professional social media platforms, such as LinkedIn (www.linkedin.com), that provide a space to engage other providers in your area. This is where the more complex, provider-driven flyer should be posted. You can also reach out to administrators of professional groups on platforms like these to start a conversation about the research that you are conducting. Keeping your own LinkedIn (or other professional social media platform) page activated and updated is invaluable here.

The key to advertising on little to no budget is creativity. If you are invited to speak at a gathering, shamelessly plug your study. Don't be afraid to call colleagues in your area to inform them of your trial and ask if you can leave a flyer or brochure in their waiting room. Contact a Facebook pet owner group and ask if you can spread the word within that group. None of these things cost money and they can go a long way.

Final note: Of all of the recruitment options available to you, face-to-face interaction with pet families or other providers will always be the most effective way to attract possible participants to your trial.

For those investigators with funds for advertising, there are a few more avenues of recruitment available.

PRINT

A recent article in Forbes focused on research that found that paper advertising is more memorable and more effective in engagement than digital advertising. It also stated that readers trust paper advertising more and that print maximizes sensory appeal (Dooley, 2016). While there is a lot of focus on digital advertising, don't forget the older standard. Print ads can vary in price depending on the medium, so take some time to research the cost of direct mail, community newspapers and larger market newspapers or local magazines. Most newspapers will charge based on size, so consider taking the very basics of your flyer and breaking it down in an appealing fractioned column format. If your study is multi-site, you might also consider advertising in a veterinary journal, but most of the time, it will behoove you to stay local and targeted in your efforts. *Below, you will see an example of a print ad* (Table 11.3).

RADIO

According to the News Generation website (www.newsgeneration.com), radio is the leading reach platform with 93% of us listening daily. Radio costs vary from market to market and also from station to station. They also vary depending on what you are looking for with different options to choose from, including time (usually 5- to 10-second increments) and time of day. Any radio advertising department will be willing to discuss peak times for advertising and it costs nothing to reach out to your local radio stations and price it out. The best case scenario is to get these numbers while you're creating your budget. If you're able to afford and utilize radio as a platform, keep your verbiage as simple as possible. For instance, "Researchers at Jefferson State University are trying to find out the causes of cancer in older dogs. Participants will be treated with care. At Jefferson State, we believe that research is the hope for tomorrow. Call us at 555-555-5555." That's a solid 15-second ad. It's simple and won't overwhelm or bore listeners. Most people need to hear the same message several times for it to "stick", so the more you can run the ad, the better.

TABLE 11.3

Example of a Print Ad Published in a Local Newspaper

Clinical Trial for Cats with Diabetes	
Minimally Invasive and Free of Charge	
Brand/logo goes here	We are offering a free-of-charge, minimally invasive treatment for cats with diabetes. Eligible cats will receive bloodwork and ultrasound to determine if your cat may respond well to the treatment.
Photo of attractive cat placed here	For full details about the study and to see if your cat may be eligible, please contact us email/phone number/fax
For more information, please visit https://xxx.xxx.edu	

METRICS

One of the most important facets in advertising your study is measuring what works. If you don't track your metrics, you are bound to make the same mistake over and over again. Carefully track how each participant came to be in your study. If you're not seeing a valuable return from an ad, cut that ad and try another tactic.

No matter what you can afford, always carefully consider your audience. From your own practice, you might be able to get a feel of what mediums could reach your particular customer base the quickest and most efficiently. For instance, if you have many elderly pet owners in your practice, take into consideration that they might not be searching the internet every day, but they could be listening to the radio or reading the local newspaper.

ONE MORE QUICK THOUGHT

If you are running an acute care study, your most valuable tool will be your patient flyer or brochure and your study staff (face to face). Don't waste money and time on advertising when a study decision needs to be made in a short window, for example, an implanted device in a pet that has recently had a stroke. Advertising works best with chronic disease.

THE RECRUITMENT PLAN

> By failing to *prepare*, you are preparing to fail.
>
> **– Benjamin Franklin**

An invaluable tool for recruitment is taking the time to come up with a solid plan with your study team. This goes beyond thinking about it and discussing it in a staff meeting. A good rule is to draft a plan and then review it with everyone who is involved in the recruitment of your trial. Recruitment plans differ from study to study and they also differ if your study is a single site vs. multi-site. This chapter section will give general tips for creating a recruitment plan for both single site and multi-site trials. The sections that could be included in a recruitment plan for a veterinary trial are as follows.

STUDY INTRODUCTION

It might feel a bit redundant to create a document that is separate from your protocol, but also contains similar introduction information. Consider this: The recruitment plan should be considered an operational document that stands the test of time. The cover page should mirror the protocol title page with the study title and logo if applicable. It should be handy for a team member to grab and reference at any time if they're trying to remember the timing of screening events and consent. The plan itself won't contain the intricacies of study visits or statistics, but should be a clear cut path to all of the stages of recruitment from screening through consent. With this in mind, the Recruitment Plan study introduction pages should contain the following:

- Quick scientific history and background of study
- Inclusion/exclusion criteria
- Schedule of events

*Reminder: A good investigator keeps in mind at the beginning of the study that most study staff will experience personnel turnover. The recruitment plan can help with the training of the study team. You should be easily able to turn the information within a recruitment plan into a training module or in-service slides. This document is created specifically for your study team to take the guess work out of recruitment.

WHERE WILL WE FIND PARTICIPANTS?

From the beginning of the trial, all personnel should have a very clear idea of where their participant pool will be coming from. For most veterinary trials, participants will be coming through vet referrals and interested pet owners. Concise methods of approach should be outlined in the recruitment plan for each recruitment pathway.

For veterinary referrals:

- Include the names and contact information of all veterinary practices that you foresee referrals coming from
- Include a telephone or email script for an introduction note to veterinary practice staff that provides basic information about your trial
- Create a protocol synopsis to send with the introduction note and attach it as an appendix
- Create a simple FAQ sheet of dos and don'ts for study staff if you are worried about professionalism with colleagues
- Attach veterinary flyer in the recruitment plan appendix

For pet owners:

- Include different advertising avenues that might bring pet owners to the study
- Include a telephone and email script for return correspondence with an interested pet family
- Create a simple FAQ sheet of dos and don'ts for study staff if you are worried about professionalism in approach
- Attach pet owner flyer in recruitment plan appendix

This section should also contain the plan for gathering metrics of recruitment platforms. Study teams will want to create a log sheet or database to capture each participant that emails or calls with interest from an advertisement that he or she has seen or heard, has been referred from a veterinary practice or has come to your study through some other route. Set the standard of metric capture early and check in often to make sure that these elements are being saved. *Below is an example of a recruitment log* (Table 11.4).

BARRIERS TO RECRUITMENT

For any trial, it's important to think through the reasons that might make enrolling patients difficult or even impossible. This looks different for a single site study vs. a multi-site study.

TABLE 11.4
Example of a Recruitment Log

Cat Diabetes Study Recruitment Log

Screen ID	Date	Time	Name	Email	Phone	Source	Comment	Participant
C-001	02.15.20	8am	Joe Smith	jsmith@ gmail. com	555-5555	Facebook	n/a	Y
C-002	03.03.20	10:30am	Jane Doe	jdoe@ aol.com	222-2222	Dr. Kind	Has two additional cases	N
C-003	04.11.20	2pm						
C-004	05.13.20	4:30pm						
C-005	07.02.20	8am						
C-006	07.26.20	8:30am						
C-007	08.27.20	1pm						
C-008	09.12.20	9am						
C-009	11.11.20	9:30am						
C-010	12.21.20	9am						

TABLE 11.5

Example of a SWOT (Strengths, Weaknesses, Opportunities, Threats) Analysis of a Clinical Trial

	Canine Cancer in Older Pets Study	
Strengths	1. Experienced study team	
	2. Large recruitment population	
	3. Nice budget for advertising	
Weaknesses	1. Short recruitment timeline	**Solutions**
	2. Short of staff	1. Set aggressive recruitment goals
		2. Arrange holiday coverage for both years
		3. Reach out to department to see if some funds can be used for new hire
Opportunities	1. Extra funding from dept. is a possibility if grant is accepted.	
Threats	1. Two study MRIs that aren't SOC	**Solutions**
		1. Detailed consent training

Single site: When trying to determine barriers to recruitment, meet with your team and others that have recruited for veterinary trials at your institution if possible. Creating a SWOT analysis could be a good idea here. SWOT stands for strengths, weaknesses, opportunities and threats and the creation of this analysis will give your team an opportunity to think through the benefits of the study, where the study is lacking, what the study has going for it and what can stop the study in its tracks. Once you've gone through these elements, it's most important to come up with solutions to the threats. Your SWOT could look like this (Table 11.5).

Multi-Site

For multi-site trials, the best approach to recognizing barriers is an easy to answer identification of barriers survey. The barriers that you face at your site might be different than the barriers faced at another. The survey can include questions based on barriers that you have identified locally and also have a section with free text room for a study team to add barriers that you might not be aware of. Once you have received the barriers from all sites, create a multi-site SWOT analysis table like the one above.

For both single site and multi-site trials, your SWOT table should be represented in your recruitment plan. More than likely, the barriers that one site might foresee will be relevant to the barriers that another site might not be expecting. Coming up with solutions beforehand will make things easier for all. *Your recruitment plan should be seen as a fluid document.* At study start-up, it might even seem light, but as issues arise, the document will grow and so will the solutions.

WHO IS YOUR TEAM?

Sitting down with your team and assigning study tasks presents a great opportunity to flush out who is doing what. Although you, as the investigator, might think that everyone is on the same page, you might be wrong. Make a list of all of the duties that might impact recruitment. Who is screening? Who is consenting the patients (see below)? Who is capturing screening and recruitment metrics? Who is creating a weekly/monthly screening report for the study team?

Every study will require different roles, so be open-minded as you create this recruitment task list. Assigning these recruitment responsibilities does not take the place of a Delegation of Responsibility log.

WHO WILL OBTAIN CONSENT?

Of all of the decisions made regarding recruitment in a trial, this could be the most important one. There are excellent Principal Investigators and terrific Research Coordinators who aren't successful at obtaining consent. This isn't an insurmountable problem! The key is to build an approach team where at least one member is completely comfortable obtaining consent. I use the word *comfortable* here because the consenting process is a highly personal one and although study staff can definitely get better at it as time goes on and with professional maturity, if a staff member isn't comfortable with the process or doesn't believe in the process, they simply shouldn't be doing it. A person who consistently can't sell your study can sink your ship quickly. This chapter sub-section will examine the elements of the consent and will offer tips and tricks to successfully consenting participants.

ELEMENTS OF CONSENT

There are several things that every consent form should offer and rights that every consent form should protect. Each consent form should make it clear who the lead investigator is, where the study is being activated, how many patients are being recruited and for how long. The form should contain an explanation of the disease being studied, what is being studied and the study questions that investigators are trying to answer – all of this information should be written in language that pet owners can comprehend. *If an investigator doubts that a pet owner understands the consent form or is not able to comprehend, that pet should not be included in the study.* The consent form should outline all procedures that will take place on this study protocol and should also include the number of visits that are expected and how long the enrollment period is. Consent forms can be tiered; for instance, if a protocol has an optional component to obtain biological samples, there can be two different areas for signature on the protocol. The pet owner might be comfortable with the study as a whole, but might not like the idea of bio samples being saved. Keep that in mind when you're designing your consent and if you would still want a pet's participation even without those samples, create a tiered consent. Risks and benefits of the trial must be included, and it must be clear that if a pet owner decides not to enroll their pet in the trial that the care and treatment of their pet will not be affected. All participation is voluntary, and it must also be explained that a participant can withdraw at any time.

Note: These elements are shared with the assumption that a trial is only being conducted within the United States.

Note: Every institution will have templates for consent creation and there is much information about creating a consent form online.

WHAT IS A STUDY TEAM'S RESPONSIBILITY IN SHARING THE CONSENT?

A study team must be honest, forthright, transparent and thorough in their consent approach. If the consent form is written well, it will cover each study procedure that will take place for the entirety of the trial and the person obtaining the consent is obligated to review each visit and procedure. *There is no need to re-consent at each visit if your study design hasn't changed and there have been no significant findings that could affect participation.*

THE ART OF THE CONSENT

Make no mistake, consenting a pet owner family isn't always easy, will require finesse and can easily be considered an art form. Below, you will find some tips and tricks to honing your consenting skills:

1. Research has shown that possible participants respond best to an investigator that is sitting down during discussions (Strasser et al., 2005, 489–497). Find a quiet spot and sit down with pet owners if at all possible.
2. Never apologize for your consent. This can be an automatic response in some. If a consent seems very long or if a protocol contains many different procedures that can present risk to the participant, some study staff might feel the need to apologize for it. This isn't necessary and could actually make a pet owner feel that there is something wrong with the protocol that is forcing study staff to apologize. Be confident, straightforward and empathetic in your approach. One example: While some imaging can present risk, it can also diagnose problems that pet owners would have never known about. When these imaging procedures are included in the protocol, this can negate the hefty cost of imaging for pet owners. While risks must be reviewed, the positives should be reviewed as well.
3. Re-consenting – Once a pet owner has consented for the entire protocol, there is no reason to re-consent because a study staff member fears that they need to be reminded of the risks. Consistently bringing up risks to pet owners could plant the seed of doubt of the safety of the protocol.

Conclude your Recruitment Plan with any other information that you think might be helpful to the study team and update as needed.

AVOIDING LOST TO FOLLOW-UPS

As wonderful as it is to consent a patient and have them participate in your trial, many trials aren't finished after one visit. Lost to follow-ups are a common hazard in research trials and careful planning during the recruitment phase of a trial might help to avoid them. Lost to follow-ups can happen to even the most diligent teams, but there are some tips and tricks to remember that can help ensure that they happen as infrequently as possible.

1. After consent send each pet owner home with an appointment card for the next visit. At the very least, the next visit should be in the books. Some study teams schedule all follow-ups during the first visit. It's really up to your team and what works for you.
2. Send out postcard reminders in advance of each follow-up appointment. Put reminders on your study schedule at approximately 2 weeks before every trial to send out these notifications. Remember to put the postcard in an envelope to ensure privacy.
3. Call and remind the pet owner 2 days before a visit occurs. It's a good idea to call at least twice and during different times of the day. If you leave a message, make it as general as possible with study contact information clearly stated.

WHEN DO YOU CONSIDER A PARTICIPANT LOST TO FOLLOW-UP?

I would consider a participant lost to follow-up 30 days after their last expected visit. Up until that moment, I would still send postcard reminders and do reminder calls, even without any contact. It's a good idea to adhere to a pre-decided contact schedule so that study staff don't feel that they need to constantly attempt contact until they get a response.

Also keep in mind that if a pet owner wants to withdraw from the study, they have every right to. If this happens, the Principal Investigator should get involved to find out the reasons why the participant is being withdrawn. This conversation should be respectful and if the pet owner still wishes to withdraw after the conversation, that participant's time in the trial is over.

As we discussed earlier in this section, your consent form should be worded to clearly convey expectations for the trial and the consent should be delivered in a way that there are no surprises to pet owners during the follow-up period. Don't gloss over the details of multiple visits, as this will only cause confusion and serve to harm participation later on in the trial.

CONCLUSION

Getting your study funded isn't the ending – it's the beginning of the journey. Get ready for the ride!

– **Krista Vermillion**

Having a career's worth of experiences simplifies making suggestions and offering tips and tricks in the area of recruitment in clinical trials. However, an investigator will never know exactly what to expect until enrollment begins. Careful planning will make this easier, but the biggest thing to plan for in recruiting for a clinical trial is constant change. Societal norms, new treatments and study staff transitions are bound to happen. With a strong recruitment foundation, different challenges that you can't possibly expect at the beginning of a trial will be easier met.

A few last tips and tricks:

1. Don't skip study team meetings. After a trial is up and running, it's easy to become complacent with meetings because of busy schedules. Canceling regular meetings can delay early awareness of possible issues.
2. In multi-site trials, check in with other study teams often in a regularly scheduled fashion. Same reasoning as above.
3. Be creative.
4. Have fun and don't lose sight of the reason behind the trial: Better treatments and faster cures.

Good luck in all of your research adventures!

REFERENCES

Dooley, Roger. "Paper Beats Digital in Many Ways, According to Neuroscience." *Forbes.* Accessed April 14, 2016. www.forbes.com/sites/rogerdooley/2015/09/16/paper-vs-digital/#53974b1e33c3.

"Radio Facts and Figures | News Generation | Broadcast Media Relations." *News Generation, Inc.* Accessed June 15, 2019. https://newsgeneration.com/broadcast-resources/radio-facts-and-figures/.

Ryan, Gemma S. "Online Social Networks for Patient Involvement and Recruitment in Clinical Research." *Nurse Researcher* 21(1) (2013), 35–39. doi:10.7748/nr2013.09.21.1.35.e302.

Strasser, Florian, J. L. Palmer, Jie Willey, Loren Shen, Ki Shin, Debra Sivesind, Estela Beale, and Eduardo Bruera. "Impact of Physician Sitting Versus Standing During Inpatient Oncology Consultations: Patients' Preference and Perception of Compassion and Duration. A Randomized Controlled Trial." *Journal of Pain and Symptom Management* 29(5) (2005), 489–497. doi:10.1016/j.jpainsymman.2004.08.011.

12 One Health
Animals, Humans, and Our Planet

Radford G. Davis

CONTENTS

ONE HEALTH—DEFINED

One Health is often defined by various stakeholders in slightly different ways, which sometimes lends a degree of fluidity and ambiguity simultaneously to the movement, allowing many nongovernmental organizations, government agencies, workers, researchers, administrators, etc., to claim a piece of the One Health pie. Including "One Health" in the title of a publication or a grant was a way to get noticed. However, getting these same stakeholders, these experts in human health, animal health, and the environment, to agree on a definition of One Health has been challenging, to say the least. One Health is not alone in its search for solid footing—Global Health, International Health, Planetary Health, EcoHealth...these fields also struggle for singular definition and unique identity. Each struggles to stand apart yet works in overlapping terrain, sometimes seeking the same objectives and outcomes. Today, however, the definition of One Health is more solid than ever, and its broad scope naturally encompasses to some degree many of these other health campaigns.

We could choose any definition of One Health from the myriad available, which vary only slightly, but for the purposes of this chapter we are going to use the definition used by the One Health Commission, which defines One Health as "...a collaborative, multisectoral, and transdisciplinary approach—working at the local, regional, national, and global levels—to achieve optimal health and well-being outcomes recognizing the interconnection between people, animals, plants, and their shared environment".[1]

It should be emphasized that One Health involves all three components, or pillars: humans, animals, and the environment, and the impact of each on the other. For many, the health of the human is the ultimate focus. For others, it may be the animal or the environment. One of the primary criticisms is that One Health research, funding, programs, and publications often focus on just two of the three components. For example, zoonoses, where the focus is on humans and animals but not the environmental component, which may significantly contribute to the risk of disease or its epidemiology. As will be emphasized throughout this chapter in our examination of the three pillars, a true One Health approach incorporates all three.

ONE HEALTH—THE EARLY YEARS

While One Health is a relatively new term, its core principles can be traced back nearly two millennia. Human health has been influenced by animals and our environment very likely dating back to the origins of humans roughly 2.5 million years ago,[2] and the divergence and eventual planetary domination of *Homo sapiens* beginning about 50,000 years ago.[2] Our relationship with our environment began to change dramatically as we adopted intentional domestication of plants approximately 11,000 years ago[3] and then the domestication of animals for food. The dog was the first animal to be domesticated, around 10,000 BCE in Southwest Asia, China, and North America.[3] This was followed by sheep, goats, and pigs around 8,000 BCE, primarily in Southwest Asia, then cows around 6,000 BCE.[3] The domestication of animals, specifically livestock, furnished humans with meat (supplanting game), milk, fertilizer, wool, leather, transportation, as well as draft power for plowing fields.[3] These things are still vital to many people today. Later, perhaps as early as 4,000 BCE, the domestication of the horse took place and became an advantageous tool in war, leading to many decisive military victories including that of the Spanish conquistador Francisco Pizarro who, with just 168 soldiers, 62 mounted on horses, conquered the Incan empire by overcoming its emperor Atahuallpa and his 80,000 soldiers in 1532.[3] As domestication of plants and animals spread and improved and the practice of intentional farming grew, more food was produced than could be gained through hunting and gathering. Human population numbers began to increase concomitantly. Humanity's footprint on the planet began to grow, for better and worse.

Aristotle (384–322 BCE) introduced the concept of comparative medicine in his examination of the common traits of animals and humans in his book series *Historia Animalium*.[4] Galen, a Greek physician who lived and worked in Rome and was born around 130 in Asia minor, dissected animals (though not humans, which was illegal[5]) and conducted animal experiments to understand the body, its functions, and to ultimately better understand disease.[6,7] Physician and veterinarian Giovanni Maria Lancisi (1654–1720) wrote about the role of the environment in the diseases of humans and animals and may have been one of the first to recommend the draining of swamps of Rome to prevent fevers (likely malaria).[4,8] Even before the concept of germ theory (the idea that microbes are responsible for infection and illness) caught on, it was recognized that poverty, crowding, and environmental conditions such as filth, foul water, dead and decaying animal carcasses, and human sewage were not good for a person. In 1348, during an outbreak of plague in Italy, early steps towards public health were taken to control plague, with the powers of authorities extending to recording of deaths, burials, marketing of food, and overseeing the sewage system, hospitals, hostelries, and even prostitution.[9] It is reported that Claude Bourgelat (1712–1779) founded the first veterinary school at Lyon, France, and with it an educational focus on animal health and human health.[4] The work of Louis-René Villermé (1782–1863) and Alexandre Parent-Duchâtelet (1790–1835) led to the creation of the veterinary specialty field of public hygiene.[4] Rudolf Virchow (1821–1902), an early pioneer in medicine, comparative pathology, and public health is given credit for noting the link between animal and human health and coining the term "zoonosis",[10] but there is some skepticism as to the authenticity of this.[11] Virchow worked out the life cycle of *Trichinella spiralis* in swine as well as its zoonotic implications.[10] He also recognized the impact that economic and social conditions could have on people's health. The beginnings of the contagion theory could be attributed to either the German Paracelsus (1490–1541) or the Italian Girolamo Fracastoro (1478–1553) in 1546, but it was Louis Pasteur (1822–1895) who in the 1860s demonstrated the existence of microbes and that disease was caused by infection with them.[6] Some of Pasteur's ground-breaking work involved zoonotic diseases, notably developing an animal vaccine for anthrax in 1881 and a human rabies vaccine in 1885. Bernhard Bang (1848–1932), a Danish veterinarian and physician, discovered the pathogen now known as *Brucella abortus* (also called Bang's disease) while investigating the cause of contagious abortion in cattle in Denmark.[12] Only later was it realized that this was also a zoonotic pathogen (Table 12.1).

In the 20th century, two veterinarians stand out as pioneers in One Health: James Steele (1913–2013) and Calvin Schwabe (1927–2006). In 1947, Steele founded a veterinary public health unit in what is today the Centers for Disease Control and Prevention and was Chief of this division.[4] Eventually, Steele took on the position as Assistant Surgeon General for veterinary affairs in 1968.[4] He was a highly regarded and skilled public health professional who worked globally on many issues and received numerous awards for his work.[13] Schwabe was a parasitologist and professor whose work on the zoonotic parasite *Echnococcus granulosus* set him on the path for examining the animal–human health connection and eventually advocating for "One Medicine" in his book *Veterinary Medicine and Human Health*.[4] Schwabe's One Medicine would later be renamed to what we know today as One Health.

ONE HEALTH—OUR CONNECTION WITH ANIMALS

Measles virus, a disease that has recently resurged in connection to low vaccination rates in some populations and the anti-vaccine movement, is one of the most

TABLE 12.1

Notable Persons in the History of One Health

Year	Name	Importance
384–322 BCE	Aristotle	Introduced concepts in comparative medicine
130	Galen	Animal dissection and experimentation to better understand the body and disease
1654–1720	Giovanni Maria Lancisi	Noted the role of environment in disease
1712–1779	Claude Bourgelat	Founded first veterinary school in Lyon, France with focus on animal and human health
1782–1863	Louis-René Villermé	Combined work helped establish the veterinary specialty of public hygiene
1790–1835	Alexandre Parent-Duchâtelet	French physician and one of the most eminent hygienists of the nineteenth century. Devoted his career to public health
1821–1902	Rudolf Virchow	Pioneer in medicine, comparative pathology, public health, and role of economic and social conditions on health. Discovered zoonotic importance of *Trichinella spiralis*
1822–1895	Louis Pasteur	Demonstrated existence of microbes and their role in animal and human diseases (the germ theory). Brought a scientific understanding to the fermentation process. Developed vaccines for rabies and anthrax
1848–1932	Bernhard Bang	Physician and veterinarian who discovered the zoonotic agent responsible for cattle abortion (*Brucella abortus*)
1913–2013	James Steele	Veterinarian and pioneer in public health. Chief of veterinary public health unit within the Centers for Disease Control and Prevention. Assistant Surgeon General for veterinary affairs, deputy assistant secretary for Health and Human Services. Pioneer in One Medicine
1927–2006	Calvin Schwabe	Veterinarian and professor. Elucidated zoonotic aspects of *Echnococcus granulosus*. Pioneer in bridging human and animal medicine and founder of the *One Medicine* concept

contagious diseases known to humanity with a reproductive number (R_0) of 12–18, meaning one active case can infect approximately 12–18 susceptible people.[14] This is far higher than that of Ebola virus, with an R_0 of around 1.5–2.5. Measles virus is in the genus Morbillivirus, a genus that also includes a number of animal viruses: dolphin and porpoise morbillivirus, phocine distemper virus, peste des petits ruminants (PPR) virus, canine distemper virus, and rinderpest virus (RPV). RPV, officially eradicated in 2011, killed hundreds of millions of livestock throughout history across Africa, Asia (including India), the Middle East, and Europe, destroying livelihoods, casting families into deep poverty, creating famines, and weakening political structures.[15,16] Measles is very closely related to RPV, with divergence of the two viruses thought to have occurred around the 11th or 12th centuries.[17] It's not hard to see how this might have happened: humans and livestock have lived close together for thousands of years,[3] and the growing settlement of people in villages, towns, and cities aided the success of measles virus.[4] Increasingly, the virus had more and more susceptible people to circulate amongst. Unfortunately, PPR, known as sheep and goat plague, has replaced rinderpest as the new scourge of livestock in Africa, Asia, and the Middle East.[18] While it doesn't infect people, it can kill 30–70% of herds and is a major threat to livelihoods, food security, and prosperity just as rinderpest was.

Livestock have always been crucial to human survival and a means of livelihood: they are a source of food, manure (used for both fertilizer and fuel), hides, fiber, and draft power. Livestock play a role in festivals and dowries and serve as an emergency fund in lean times, as collateral for credit, and in some cultures as indicators of status or wealth. Some families greatly look forward to the dowry of livestock they will receive when their daughter is married, which unfortunately is sometimes the impetus for marrying off a daughter at a young age. Livestock contribute 40% of the global value of agricultural output and support the livelihoods of 1.3 billion people, including many living in poverty.[19] The UN Food and Agriculture Organization (FAO) estimates that there are approximately 752 million poor livestock keepers worldwide, a figure that has been increasing about 1.4% per year, with 85% of the poor livestock keepers in sub-Saharan Africa living in extreme poverty.[20] To many, livestock is a vital lifeline.

Unfortunately, in addition to the benefits livestock provide for humanity, they also impose significant negative impacts on our environment that can impact human health. Livestock is the world's largest user of land, accounting for nearly 80% of all agricultural land when we consider pasture and cropland dedicated to growing of livestock feed.[19] Pasture requirements alone for livestock account for 26% of the Earth's ice-free land.[19] Clearing forest, often by burning, to graze cattle (as of late 2019, vast swaths of Brazilian rainforest continue to be burned for grazing cattle[21]) or grow crops destined for livestock feed can lead to land degradation, air pollution, water contamination, increased flood risks, a decline in animal and plant biodiversity, and much, much more. As we will see later in this chapter, drastically altering an ecosystem can ultimately lead to an increase in human–wildlife encounters and the emergence of diseases that threaten humans the world over.

Approximately 80% of the world's extreme poor (living on $1.90/day or less) live in rural areas and depend a great deal on agriculture, often either owning a farm or working in agriculture for a wage.[22] Such wage workers and also pastoralists are highly likely to be extremely poor.[22] There are anywhere from 200 million to 500 million pastoralists worldwide, the large majority living in sub-Saharan Africa. About 85% of pastoralists and 75% of agro-pastoralists live in extreme poverty.[22] In 2017, of the 753 million people living in extreme poverty, 59% were living in countries affected by fragility or environmental vulnerability or both.[23] As global extreme poverty rates decline, the extreme poor will be increasingly concentrated in contexts of institutional fragility and conflict, mostly in sub-Saharan Africa.[22]

From a One Health perspective, the keeping of livestock in a responsible manner can be accomplished within the framework of the Sustainable Development Goals (SDGs),[24] and can even help in achieving most of these goals. For example, improving the health of food animals means they more readily gain weight, produce milk (or eggs if we consider chickens), produce healthy offspring, and generally thrive, generating income (SDG 1, no poverty) for the family and a secure source of food (SDG 2, zero hunger). Extra income and food can mean improving family health (SDG 3, good health and well-being) and child education (SDG 4, quality education). Livestock, especially smaller animals, such as pigs, chickens, sheep, and goats, are also important assets for empowering rural women (SDG 5, gender equality), who can earn income that remains under their control and therefore become a more independent contributor to household income and food security.[20] Better management and policies surrounding livestock can reduce the zoonotic disease burden, foodborne illnesses, and water contamination and hence the waterborne disease burden (SDG 6, clean water and sanitation). Biofuel derived from manure fermentation can be used to bring clean fuel to those without and replace dirty, polluting solid forms of fuel such as wood, coal, or charcoal (SDG 7, affordable and clean energy). We could go on with the remaining eight goals, but the line of evidence and the positive trends in fulfilling the SDGs by 2030 continue.[24]

On a more intimate human–animal relationship scale, a large body of evidence today supports that owning pets is not only beneficial to our health but to our emotional state as well. Walking a dog provides exercise needed to keep both owner and pet healthy and gets neighbors meeting and conversing, creating a more friendly, social feel to the neighborhood as well as improving the quality of life for its residents.[25] Dog ownership has been associated with lower blood pressure, cholesterol, and triglyceride levels, among other health benefits, and dog owners tend to make fewer nonroutine appointments with their physician.[25] Dog ownership has also been associated with a reduction in sensitization to allergens in early childhood, and prenatal exposure to household pets has been linked to a lowered risk for allergic disease in offspring.[26] Exposure to pets pre- and postnatal has been connected to a greater richness of beneficial gut microbiota in children, which appear to be associated with a reduction in the risk of obesity and in protecting against atopy.[26] In 1860, Florence Nightingale, an English woman credited with laying the foundations of modern nursing, but also a prodigious writer, statistician, and social reformer, was one of the first people to recognize the positive impacts companion animals had on those who suffered from chronic illness.[27] The first documented use of pets for therapeutic reasons, however, was well before Nightingale's time, at the Quaker Retreat in York, England, in 1792.[28] Today, pets are widely used in animal-assisted activity (AAA) by providing nursing home patients, school children, shut-ins, prison inmates, and others periods of comfort, companionship, and distraction.[25] Animal-assisted therapy (AAT) is used in a more goal-directed manner involving the pet as part of the patient's treatment plan in coordination with the health care professional. The goals of therapy may be physical, such as improving the motor skills and coordination in a stroke victim through petting the animal or throwing a ball, or emotional, as with someone who has suffered abuse or posttraumatic stress disorder (PTSD).[25] AAA has been associated with the reduction in pain and pain medication intake in adults, lower post-surgical pain in children, and decreased anxiety and epinephrine levels in patients with heart failure.[25]

ONE HEALTH—ANIMALS AS SENTINELS AND COMPARATIVE MEDICINE

Soon after domestication, the dog was used, as it continues to be used today, as an early warning system for invasion or attack.[29] This is a marvelous historical example of how animals serve as sentinels for human health and safety.[30] To a great extent, wildlife, food animals, pets, and humans share the same environment—the same land, air, and water, and potentially the same toxic and infectious exposures. Of course, in some situations this can be reversed—humans can be sentinels for exposures or diseases that affect animals (e.g., influenza).

DDT was developed in the 1940s to combat malaria, typhus, and other insect-borne diseases to significant success, but its indiscriminate use, environmental persistence, and its negative impact on wildlife brought a ban on its use in 1972 in the United States. DDT is now one of 12 chemicals identified as persistent organic pollutants, which are restricted in production and use across the world under the Stockholm Convention on Persistent Organic Pollutants. It should be noted that the World Health Organization still supports the use of DDT in controlled, indoor applications for combating malaria (the spraying of walls and ceilings where mosquitoes will land), in part because of its long residual efficacy.[31]

Some animals, because of their greater susceptibility and shorter life span, prove to be excellent sentinels for threats to human health. For example, the historical use of canaries, with their rapid metabolism and heart rate, in coal mines to warn of the presence of toxic gases such as carbon monoxide and methane.[29,30] The death of cattle at a livestock show in England in 1873 was associated with a dense industrial fog and occurred before the human health effects of air pollution were well known.[32] Livestock have also been natural sentinels for ergot-contaminated grain for centuries. And the environmental health effects of many toxins (dioxin, aflatoxin, organic mercury, chlorinated naphthalene) were first identified in domestic animals.[32] Pets and people can be affected by the same toxins in the home: carbon monoxide, lead, mercury. Perfluoroalkyl substances (PFAS) are ubiquitous chemicals associated with multiple adverse health outcomes in people as well as demonstrated toxicity in laboratory animals. Routes of human exposure are uncertain, but the use of PFAS in household products such as nonstick cookware and anti-stain products for textiles point toward indoor exposures.[33] A positive association in cats between disease (thyroid, liver, respiratory) and PFAS levels has been found. It seems unsurprising then, given what we know of the ability of animals to serve as sentinels, that cats, indoor cats particularly, have proven to be good sentinels for environmental PFAS exposure and the consequential health risks in humans.[33]

Animals are also sentinels for naturally occurring diseases, known or unknown, as well as for pathogens released via bioterrorism attack.[34–37] Today we surveil animal populations or individual animals to monitor the epidemiology of a disease and to better assess the risk to humans. We surveil animals for influenza, West Nile virus, rabies, plague, brucellosis, Middle East Respiratory Syndrome coronavirus (MERS-CoV), Ebola virus, and many other pathogens, as well as for almost every new disease that emerges. Global surveillance networks have been established for many of these diseases, reporting on animal and human cases and disease spread. When a new disease makes itself known, the source is sought, and today, more often than not, new diseases that threaten human health tend to come from wildlife.

The threats to human health for which animals serve as sentinels are not limited to toxins and infectious diseases. By studying the health of pets, their diseases, conditions, their responses to treatments, we can develop a better, broader approach to combating human disease. Animals and human share considerable overlap in physiology and anatomy, depending on the species we are considering, of course. We know, for example, that mountain gorillas (*Gorilla beringei beringei*) share a 98.4% genetic makeup with humans, and their anatomy and physiology is nearly identical to ours.

Humans have benefited greatly from the many discoveries derived from the study of animals under observational or experimental conditions. The use of animals in research dates back to Erasistratus of Ceos (304–258 BCE), who studied under Aristotle and correctly identified the heart as the distributor of blood.[38] While controversial to some, the use of laboratory animals for medical research has been responsible for significant advances in human and animal health. The use of animals in research has broadened our understanding of important zoonotic diseases such as yellow fever, anthrax, Ebola virus, plague, rabies, influenza, leptospirosis, typhus, brucellosis, as well as HIV, which is not zoonotic but has zoonotic origins in simian immunodeficiency viruses that were acquire by humans from nonhuman primates long ago.[38] The use of animals in research has allowed us to create human vaccines that have prevented death and disability in perhaps hundreds of millions of people from such diseases polio, rabies, smallpox, influenza, and as of 2016 Ebola virus.

Comparative medicine can provide insights and advances in fighting disease and improving health and increasing life span. For example, dogs are excellent models for studying respiratory cancers of humans because of their exposure to such things as in-home tobacco smoke, radon and asbestos.[32] Cancer in companion animals is very common (estimates put canine cancer deaths at 40–50% of those over the age of 10 years), and remarkably similar to cancer in humans in many ways that mouse models cannot capture.[39] This has brought significant attention to the value of spontaneous canine cancer in drug discovery and validation that can benefit companion animals as well as humans.[39] This has been coined "comparative oncology". By tapping into a comparative medicine approach—a One Health approach—we can greatly expand our understanding of diseases, and through clinical trials learn how effective therapies in animals can benefit humans, and vice versa.

ONE HEALTH—DISEASES OLD AND NEW

In the last few decades the world has experienced a tremendous decline in the health burden due to infectious diseases.[40] From 2000 to 2012, the percentage of all deaths due to infectious diseases decreased from 23% to 17%.[40] Amongst these diseases linger zoonoses, which make up an estimated 61% of known human pathogens, and roughly 60% of emerging diseases events are attributed to zoonoses, most of which derive from wildlife.[41] HIV-1 and 2, while not zoonotic, have their origins in simian immunodeficiency viruses (SIV), which people almost certainly acquired through contact with tissues, blood, and various body fluids during the hunting, handling, and eating of nonhuman primates.[42] Since 2000, the incidence of HIV and the number of deaths on a global scale continues its downward trend, as it does for tuberculosis and malaria,[40,43] though there was virtually no reduction in malaria between 2015–2017.[44] Of course, where a person lives makes a difference in what they are most likely to die from: only one infectious disease can be counted in the top ten causes of death in high-income countries, yet low-income countries can count five.[45] We've had notable successes in battling infectious diseases—witness the eradication of smallpox in 1980 and rinderpest in 2011. While noncommunicable disease such as ischemic heart disease, stroke, chronic obstructive pulmonary disease, and diabetes are on the rise and garner a much bigger burden of disease today than they did in 1990, we have not yet finished with infectious diseases. As low- and lower-middle income countries move into the middle-income bracket and gain greater wealth, they will, for a significant period of time, continue to face the familiar burden of the same communicable diseases that haunted them for so long, but also a rise in obesity and all of the noncommunicable diseases that come with it, such as diabetes. Such countries face a daunting double burden.

One Health has gained recognition and traction as a movement thanks in part to the dozens of zoonotic outbreaks that have occurred across the globe since the mid-20th century. The role of animals, particularly wildlife, and the resultant human morbidity and mortality connected to these outbreaks have been made clear, and are frightening. But we cannot ignore the environmental component and the human-centric abuse of our environment that contribute to many of these outbreaks: a growing human population and a push into once previously remote areas brings wildlife, domestic animals, and humans into closer contact, offering more opportunities for disease sharing.[46] Deforestation for agriculture expansion, the fragmentation of wilderness, the fragmentation of rivers by dams, and climate change all assist in the emergence of new pathogens, and the re-emergence of ones forgotten or neglected.[46] Such threats and their spread is guaranteed by a growing demand in air travel, international maritime shipping, socioeconomic conditions, health and wealth inequalities, conflict, political neglect, and corruption, in addition to the environmental and ecological factors.[40] The Ebola outbreaks in West Africa (2014–2016) are an excellent example of how many of these factors contribute to disease emergence.

Ebola virus disease (EVD) was first recognized in 1976 in two separate outbreaks that occurred in the Democratic Republic of Congo (DRC) and what is now known as South Sudan.[47] There is some evidence that implicates fruit bats of the Pteropodidae family as the reservoir host of this virus, and initial infection in humans is through close contact with bats or other infected animals, such as chimpanzees, gorillas, monkeys, forest antelope, and porcupines.[48] Once infection in a person takes hold, person-to-person transmission is easily accomplished through close contact with blood, vomitus, sweat, urine, and other secretions and body fluids.[49] The first case in the massive 2014–2016 outbreak that resulted in over 28,000 cases and 11,000 deaths is thought to have been an 18-month-old boy from a remote village in Guinea, who is speculated to have had contact with a bat.[50,51] Further evidence of the role of bats in Ebola virus comes from the outbreak in the DRC in 2007, which was linked to people buying fresh-killed fruit bats to eat, bats that had migrated in large numbers and settled in fruit trees and palm trees of an abandoned plantation.[52] Ebola virus was discovered in a bat in Liberia in 2018,[53] and a new strain of Ebola (Bombali virus) was discovered in a bat in Sierra Leone in 2018,[54] as well as in bats in Kenya and Guinea in 2019.[55,56]

For many people in African countries eating the meat of wildlife—a.k.a. bushmeat—is part of their culture, their everyday existence; this includes the eating of bats. Sierra Leone, Guinea, and Liberia, where the Ebola outbreak was centered, lack well-developed health care and public health infrastructure. Physicians are scarce, ambulances even more so. Sierra Leone and Guinea were previously colonized by Britain and France, respectively, which left the countries struggling to find stable democratic footing after their independence. Since then, all three countries have suffered from some combination of civil war, authoritarian government, corruption, and questionable election practices.[57] The countries continue to suffer from low adult literacy rates (30–47%) and low GDP per capita ($1,600–$2,200/yr.).[57] In Sierra Leone, it is estimated that 52% of the population lives in extreme poverty, Liberia 38%, and Guinea 35%.[58] The majority of people in these countries are employed in the agricultural sector. Poverty drives desperation to survive, forcing people deeper and deeper into forests to find food, hunt, extract minerals, and cut wood to make and sell charcoal.[59] In addition, forests are cleared for logging, to grow crops such as palm for palm oil, and to graze livestock. All of these activities promote greater direct and indirect contact between humans and animals and pathogens (Figure 12.1).

Between 1990 and 2010, Africa lost 10% of its forests.[60] The Guinea forest region has been heavily deforested for logging and agriculture, and this forest shares borders with Sierra Leone, Liberia, and Côte d'Ivoire, a country which has destroyed nearly 80% of its forests in order to grow cocoa.[61] In fact, a large swath of forest runs across West and Central Africa, called the "Ebola forest belt" by some.[51] Deforestation influences bat movement and abundance, and Ebola outbreaks in Africa have been significantly associated with deforestation along rainforest biomes.[62] The 2014–2016 Ebola outbreak was ecologically linked to poverty, and that poverty in turn was, and still is, largely due to the overall failure

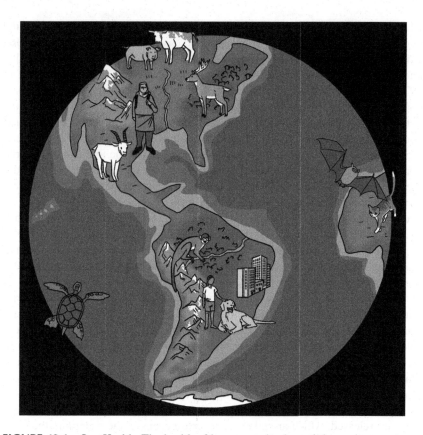

FIGURE 12.1 One Health: The health of humans, animals, and the environment cannot be easily separated. Wildlife, humans, and domestic animals frequently share the same territory, impacting one another and their environment. Where they overlap is where conditions and diseases are most likely to emerge that will affect health and where One Health strategies will be needed most. Climate change influences all land, air, water, and life within our biosphere. It impacts health, food security, biodiversity, where we live, social welfare, livelihoods, disease transmission, and much more.

of each nation on a broad scale. Authoritarian governments or oligarchies extract what they can from their people and their country's resources and rarely make legislation or policies that put their position of power and wealth at risk.[63] Corruption continues along the lines of succession. Money that could improve and support education, hospitals, public health, the training of health care workers, the opening up of free markets, granting greater land rights, and promoting innovation instead is diverted to inflate bank accounts and a comfortable way of life for a select few.[63] Or the country may be more at the mercy of warring factions, clans, or tribes that vie for power in deadly ways with little or no central democratic government of any power. Such is the case in the Democratic Republic of Congo, where the second-largest Ebola outbreak in history is still occurring as of the beginning of 2020, with approximately 3,300 cases and 2,200 deaths. The DRC gained its independence from Belgium in 1960, and conflict, political instability, and poverty have plagued the country ever since, and Ebola, first seen there in 1976, was not far behind. The DRC is rich in oil, cobalt, coltan, gold, diamonds, copper, and other natural resources, but is unable to realize their value for the betterment of the nation and its people in large part because of the corruption and anarchy that reigns. Newly minted, struggling democracies that might break the extractive mold of an authoritarian government struggle to break the in-bred corruption or may utilize machinations to install an authoritarian leader under the guise of a "free" election. It must be pointed out that the social and political structure of a country, the free will of the people, and shared governance play an overarching role in where people live, where they work, how much money they make, what they eat, whether they have access to quality health care, what risks they face to their health, and what policies the government makes, or doesn't, regarding agriculture, water, pollution, and the environment as a whole. These are One Health matters.

In 2020, we sit on the brink of the eradication of polio and Guinea worm, with just a few dozen cases each. Guinea worm (*Dracunculus medinensis*) epitomizes One Health and the trifecta of human, animal, environment in its epidemiology and the solutions it will take to eradicate it. People are infected with *D. medinensis* when they drink surface water containing tiny infected crustaceans. Once inside a human, *D. medinensis* larva mature into adults, with fertilized females up to 3 feet in length migrating to the surface of the skin a year later and emerging in a blister. If the worm protruding from the blister contacts water then eggs are released, which are taken up by crustaceans in the water and the cycle repeats itself.[64] South Sudan, Mali, Chad, Ethiopia, and Angola are considered endemic for Guinea worm, with Chad documenting 24 cases and Angola one case in 2019.[65] This is a remarkably low number considering there were 3.5 million cases in 1986. What was once a fairly straightforward disease, however, has become complicated almost overnight by the discovery in 2012 that dogs can also be infected and serve as a source for continuing the parasite's life cycle. Dogs are infected when they consume discarded raw fish or fish entrails.[64,65] Chad had 1,567 infected dogs in 2019, Ethiopia six, Mali two, and Angola one. South Sudan has reported only one infected dog, that being in 2015.[65] It turns out, however, that dogs are not the only animal capable of being infected. In 2018, in addition to 11 infected dogs, Ethiopia reported five infected cats and one baboon. Mali had 16 infected dogs and two cats.[65] This is truly a One Health zoonotic problem requiring a One Health solution. Eradicating this disease involves mobilizing communities where Guinea worm occurs to take action, case detection and containment for both humans and animals, and educating the people about transmission and prevention measures such as preventing people with emerging worms from entering a body of water, chemically treating surface water with temephos to kill the crustacean, filtering or boiling water prior to drinking, drinking only from protected wells, and burying fish and fish entrails to prevent dogs from scavenging.[66]

ONE HEALTH—BIODIVERSITY AND OUR PLANET

Biodiversity encompasses the diversity of all living things: animals and plants, microbes, their genes, and their ecosystems—terrestrial, marine, or other aquatic ecosystems—to include the diversity within and between species and ecosystems.[67–69] It is the "web of life".[68] Intact functioning ecosystems provide us with numerous benefits such as food, raw materials (e.g., timber), and medicines. It's estimated that as much as 80% of people living in rural areas of developing countries rely on plant-based traditional medicine and that three-quarters of top-ranking prescription drugs contain plant-derived compounds.[70] Ecosystems act as a carbon sink to combat rising global CO_2 levels. They provide us with fresh water, filtering it and regulating its flows, and aid in drought resistance.[67] Ecosystems moderate extreme weather events, provide air and climate regulation, nutrient cycling, photosynthesis, support soil formation, reduce erosion, and promote pollination. We obtain significant mental, aesthetic, spiritual, recreational, and physical benefits from natural places.[71] No matter how large or miniscule the species, the complex interactions between them create successful ecosystems on which we are dependent. Such rich biodiversity and healthy ecosystems are imperiled by human-driven exploitation and transformation.

Forests cover nearly 31% of the Earth's surface and are home to more than 80% of all terrestrial species of animals, plants, and insects, including pollinators, which affect about one-third of the global food supply.[69] Approximately 1.6 billion people rely on forests for their livelihood, and poor, rural women are heavily impacted by their disappearance.[70] Still, deforestation and land degradation persist, with an estimated 20% of Earth's land degraded between 2000 and 2005.[70] Today, it is estimated that 52% of agricultural land is moderately or severely affected by soil degradation.[72] Other threats to biodiversity include the fragmentation of natural habitats (forests and rivers), overexploitation of our natural resources (such as overfishing), water and air pollution, invasive species, climate change, and ocean acidification.[60,69] Increasing human populations and our extractive tendencies have contributed to unprecedented losses in biodiversity.[67] Because of these, the abundance of native species in most major land-based habitats has fallen approximately 20% since 1900,[73] and between 1970 and 2014 our world experienced a decline of 60% in vertebrate population sizes.[68] Since the 16th century, at least 680 vertebrate species have gone extinct, and 9% of domesticated breeds of mammals used for food and agriculture have become extinct just since 2016.[73] Today, we have less than 13% of the wetlands we had a few centuries ago, and we have lost nearly half of our living coral reefs, which are important to approximately 350 million people throughout the world by providing coastal protection and habitat for fish, not to mention the tourism industry of some countries such as Australia.[74] Around 1 million species of animals and plants face extinction in the coming decades unless we reduce and reverse biodiversity loss.[75]

There is evidence that areas with high wildlife biodiversity also harbor high pathogen diversity, a potential risk to global health,[76] but that intact ecosystems can help regulate diseases and disease-carrying arthropods.[69] A greater diversity of disease host species may result in a lower or higher likelihood of pathogen transmission.[67] For example, when there are nonhost snails present, there appears to be a lower risk of transmission to humans with *Schistosoma mansoni* since this organism is more likely to invade a snail unsuitable for human transmission compared to a setting with a more homogenous snail population.[67] The probability of hantavirus transmission between rodents in Utah is lower when rodents live amongst a diverse population of mammals.[67] It's been argued that high biodiversity in areas where Lyme disease occurs could protect humans from infection since there is a dilution of the animal reservoir and thus an increase in noncompeting hosts leading to a lower prevalence of infection in ticks.[77] But the evidence for a link between biodiversity and proportion of competent hosts (and hence the "dilution effect") is not fully proven.[77] The loss of biodiversity may increase pathogen transmission if it results in reduced predation and competition on reservoir hosts, resulting in an increased density of these pathogen-carrying hosts.[67] So whether a reduction in biodiversity results in higher or lower pathogen transmission depends a good deal on how resilient the competent host is and if it will thrive with the loss of life around it, or whether the host is one of the casualties of biodiversity loss and the risk of transmission therefore drops.[67] The primary hosts for Lyme disease, West Nile, hantavirus pulmonary syndrome, and bartonellosis appear to increase in abundance as biodiversity and hence competing hosts, which can serve as buffers, decline.[67] In reality there is a high degree of "...complexity and scale dependence of the biodiversity-disease relationship and...the relationship might be negative, positive, or neutral, depending on the context".[77] For the most part, biodiversity seems to protect against disease transmission,[67] but the degradation of habitats and biodiversity, along with human encroachment into wildlife habitats, adds to disease exposure and transmission.[60,67,78] Knowing what we do about biodiversity, we can see that it is a One Health issue, but it is also an economic, developmental, security, social, and a moral issue.[73] The loss in biodiversity threatens livelihoods, water supply, availability of and access to food, our resilience to extreme weather, and much more.[74]

It has been estimated that nearly half of the world's emerging disease events (over 300)[41] that occurred between 1940 and 2005 were the result of changes in land use, agriculture practices, and food production practices.[67] These activities increased the rates of contact between humans and animals and therefore pathogen transmission.[67] In 2018, NASA reported that the accelerated destruction of Borneo's forest contributed to the largest single-year increase in carbon emissions in 2,000 years, making Indonesia the fourth-largest source for such emissions.[79] The clearing of forests to grow palm trees and the building of hydroelectric dams are in turn contributing to the rise of zoonotic malaria (*Plasmodium knowlesi*) from long- and pig-tailed macaques in Malaysian Borneo, where it has become the leading cause of malaria hospitalizations.[78,80] In the summer of 2019, palm oil farmers set illegal fires in Indonesia, burning an area larger than the state of Rhode Island, destroying even more habitat of the endangered orangutans in Borneo and forcing Malaysia to shut hundreds of schools and distribute half-a-million face masks in response to the pollution.[81]

The emergence of Nipah virus and its animal and human impact is an excellent lesson in how altering the landscape for agriculture purposes and changes in biodiversity allow for diseases to emerge. Nipah virus was first discovered during an outbreak in 1998 in Malaysia when large numbers of pigs developed respiratory and neurological signs.[82] High densities of pigs on farms aided the pig-to-pig transmission,[67] and pig-to-human transmission resulted in 265 cases of encephalitis and 105 deaths.[83,84] Over 1 million pigs were killed to contain the outbreak. Nipah virus has since caused outbreaks in India and Bangladesh, which were traced not to pigs but to the consumption of date palm fruit, palm sap, or raw date palm juice contaminated with bat urine or saliva.[85,86] Person-to-person transmission has also been reported. It turns out that fruit bats, particularly pteropid bats (flying foxes) are the reservoir of Nipah and like to roost in date palm trees. And it shouldn't come as a surprise that those villages in Bangladesh that experienced Nipah outbreaks were more likely to have a higher human population density, but what was surprising was that the bats thrived in more fragmented forests compared to control villages.[86] There were more bat roosts in villages with fragmented forests, and bats had access to a greater diversity of trees since many of the villagers planted trees in their home gardens, trees that offered the bats alternative food sources when fruit was scarce.[86] This adaptation of bats may portend a growth in bat populations in the future, along with the threat of Nipah virus, alongside humans and their gardens.[60]

Bats are also speculated to be the reservoirs of several other zoonotic diseases, particularly coronaviruses (CoVs) such as Severe Acute Respiratory Syndrome (SARS),[87] a coronavirus which emerged in China in 2002 and resulted in over 8,000 human illnesses and 774 deaths worldwide;[88] and Middle East Respiratory Syndrome coronavirus (MERS-CoV), which emerged in Saudi Arabia in 2012 and has resulted in nearly 2,500 cases and over 850 deaths. MERS-CoV was likely transmitted by bats to dromedary camels in the distant past and is now moving camel-to-person as well as person-to-person.[89] Hendra virus, which causes severe and fatal disease in horses and humans in Australia, also has the bat as its reservoir.[90]

The current trends in loss of biodiversity and ecosystems will hinder the progress of an estimated 80% of the assessed targets of the 2030 Sustainable Development Goals, the 2020 Aichi Biodiversity Targets, as well as the Paris climate agreement.[73] Unfortunately, a growing human population with unchecked, unsustainable consumption and production will only continue or worsen the negative trends in the losses of biodiversity and ecosystem functions unless broad political support and action are achieved. [73]

ONE HEALTH—FORCED MIGRATION, URBANIZATION, AND CLIMATE CHANGE

The UN Refugee Agency (UNHCR) estimates there are nearly 71 million people who have been forcefully displaced, with 37,000 people a day being forced to flee their homes because of conflict and persecution.[91] Mass forced migration and the refugee camps that often go along with migration are frequently accompanied by a multitude of health concerns, including disease outbreaks. Infectious diseases are opportunists that always exploit overcrowding, poverty, and unhygienic conditions; conditions found in nearly all refugee camps. Conflict, an overwhelming cause of forced migration, harms infrastructure, access to health care, institutions, natural resources, livelihoods, social capital, and many more things. People forced to flee their homes become vulnerable to disease, malnutrition, climate change,[92] and exploitation. In August of 2017, about 700,000 Rohingya fled Myanmar into Bangladesh to escape large-scale ethnic cleansing, some taking cattle, buffalo, sheep, and goats with them. Among the diseases that emerged was diphtheria, a childhood disease which is preventable with a vaccine. Diphtheria can be caused by the bacteria *Corynebacterium diphtheriae*, *C. ulcerans*, or *C. pseudotuberculosis*, these last two less common globally and associated with animal contact and consuming raw dairy products.[93] Interestingly, in the UK *C. ulcercans* is now reported more often than *C. diphtheriae*.[93–95] The Rohingya diphtheria outbreak may well have had cattle origins, especially given that test results on cases were not that helpful in pinpointing the pathogen.[94] This is a unique One Health situation, a teachable moment that forces us to realize not just the importance of medical professionals and public health experts in tackling refugee health and safety, but also to recognize that other disciplines and sciences, including veterinarians, can play a role. A better understanding of the One Heath issues and consequences related to conflict and the large-scale movement of people and animals is important to protecting the health of all involved.

The world's population is expected to reach nearly 11 billion by 2100.[96] What the actual number will be will depend upon the total fertility rate of the world and whether it declines, or not, and how quickly it declines. People move from rural life to the cities for better jobs, higher pay, better education systems for their children, and for an overall chance at a better life. As of early 2020, just over 55% of the world lives in cities. By 2050 that will be 68%, and nearly 90% of this increase will take place in Asia and Africa,[97] regions where many countries still struggle with high levels of poverty and high fertility rates. In Africa, only 43% of its population now live in cities, in contrast to 82% in North America.[97] The size of most cities continues to grow, as does their population density. By 2030, we will have 43 megacities—cities with more than 10 million inhabitants.[97] With more people there comes a need for more everything: more hospitals, more fresh water, a larger sanitation network, more schools, more food, more housing, more jobs, more energy. And with a greater population density comes the greater likelihood of sharing communicable diseases. Cities are an economic, social, and environmental challenge. Urbanization means green space is minimal. There is greater pollution in an automobile-centric society where people exercise less, sit in their cars and offices more, and the noncommunicable disease (obesity, diabetes, heart disease, cancer, etc.) burden grows. There are arguments that cities deprive us of exposure to an array of microbes, limiting the biodiversity of microbes we are exposed to resulting in higher levels of asthma, eczema, and allergies later in life.[69] Returning to the Ebola outbreak of West Africa, this outbreak was unique in that it hit major cities, as compared to previous outbreaks in other countries that were more rural in their impact and more easily controlled. The West Africa outbreak highlighted the dangers of cities lacking the basic necessities to meet the needs of their people. When Ebola hit, Sierra Leone, Liberia, and Guinea had too few physicians and other health care workers, too few hospitals, poor health care infrastructure, little to no functional public health, and poor sanitation. A deadly zoonotic disease was able to circulate, kill, and terrorize the capitals of these countries,[98,99] and frighten the rest of the world.

Climate change impacts health in the following ways: 1) directly via morbidity and mortality due to extreme weather events such as heat waves, floods, and drought; 2) indirectly via impacts from environmental and ecosystems changes such as alterations in patterns of disease vectors, increases in waterborne diseases, and increased pollution; and 3) through human (societal) systems such as undernutrition and mental illness due to things such as food insecurity or violent conflict; or economic losses, damage to healthcare systems by extreme weather events, and other environmental stressors.[92] Heat-related mortality has risen and cold-related mortality fallen in some areas of the world as a result of global warming.[92] Climate-related extremes such as wildfires, hurricanes, floods, and heat waves expose the vulnerability of ecosystems and some human systems.[92] The Intergovernmental Panel on Climate Change (IPCC) points out that while diseases may spread as our climate changes, it is believed that, until about mid-century, climate change will mostly exacerbate the health problems that already exist.[92] Changes in landscape and land use, including urbanization and climate change, are connected and feedback on one another.[100] Cities account for more than 70% of global CO_2 emissions.[101] In late 2019, in a speech at the World Mayors Summit in Copenhagen, the UN Secretary-General António Guterres said "Cities are where the climate battle will largely be won or lost".[101] Deforestation and converting land to other purposes, such as agriculture, contributes about 25% of global greenhouse gas emissions.[74] Such land, depleted of robust ecosystems and biodiversity, is now less resilient to climate change, extreme weather, and other disturbances.[74]

Climate change will limit the transmission of some pathogens and enhance that of others, particularly vectorborne and waterborne agents, as temperatures and precipitation change.[102,103] Human exposure to diarrheal disease has already been associated with warmer temperatures (to include *Salmonella* and *Campylobacter*)[92] and increased rainfall.[102] From 2004 to 2016, the United States experienced a tripling of human vectorborne disease cases and documented nine new vectorborne diseases.[104] How much of this trend was due to climate change is not known, but it sets a worrying trend. The *Aedes aegypti* mosquito, capable of transmitting Zika, chikungunya, dengue, and yellow fever is increasingly being discovered in countries and US states previously known to be free of it. Warming temperatures aid in growing the mosquito population, but so does inadequate waste systems, piling up of trash, and stagnant or stored water. Add to these factors the swelling urban populations and we see why dengue is now at an all-time high.[105] Roughly 40% of the world's population lives where dengue occurs, causing at least 100 million illnesses each year.[106] In the past 50 years, dengue incidence has increased 30-fold across the globe.[92] This growing threat can also be blamed in part to our unceasing love affair for air travel, which carries mosquitoes and infected travelers to naïve exotic places. The impact of climate change on mosquito-borne diseases can be challenging to assess because things such as poverty, social factors, health care infrastructure, vector-control, access to antimicrobials, and other things play such a heavy role in the burden of these diseases.[102]

In 2018, while we were exploiting the Earth's resources at a rate 1.7 times faster than our planet's ecosystems could replenish,[107] we were setting a milestone as the fourth warmest year on record.[108] Since 1969, we've been steadily increasing our extraction and demands on nature so that we consume our planet's resources earlier and earlier each year. Humanity's demand for more food, timber, fossil fuels, roads, automobiles, mobile phones, laptops, and big screen TVs knows no boundaries. Earth Overshoot Day is projected each year, and in 2018 we fully consumed our planet's natural capital for that year by August 1st (a new record), meaning that for 5 months until the end of the year we were taking more than what our world could naturally give.[107] This is our global ecological footprint, and 60% of this ecological footprint comprises our carbon footprint.[107] The full measure of climate change is a process of never-ending discovery, as is discerning the health burden on humans and animals and the impact on our environment. Climate change is already contributing to species extinction, directly and via infectious diseases.[92,102] Species have shifted their geographic ranges, seasonal activities, migration patterns, and species interactions due to climate change.[92] Milder winters and an increase in planting of exotic plants have allowed monarch butterflies to breed year-round in the United States, resulting in greater rates of infection compared to migratory monarchs.[102] Expansion of hosts and parasites into the Arctic, for example, along with the emergence of disease in tandem with climate warming or extremes has been connected to the decline of Arctic species.[102] Such an impact on wildlife, if significant enough, could put indigenous people's way of life in jeopardy.

Ecological overspending brings negative climate change and ecological impacts such as forest die-offs, collapsing fisheries, fresh-water scarcity, soil erosion, and biodiversity loss.[107] We've already seen what happens with biodiversity loss. Climate change related events, such as drought, flooding, and severe storms, disproportionately affect rural communities living in extreme poverty who lack resources and have low adaptive capacity to cope with the impacts of climate stresses and shocks.[22] This will affect human settlements, promote population migration, and alter the spread of diseases. These events could push an additional 100 million into poverty if inadequate action is taken and aggravate food insecurity and undernutrition.[22,100] Technological innovations (antibiotics, insecticides, etc.) can mask the true effect of climate change on human diseases, but this is less possible with wildlife and plants, making climate change easier to detect in those life forms.[102] Livestock, particularly the unregulated growth of livestock populations, can generate a number of negative outcomes: zoonotic diseases, water and soil pollution, deforestation, loss of biodiversity, and unsustainable use of land resources for feed grain production.[20] The livestock sector is also responsible for approximately 14.5% of all human-induced greenhouse gas emissions (GHGs), with cattle accounting for about 65% of this.[109] Food consumption accounts for 13% of GHGs, with meat and dairy consumption accounting for 75% of that total.[101]

Without altering course, climate change will mean a greater risk for injury, disease, and death from heat waves and fires, a higher risk of undernutrition from lower food production (especially in poorer regions), more lost work and productivity in vulnerable populations, and a higher risk for foodborne, waterborne, and vectorborne diseases.[92] Any positive effects we will see in a reduction of cold-related mortality, opening up of new regions to food production, and reduced capacity of disease vectors due to temperatures being too hot will increasingly be outweighed by the global negative impacts.[92]

ONE HEALTH—CONCLUSION

One Health is not a new approach, but it has nonetheless struggled for a firm definition. The recognition of its primary pillars—humans, animals, and the environment—and their interconnectedness go back hundreds to thousands of years, but all too often only two of the three pillars are accepted as adequate in meeting a One Health approach. While there is considerable influence, connection, and feedback between any two of the three pillars, true One Health involves considering all three simultaneously. This chapter has laid out the many ways in which humans, animals, and our environment are connected and influence each other, for good or bad. It is said that in 1848, to address the typhus epidemic in Upper Silesia, Virchow suggested that the implementation of political, economic, and social reforms would be needed.[100] Virchow was ahead of his time in recognizing the many causes of poor health and how they accentuate and feed off one another, and the need for a multiprong approach to solving a complex health problem. We've seen how poverty plays a role in the emergence of disease, how authoritarian governments, corruption, and conflict worsen poverty, worsen the health of humans and animals, and lay waste to the environment. Our world is changing. Humanity threatens its own existence through deforestation, water and air pollution, the annihilation of species, and climate change. Despite losing upwards of 75–90% of all species more than once in five mass extinction events over the last 485 million years,[110] the Earth recovered, and new species evolved to fill in the gaps and flourish. Our planet will recover from a sixth extinction event, but very likely without humans. Preventing further loss of biodiversity and ecosystem destruction and reversing the damage done will help in reducing emerging zoonoses, slow climate change, reduce the burden of infectious and noncommunicable diseases, and protect the ecosystem services that are necessary for human existence and vital to life on Earth. In the short term, a One Health approach is a means to accomplish most of the SDGs by 2030, if we put in a solid effort and have the political will. In the long term, One Health is a way to solve some of our most vexing problems and to mitigate against new ones, perhaps even prevent them entirely. We must seek a sustainable way to maintain the health of humans, animals, and our environment, and to value our planet for more than the economic gains we derive from it, because that is not a sustainable way to live.

REFERENCES

1. One Health Commission. What is one health? www.onehealthcommission.org/en/why_one_health/what_is_one_health/ Accessed October 20, 2019.
2. Harari YN. *Sapiens.* New York: HarperCollins Publishers; 2015.
3. Diamond J. *Guns, Germs, and Steel.* New York: W. W. Norton & Company; 1999.
4. Evans BR, Leighton FA. A history of one Health. *Revue Scientifique et Technique.* 2014;33(2):413–420.
5. Kiple KF, Ornelas KC. Experimental animals in medical research: A history. In: Paul EF, Paul J, eds. *Why Animal Experimentation Matters.* New Brunswick: Transaction Publishers; 2001, 23–48.
6. Golub ES. *The Limits of Medicine: How Science Shapes Our Hope for Cure.* New York: Random House; 1994.
7. Nuland SB. *Doctors: The Biography of Medicine.* New York: Random House; 1989.
8. Giovanni Maria Lancisi (1654–1720)--cardiologist, forensic physician, epidemiologist. *Jama,* 1964;189:375–376.
9. Golub ES. *The Limits of Medicine.* New York: Random House; 1994.
10. Schultz M. Rudolf Virchow. *Emerging Infectious Diseases.* 2008;14(9):1480–1481.
11. Woods A, Bresalier M, Cassidy A, Dentinger RM. Wellcome Trust-funded monographs and book chapters. In: *Animals and the Shaping of Modern Medicine: One Health and Its Histories.* London, UK: Palgrave Macmillan; 2017.
12. Cox F. Brucellosis. In: F Cox, ed. *The Wellcome Trust Illustrated History of Tropical Diseases.* London, UK: The Wellcome Trust; 1996.
13. Carter C, Hoobler C. *One Man, One Medicine, One Health: The James H. Steele Story.* Charleston, SC: Craig Carter; 2009.
14. Lamb E. Understand the measles outbreak with this one weird number: The basic reproduction number and why it matters. In: *Roots of Unity.* Scientific American; 2015.
15. Barrett T, Rossiter PB. Rinderpest: The disease and its impact on humans and animals. *Advances in Virus Research.* 1999;53:89–110.
16. Roeder P, Mariner J, Kock R. Rinderpest: The veterinary perspective on eradication. *Philosophical Transactions of the Royal Society of London Series B, Biological Sciences.* 2013;368(1623):20120139.
17. Furuse Y, Suzuki A, Oshitani H. Origin of measles virus: Divergence from rinderpest virus between the 11th and 12th centuries. *Virology Journal.* 2010;7:52.
18. UN Food and Agriculture Organization. Peste des petits ruminants. www.fao.org/ppr/en/. Accessed November 1, 2019.
19. UN Food and Agriculture Organization. FAOs role in animal production. www.fao.org/animal-production/en/. Accessed September 3, 2019.
20. UN Food and Agriculture Organization. Pro-poor livestock policy initiative. Livestock sector development for poverty reduction: An economic and policy perspective. 2012. www.fao.org/3/i2744e/i2744e00.pdf. Accessed August 30, 2019.
21. Krauss C, Yaffe-Bellany D, Simões M. Why Amazon fires keep raging 10 years after a deal to end them. *New York Times,* 2019.
22. UN Food and Agriculture Organization. The role of agriculture and rural development in achieving SDG 1.1. 2019. Accessed August 30, 2019. www.un.org/development/desa/dspd/wp-content/uploads/sites/22/2019/03/FAO-ending-extreme-rural-poverty-1.pdf.

23. Development Initiatives. *Global humanitarian assistance report:2018*, 2018.
24. UN Food and Agriculture Organization. Measuring the role of livestock in the household economy. 2016. www.fao.org/3/a-i6739e.pdf. Accessed September 3, 2019.
25. Johnson R. The human-animal bond and animal-assisted therapy. In: Davis RG, ed. *Caring for Family Pets: Choosing and Keeping Our Companion Animals Healthy.* Santa Barbara, CA: ABC-CLIO; 2011, 29–41.
26. Tun HM, Konya T, Takaro TK, et al. Exposure to household furry pets influences the gut microbiota of infant at 3–4 months following various birth scenarios. *Microbiome.* 2017;5(1):40.
27. Braun C, Stangler T, Narveson J, Pettingell S. Animal-assisted therapy as a pain relief intervention for children. *Complementary Therapies in Clinical Practice.* 2009;14(2):105–109.
28. Pandzic I. *Animal-Assisted Therapy and PTSD.* San Diego, CA: Naval Center for Combat & Operational Stress Control; 2012.
29. Schmidt PL. Companion animals as sentinels for public health. *Veterinary Clinics of North America Small Animal Practice.* 2009;39(2):241–250.
30. Rabinowitz PM, Scotch ML, Conti LA. Animals as sentinels: Using comparative medicine to move beyond the laboratory. *ILAR Journal.* 2010;51(3):262–267.
31. World Health Organization. *The use of DDT in Malaria Vector Control. WHO Position Statement,* 2011.
32. Bukowski JA, Wartenberg D. An alternative approach for investigating the carcinogenicity of indoor air pollution: Pets as sentinels of environmental cancer risk. *Environmental Health Perspectives.* 1997;105(12):1312–1319.
33. Bost PC, Strynar MJ, Reiner JL, et al. U.S. domestic cats as sentinels for perfluoroalkyl substances: Possible linkages with housing, obesity, and disease. *Environmental Research.* 2016;151:145–153.
34. Davis R. Companion animals as sentinels for emerging diseases. *Clinician's Brief.* 2014;12:11–13.
35. Davis RG. The AbCs of bioterrorism for veterinarians, focusing on Category B and C agents. *Journal of the American Veterinary Medical Association.* 2004;224(7):1096–1104.
36. Davis RG. The ABCs of bioterrorism for veterinarians, focusing on Category A agents. *Journal of the American Veterinary Medical Association.* 2004;224(7):1084–1095.
37. Rabinowitz P, Gordon Z, Chudnov D, et al. Animals as sentinels of bioterrorism agents. *Emerging Infectious Diseases.* 2006;12(4):647–652.
38. Kiple KF, Ornelas KC. Experimental animals in medical research: A history. In: Paul EF, Paul J, eds. *Why Animal Experimentation Matter. The Use of Animals in Medical Research.* New Brunswick, NJ: Social Philosophy and Policy Foundation; 2001, 23–48.
39. Garden OA, Volk SW, Mason NJ, Perry JA. Companion animals in comparative oncology: One Medicine in action. *Veterinary Journal (London, England: 1997).* 2018;240:6–13.
40. World Health Organization. *Health in 2015: from MDGs to SDGs,* 2015.
41. Jones KE, Patel NG, Levy MA, et al. Global trends in emerging infectious diseases. *Nature.* 2008;451(7181):990–993.
42. Kalish ML, Wolfe ND, Ndongmo CB, et al. Central African hunters exposed to simian immunodeficiency virus. *Emerging Infectious Diseases.* 2005;11(12):1928–1930.
43. United Nations. *The Sustainable Development Goals Report 2018,* 2018.
44. World Health Organization. *World Malaria Report 2018,* 2018.
45. World Health Organization. The top 10 causes of death. www.who.int/news-room/fact-sheets/detail/the-top-10-causes-of-death. Accessed October 21, 2019.

46. Centers for Disease Control and Prevention. One health basics. 2019. www.cdc.gov/onehealth/basics/index.html. Accessed July 1, 2019.
47. Centers for Disease Control and Prevention. History of Ebola virus disease. www.cdc.gov/vhf/ebola/history/summaries.html. Accessed October 16, 2019.
48. World Health Organization. Ebola virus disease. www.afro.who.int/health-topics/ebola-virus-disease. Accessed October 21, 2019.
49. Centers for Disease Control and Prevention. Ebola transmission. www.cdc.gov/vhf/ebola/transmission/index.html. Accessed October 16, 2019.
50. Centers for Disease Control and Prevention. Ebola: 2014–2016 Ebola outbreak in West Africa. www.cdc.gov/vhf/ebola/history/2014-2016-outbreak/index.html. Accessed October 16, 2019.
51. Meseko CA, Egbetade AO, Fagbo S. Ebola virus disease control in West Africa: An ecological, one health approach. *The Pan African Medical Journal.* 2015;21:6.
52. Leroy EM, Epelboin A, Mondonge V, et al. Human Ebola outbreak resulting from direct exposure to fruit bats in Luebo, Democratic Republic of Congo, 2007. *Vector Borne and Zoonotic Diseases (Larchmont, NY).* 2009;9(6):723–728.
53. Grady D. Deadly Ebola virus is found in liberian bat, researchers say. *New York Times,* January 24, 2019.
54. Goldstein T, Anthony SJ, Gbakima A, et al. The discovery of Bombali virus adds further support for bats as hosts of ebolaviruses. *Nature Microbiology.* 2018;3(10):1084–1089.
55. Forbes KM, Webala PW, Jaaskelainen AJ, et al. Bombali virus in Mops condylurus Bat, Kenya. *Emerging Infectious Diseases.* 2019;25(5).
56. Karan LS, Makenov MT, Korneev MG, et al. Bombali virus in Mops condylurus Bats, Guinea. *Emerging Infectious Diseases.* 2019;25(9).
57. Central Intelligence Agency. World fact book. www.cia.gov/library/publications/resources/the-world-factbook/. Accessed October 22, 2019.
58. The World Bank. Poverty headcount ratio at $1.90 a day (2011 PPP) (% of population). https://data.worldbank.org/indicator/SI.POV.DDAY?end=2015&start=1981&view=chart. Accessed October 22, 2019.
59. Bausch DG, Schwarz L. Outbreak of Ebola virus disease in Guinea: Where ecology meets economy. *PLoS Neglected Tropical Diseases.* 2014;8(7):e3056.
60. Whitmee S, Haines A, Beyrer C, et al. Safeguarding human health in the Anthropocene epoch: Report of the Rockefeller Foundation-Lancet Commission on planetary health. *Lancet (London, England).* 2015;386(10007):1973–2028.
61. Pearce F. The Real price of a chocolate bar: West Africa's rainforests. *Yale Environment 360,* February 21, 2019.
62. Olivero J, Fa JE, Real R, et al. Recent loss of closed forests is associated with Ebola virus disease outbreaks. *Scientific Reports.* 2017;7(1):14291.
63. Acemogu D, Robinson J. *Why Nations Fail: The Origins of Power, Prosperity, and Poverty.* New York: Crown Publishing; 2013.
64. Centers for Disease Control and Prevention. Guinea worm: Biology. www.cdc.gov/parasites/guineaworm/biology.html. Accessed October 16, 2019.
65. The Carter Center. Guinea worm eradication program. www.cartercenter.org/health/guinea_worm/index.html. Accessed October 21, 2019.
66. Centers for Disease Control and Prevention. Guinea worm: Prevention and control. www.cdc.gov/parasites/guineaworm/prevent.html. Accessed October 16, 2019.
67. Keesing F, Belden LK, Daszak P, et al. Impacts of biodiversity on the emergence and transmission of infectious diseases. *Nature.* 2010;468(7324):647–652.
68. World Wildlife Fund. *Living Planet Report 2018.*

69. Romanelli C, Cooper HD, de Souza Dias BF. The integration of biodiversity into one Health. *Revue Scientifique et Technique.* 2014;33(2):487–496.
70. United Nations. Sustainable development goals –15 life on land. www.un.org/sust ainabledevelopment/biodiversity/.
71. World Wildlife Fund. *Living Planet Report 2016.*
72. United Nations. Sustainable development goals - 15, life on land. www.un.org/sust ainabledevelopment/biodiversity/. Accessed December 12, 2019.
73. Intergovernmental Science-Policy Platform on Biodiversity and Ecosystem Services. *Report of the Plenary of the Intergovernmental Science-Policy Platform on Biodiversity and Ecosystem Services on the Work of its Seventh Session. Summary for Policymakers of the Global Assessment Report on Biodiversity and Ecosystem Services of the Intergovernmental Science-Policy Platform on Biodiversity and Ecosystem Services,* May 2019.
74. The World Bank. Biodiversity. www.worldbank.org/en/topic/biodiversity#1. Accessed December 12, 2019.
75. Diaz S, Settele J, Brondizio E, et al. *Report of the Plenary of the Intergovernmental Science-Policy Platform on Biodiversity and Ecosystem Services on the Work of Its Seventh Session. Summary for Policymakers of the Global Assessment Report on Biodiversity and Ecosystem Services of the Intergovernmental Science-Policy Platform on Biodiversity and Ecosystem Services,* 2019.
76. Langlois EV, Campbell K, Prieur-Richard AH, Karesh WB, Daszak P. Towards a better integration of global health and biodiversity in the new sustainable development goals beyond Rio+20. *EcoHealth.* 2012;9(4):381–385.
77. Wood CL, Lafferty KD. Biodiversity and disease: A synthesis of ecological perspectives on Lyme disease transmission. *Trends in Ecology and Evolution.* 2013;28(4):239–247.
78. Fornace KM, Alexander N, Abidin TR, et al. Local human movement patterns and land use impact exposure to zoonotic malaria in Malaysian Borneo. *Elife.* 2019;8.
79. Lustgarten A. Palm oil was supposed to help save the planet. Instead it unleashed a catastrophe. *The New York Times Magazine: New York Times,* 2018.
80. Beaubien J. You don't want to monkey around with monkey malaria. *NPR: Goats and Soda,* December 11, 2014.
81. Mellen R. Wildfires in Indonesia have ravaged 800,000 acres. Palm oil farmers are mostly to blame. *The Washington Post,* September 18, 2019.
82. Lam SK, Chua KB. Nipah virus encephalitis outbreak in Malaysia. *Clinical Infectious Diseases: An Official Publication of the Infectious Diseases Society of America.* 2002;34(Suppl 2):S48–51.
83. Yob JM, Field H, Rashdi AM, et al. Nipah virus infection in bats (order Chiroptera) in peninsular Malaysia. *Emerging Infectious Diseases.* 2001;7(3):439–441.
84. Hsu VP, Hossain MJ, Parashar UD, et al. Nipah virus encephalitis reemergence, Bangladesh. *Emerging Infectious Diseases.* 2004;10(12):2082–2087.
85. World Health Organization. Nipah virus. www.who.int/news-room/fact-sheets/d etail/nipah-virus. Accessed October 25, 2019.
86. Hahn MB, Gurley ES, Epstein JH, et al. The role of landscape composition and configuration on Pteropus giganteus roosting ecology and Nipah virus spillover risk in Bangladesh. *The American Journal of Tropical Medicine and Hygiene.* 2014;90(2):247–255.
87. Wang LF, Shi Z, Zhang S, Field H, Daszak P, Eaton BT. Review of bats and SARS. *Emerging Infectious Diseases.* 2006;12(12):1834–1840.

88. Centers for Disease Control and Prevention. Severe acute respiratory syndrome (SARS): Frequently asked questions about SARS. www.cdc.gov/sars/about/faq. html. Accessed October 16, 2019.

89. World Health Organization. Middle East Respiratory syndrome coronavirus (MERS-CoV). World Health Organization. www.who.int/en/news-room/fact-sheet s/detail/middle-east-respiratory-syndrome-coronavirus-(mers-cov). Accessed October 23, 2019.

90. World Health Organization. Hendra virus (HeV) infection. www.who.int/emergenc ies/diseases/hendra-virus/en/. Accessed October 21, 2019.

91. UN Refugee Agency. Where the world's displaced people are being hosted. www.u nhcr.org/en-us/figures-at-a-glance.html. Accessed October 27, 2019.

92. Intergovernmental Panel on Climate Chage (IPCC). *Climate Change 2014. Impacts, Adaptation, and Vulnerablity. Part A: Global and Sectoral Aspects*, 2014.

93. Wagner KS, White JM, Crowcroft NS, De Martin S, Mann G, Efstratiou A. Diphtheria in the United Kingdom, 1986–2008: The increasing role of Corynebacterium ulcerans. *Epidemiology and Infection.* 2010;138(11):1519–1530.

94. Flowra MT, Asaduzzaman M. Resurgence of infectious diseases due to forced migration: Is planetary health and one health action synergistic? *The Lancet Planetary Health.* 2018;2(10):e419–420.

95. Moore LSP, Leslie A, Meltzer M, Sandison A, Efstratiou A, Sriskandan S. Corynebacterium ulcerans cutaneous diphtheria. *The Lancet Infectious Diseases.* 2015;15(9):1100–1107.

96. UN Department of Economic and Social Affairs. World population prospects 2019. https://population.un.org/wpp/Graphs/Probabilistic/POP/TOT/900. Accessed October 29, 2019.

97. UN Department of Economic and Social Affairs. 68% of the world population projected to live in urban areas by 2050, says UN. www.un.org/development/desa/en /news/population/2018-revision-of-world-urbanization-prospects.html. Accessed October 28, 2019.

98. Rico A, Brody D, Coronado F, et al. Epidemiology of epidemic Ebola virus disease in Conakry and surrounding prefectures, Guinea, 2014–2015. *Emerging Infectious Diseases.* 2016;22(2):178–183.

99. Ratto J, Ivy W, 3rd, Purfield A, et al. Notes from the field: Ebola virus disease response activities during a mass displacement event after flooding--freetown, Sierra Leone, September-November, 2015. *MMWR Morbidity and Mortality Weekly Report.* 2016;65(7):188–189.

100. Black PF, Butler CD. One Health in a world with climate change. *Revue Scientifique et Technique.* 2014;33(2):465–473.

101. United Nations. Guterres: "Cities are where the climate battle will largely be won or lost". https://unfccc.int/news/guterres-cities-are-where-the-climate-battle-will-l argely-be-won-or-lost. Accessed October 29, 2019.

102. Altizer S, Ostfeld RS, Johnson PT, Kutz S, Harvell CD. Climate change and infectious diseases: From evidence to a predictive framework. *Science (New York, NY).* 2013;341(6145):514–519.

103. Watts N, Amann M, Arnell N, et al. The 2018 report of the Lancet Countdown on health and climate change: Shaping the health of nations for centuries to come. *Lancet (London, England).* 2018;392(10163):2479–2514.

104. Rosenberg R, Lindsey NP, Fischer M, et al. Vital signs: Trends in reported vector-borne disease cases - United States and territories, 2004–2016. *MMWR. Morbidity and Mortality Weekly Report.* 2018;67(17):496–501.

105. Newey S. A 'perfect storm': The steady rise of dengue fever worldwide. *The Telegraph*, August 8, 2019.
106. Centers for Disease Control and Prevention. About dengue: What you need to know. www.cdc.gov/dengue/about/index.html. Accessed November 6, 2019.
107. UN Framework Convention on Climate Change. Earth's annual resources budget consumed in just 7 months. https://unfccc.int/news/earth-s-annual-resources-budget -consumed-in-just-7-months. Accessed October 28, 2019.
108. Berkeley Earth. Global temperature report for 2018. http://berkeleyearth.org/2018- temperatures/. Accessed October 29, 2019.
109. UN Food and Agriculture Organization. Tackling climate change through livestock. 2013. www.fao.org/3/i3437e/i3437e.pdf. Accessed September 3, 2019.
110. Greshko M. What are mass extinctions, and what causes them? *National Geographic*; 2019.

13 Communication and Expectations

Kristen V. Khanna and Karen Gozdan-Aiken

CONTENTS

GETTING THE WORD OUT

Efforts to conduct research in comparative medicine, as described in this book and elsewhere, are the result of relationships and synergies that started with individuals who recognized the opportunity to understand health and disease in a broader sense and to integrate and inform the biology of disease to the fullest extent possible. If exposure to clinicians and scientists who have this view is the first step to expanding the reach of comparative medicine, then "getting the word out" by and about those people is essential.

WHAT'S THE WORD?

We may start with the question: which word should we use? The basics of communicating the possibilities of breaking down the barriers between human and veterinary sciences in an effort to hasten the pace of medical discovery would benefit from the development of consistent terminology. A brief search of "translational medicine" results in discussions of bench to bedside innovation, rather than bidirectional knowledge shared between the human and animal health fields. While "One Health" often takes on more of a zoonotic focus when defined as an integrative effort to attain optimal health for people, animals and the environment. Perhaps it is a combination of these two ideas, and the language has not been sufficiently developed to describe the ability to model disease in different species in an attempt to move forward in a more expeditious, and mutually beneficial, manner. This may require more thought, but something as simple as "species-agnostic medicine" (Nahama 2019) could be considered a subset of translational medicine; one in which a single molecule is moved from the bench, through clinical trials without a preference for which species the data and insights are derived from so long as the study design is well justified and relevant species-specific considerations are made. This could be followed by a segue to human trials. Or these studies could be conducted in different species in parallel, designed to mutually inform.

TRAINING VETERINARY SCIENTISTS TO INTEGRATE INTO HUMAN RESEARCH TEAMS

Creating the right conditions for a productive translational research environment has been accomplished to date by training veterinarians who could be described as having the ability to speak more than one language and placing them in human research settings. A knowledge gap is filled by "speaking" both veterinary and human medicine. Veterinarians receive diverse, multi-species training, combined with a deep understanding of evolutionary biology, requiring a mindset of making comparisons and understanding contrasts. Training in human medicine is focused on a single species, with less focus on compare-and-contrast, yet individuals in that research setting are routinely expected to make even larger leaps between data generated in a rodent or pig and what those data might mean for human patients. The language of these animal models is inherently more anatomical and less physiological and/or pathobiological, and still even less about spontaneously occurring disease. A real professional dichotomy exists between these clinician-scientists trained in human medicine, who may understandably be less comfortable working on naturally occurring disease, in their species of interest (humans), let alone in companion animals. First and foremost, by its very definition, veterinary clinical research involves interacting with a patient and an owner. Some have compared it to working with a pediatric patient and a parent. Understanding the value of data collected in this setting is something that is a conventional component of veterinary residency training, regardless of specialty, and transfers well into research in the comparative setting.

One principal investigator from a large US-based research university has incorporated the conduct of clinical research in pets in his laboratory by specifically seeking out veterinarians at the completion of their residencies. This individual felt it was far more successful to integrate veterinary scientists into human clinical research teams rather than to train human scientists in the conduct of research involving companion animals. A recent project, which was fully funded and meant to be conducted in purpose-bred dogs (i.e., not client-owned pets), could not be completed as originally planned because participating scientists were uncomfortable working with dogs. The individuals working on the project had been trained in laboratory animal residencies; a clinical veterinarian was able to consult and thereby move the project forward.

This investigator's future study of naturally occurring disease may be facilitated by establishing connections between the basic scientists who typically (but not always), make up the backbone of the research team; the medical doctors who rotate through the lab and bring a unique view of the bedside and unmet needs in human medicine; the laboratory animal veterinarians who have an understanding of scientific interpretation; and clinical veterinarians, who are trained in the care of the patient. Individually, each is looking for and contributes to the opportunity to inform human and animal health in a unique way. Establishing a clearing house for funded collaborations, with equal footing in the medical and veterinary schools, creating and highlighting opportunities between veterinary residencies, human medicine residency programs and their respective laboratory science counterparts, would be an ideal place to start getting the "right" people working together in the "right" clinical and scientific ecosystem.

INCREASING AWARENESS

Because veterinarians are already comparative scientists by training, awareness of this unique capability would be a large step forward. We should make clear to veterinarians that a future in a laboratory or human research setting is a viable option, work to make sure those positions are available, and provide a viable career path for those who are interested. To the extent we can provide opportunities for veterinarians, physicians and researchers to work together and provide a venue for them to hear each other's questions, this could shape the future of what this field can accomplish.

Industry can raise awareness by creating jobs that define this knowledge base as a marketable skill set. Hiring veterinarians and placing them in clinical development programs will expand career options for individuals trained in veterinary medicine, thereby making an impact on all medicine, truly helping to achieve "One Health." In the sponsored research realm at a University, a sponsor company may also provide financial support for positions in comparative clinical medicine. Companies and contract research organizations (CROs) could engage veterinarians as consultants or employees, to bring their training to bear on research questions that could be answered in pet animals (see also Chapter 6).

Conferences and workshops are an ideal time to highlight these opportunities, whether as the topic of the event, an adjacent meeting or the side benefit of bringing like-minded people together. In fact, the concept of the CRO currently led by one of the chapter's authors (KK) was first hatched in a bar while in attendance at a conference. Most veterinary students advance through school with clinical practice as the endgame because opportunities to explore alternative options may not have been sufficiently presented to those students.

Drawing specific attention to the field, in the spring of 2015, the Office of Research Infrastructure Programs (ORIP) at the National Institutes of Health (NIH) sponsored a workshop called, "One Health: Integrating the Veterinarian

Scientist into the Biomedical Research Enterprise." The purpose of the workshop was to identify how the concept of One Health can advance the NIH mission with regard to both basic and applied research, including training of the biomedical work force and concentrating on the veterinarian scientist.

Also in 2015, Dr. Cheryl London produced a TED Talk (TEDx OhioStateUniversity) titled, "Of Mice and Men," on the promise of comparative oncology and the place for pets in this research endeavor. To Dr. London's point in her Talk, conducting clinical trials in companion animals, which are comparatively more similar to humans than mice, drugs with an insufficient margin of safety or effectiveness can be removed from the pipeline earlier. This results in a subsequent decrease in expense for the industry. As of this writing the Talk has had thousands of views. But we can and should ask ourselves how we can grow viewership exponentially, thereby exposing current veterinarians and veterinary students, as well as laboratory veterinarians and scientists, to the fact that this is a way to work cooperatively.

Last, there have been many "local news" stories published on the topic of a clinical study or a pet receiving investigational treatment that may inform a human clinical development program. Pet owners nearly universally react positively to the notion that their pet might impact the treatment of the future for animals and people. These stories are more than just "feel good news" to the owners, veterinarians and scientists working together to advance treatment options for pets and people, and they serve to educate the general public.

BARRIERS TO SUCCESS THAT CAN BE AVOIDED OR OVERCOME WITH COMMUNICATION

There are several key barriers to progress in the field that are likely to benefit from an articulate, cohesive and inclusive communications approach: (i) concern about the impression on a regulator (e.g., FDA or USDA) of the impact of animal studies on the status of a human drug; (ii) funding, and more specifically a perception that the cost of studies in pets should be much less than studies in humans (this can be true but is not always true, depending on the protocol and the intent of the study); (iii) the pharmaceutical industry may have concerns that a human drug available to the veterinary market may negatively impact the possible upside potential in the human market; (iv) those in the human medical profession may view veterinary training as "less than" rather than different and value-added; and (v) developing a sense of trust within a study team (e.g., how does a veterinarian know that a medical doctor has the best interest of their companion animal patient and how do we prevent the veterinary team from feeling "used" by the medical team?).

SPONSOR AND FUNDING AGENCY COMMUNICATION

One cannot overestimate the importance of communication between a sponsor and the institution, clinic or entity (such as a CRO) managing and/or conducting the research or a clinical trial. There are formal methods of communication and delegation of responsibilities, such as a contract, statement of work and budget or estimate for the cost of the work; there are best practices of communication such as standing meetings and regularly scheduled exchange of documents that provide progress updates; and there are informal communications, including phone, email, chat systems or daily briefings, that deepen the relationships between the parties and ultimately serve the integrity of the project, particularly during times of strain or crisis.

CONTRACTS AND AGREEMENTS

Sponsors engage an institution or entity with a legally binding contract nearly without exception. The agreement may be a Master Service Agreement (MSA) to stipulate general terms and a separate exhibit (e.g., Statement of Work (SOW) or Work Order (WO)) that stipulates the specifics of a particular study or project. This is most common when the relationship between the sponsor and entity is such that multiple projects are expected. Alternatively, a one-time service agreement may be used. In a regulated setting, these documents serve to formally and in most cases legally delegate the responsibility of the sponsor to the other party. In a non-regulatory setting, while not a delegation of duties in the strictest sense of the phrase, these documents still provide the legal context for the description of the work to be completed.

While not an exhaustive list, MSA or stand-alone service agreements are likely to include clauses related to:

- A comprehensive description of the services and the exchange of related materials
- Deliverables and timelines
- Mechanisms of termination and downstream expectations following a standard or an early termination
- Allowance (or not) for the use of subcontractors
- Compensation for the work, definitions of expenses and a mechanism for amending the scope of work and corresponding payment (i.e., a change order)
- Terms of maintaining confidentiality
- Ownership of data
- The status of existing intellectual property (IP) related to the work and the potential creation of new IP (and ownership thereof)
- Standards of performance and remedies for defective or problematic work
- Indemnification
- Regulatory standards, compliance and related matters, if applicable
- Representations
- Legal conditions and terms (e.g., state laws that preside over the contract and would be used to litigate or arbitrate in the event of a breach of contract)

In most cases a cost estimate for the study is provided in advance. A sponsor may elect to fully fund a project, such that the pet owners do not pay out of pocket; this is most common for regulatory studies where the protocol demands that procedures be performed on a prescribed schedule. In this setting, sponsors most often will compensate the veterinary clinic for the services it provides in the management of any medical needs during the study, and possibly for pre-determined time after the completion of the study. The sponsor may also choose to bear financial responsibility for access to the study drug, leaving the owner to be financially responsible for any other medical expenses. Regardless of the split on fees between sponsor and pet owner, a schedule of costs per activity is agreed upon at the start of a study, recognizing some fluidity in the actual charges incurred. Perhaps some site visits will not occur according to schedule (e.g., a dog withdraws from the study early, an owner has to delay a visit due to a conflict or a patient needs to be seen on an emergency basis). Reimbursement (i.e., payment) of clinical care and study-related documentation by the site in the setting of a clinical trial typically will occur according to a pre-ordained schedule once appropriate documentation has been filed with the sponsor or designee. Clearly setting these expectations and the communication around them at the beginning of a study helps to manage unforeseen issues, some of which may be handled with the aforementioned change order, or amendment, and others of which may be handled informally, often if simply agreed upon in writing by both parties, per the study contract.

REGULARLY SCHEDULED AND INFORMAL COMMUNICATION

The scheduling of routine updates and opportunities for communication during a study is common sense and a Communication Plan is a study document that may be created to outline expectations for communication. The Plan could include routine meetings, but also details how to instruct an investigator to communicate if they have a problem, or how to relay that one of the study sites has encountered something unexpected. A Communication Plan should provide for an alternative line of communication in the event there is a breakdown between the investigator and the oversight team. Communication plans such as these may also protect the sponsor or others from misguided or accidental communication that results in an unmasking (i.e., unblinding) of a patient that has been randomized to receive a certain study treatment, particularly in the case of a completely masked study team.

Informal communication serves the purpose of keeping lines of communication open and keeping team members and investigators quickly informed of new developments or works in progress. Being mindful that in certain studies where documentation of communication is a component of quality study conduct, informal study-related communication in the form of phone calls, texts, chat groups or teams may be kept to a minimum, is reserved solely to serve a defined purpose or, in most cases, such as in a GCP study, is documented just as any other correspondence or communication would be, no matter how informal.

COMMUNICATION WITH THE PURPOSE OF RECRUITING RESEARCH PARTICIPANTS

Recruitment is different for every single study, but one of the most important elements of a clinical trial no matter the research area, is the recruitment of the correct candidates for enrollment. There are numerous agencies that explicitly deal with clinical trial recruitment on the human side, while it could still be considered a developing skill set in veterinary clinical trials. No matter the purpose of the study, the objective of recruitment is to pair the most medically qualified study participants with investigators. A good recruitment campaign will attract and limit the candidates to those that best qualify, without over-restricting the pool and potentially eliminating possible candidates.

Getting the word out to potential pet owners and veterinarians, by creating an awareness of the trial or research program, is an important step in recruitment. The recruitment campaign should be as customized and unique as the enrollment criteria. Reaching pet owners may include various permutations of sourcing from primary veterinary hospitals, referral clinics, dog breeders, pet stores, groomers, breed clubs and social media groups. Each recruitment source will require a unique set of communication tools, including written materials, website landing pages, a mix of social media platforms, call centers, advertising, personalized communication with local hospitals, continuing education meetings and more. (For additional information on recruitment and advertising, see Chapter 11.)

It is a good feeling when interest in a study is high, but it needs to be interest from the population described above, namely medically appropriate owners and their pets. It is worth spending time and resources training staff to adequately pre-screen patients, thereby avoiding bringing in the wrong patients for screening visits and eliminating early study withdrawals, both of which can be costly, time-consuming and disappointing to all involved. The pet owner is truly a unique factor in companion animal clinical trials when compared to human studies. Pre-screening will not only eliminate enrollment of animals that are not medically a good study match, but also may eliminate pet owners that are not committed to completing the rigorous requirements of some studies. Owners can also be advocates beyond what would be considered appropriate during a clinical trial and there is a need to train them about their communication and use of social media, etc.

No matter how a recruitment campaign is structured, the goal is to meet enrollment as quickly as possible, so resources are not wasted. Appropriate and timely enrollment is one of the greatest challenges in the conduct of clinical trials, making communication related to enrollment essential to this work.

PET OWNER COMMUNICATION

Communication in a veterinarian–client relationship differs from that of the human physician–patient relationship in that the communication is, of course, not directed at the actual patient, but to the patient's decision maker. A veterinarian's ultimate goal is to provide his or her patient with the best quality of life, while communicating with the pet owner regarding how clinical trial plans can inform a diagnosis and/or treat a particular condition. There are important nuances in the veterinarian–pet owner discussion of clinical trial enrollment. The concept that human medicine may benefit from studies in companion animals is something that should be explained to pet owners. Owners may feel their contribution to the future of veterinary medicine and human medicine is one of the most important reasons to participate in a clinical study. The knowledge that the work is being done by a team or consortium of doctors, veterinarians and scientists in some cases helps owners to accept their pet's condition with greater ease.

First, while it may seem simple, the most difficult task of communication with a pet owner is to be sure they have heard and understand the intent of the research and what the investigator has said. Partners for Healthy Pets, a collaborative alliance led by the American Animal Hospital Association (AAHA) and the American Veterinary Medical Association (AVMA), analyzed perceived communications between veterinary staff and pet owners over a 5-year period. Following preventive care visits, both staff and owners completed a survey regarding their time in the exam room, and in particular, what services were provided. In one example, 73% of the practice staff said a pain assessment was performed, while only 45% of clients were aware that the assessment was performed. This disparity highlights the experience of disconnect in communication between veterinarians and their clients.

Second, while veterinary staff have been trained to discuss preventive care, diagnostics and treatment with pet owners, they may lack proficiency in explaining details of a clinical trial. Veterinary staff can explain the benefits of an approved medication for a particular indication but may not be trained in conveying the benefits of enrolling their pet in a trial for a treatment that is unproven, may result in unknown side effects, and, for which in some cases, the pet may go through the treatment process without ever receiving the actual medication being tested.

The Rule of Seven, a time-tested marketing concept, says that a buyer needs to hear or see a message seven times before they buy something. Although the number is less important, the message of repetition is very important in this case. In a clinical trial, veterinarians are essentially promoting participation in a study and potential exposure to an investigational product to the pet owner based on the perceived benefits to their pet of entering into the trial. Added to that is the fact that people are different types of learners or communicators, whether it be verbal, non-verbal, written or visual. Together this means that in communicating the messaging behind the clinical trial, it is important to get that message out to the owner multiple times, while implementing a variety of communication techniques, and repeating that message to avoid miscommunication.

Compliance is key to the success of a clinical trial. And great communication between veterinary staff and pet owners is crucial to good compliance. Below is a list of some communication tools that are essential for the clinical trial "toolbox" for both the pet owner and the investigator.

PET OWNER DIRECTED

1. Written – a written overview of the trial that pet owners can review in the exam room and take home with them. This should include the aim of the trial, qualifications required of the pet, time commitment, potential complications, what the owner/dog receive if they qualify and the benefits of enrolling.
2. Visual – a more detailed description of the trial that uses visual descriptors (tables, graphs, sketches, etc.) that the investigator and his or her staff can use to help review the specifics of the trial in the exam room.
3. Website – two parts (written and visual):
   a. For pet owners who have already discussed the clinical trial with their veterinarians – providing a more complete description of the trial that pet owners can review in their homes, and with other decision makers.
   b. For pet owners directed to site for first time – these pet owners may have reached the site through social media or a handout at the clinic; this allows them to review the trial and sign up for more information or directs them to a local investigator for an initial interview.

INVESTIGATOR/STAFF DIRECTED

1. Frequently Asked Questions – this provides investigators with the framework to answer the more commonly asked questions. It may be helpful to keep a running list of questions from investigators that can be added to the FAQs.
2. Video – depicting an investigator/staff member walking a client through the discussion of the clinical trial, again providing the framework for the staff prior to discussing the trial with the owner.

While developing a really good set of communication tools for each trial can be indispensable, it is also important to understand that veterinarians and pet owners are individuals and have their own unique ways of communicating. Developing a system that provides support when needed is as important as allowing for room to individualize the methods. The benefits of a pet's participation in a clinical trial will most likely be one of the most important determining factors for an owner and can include access to treatment their pet may otherwise not receive and the ability to help advance both human and veterinary medicine and treatments for future patients. It is also important to convey to investigators the importance of not imbuing owners with any sense of false hope. Discussions with pet owners need to be up front and honest, covering both the benefits and the potential downsides of participation.

Recognition of the intertwining nature of health, disease and all the people involved makes communication more important than ever. The ultimate goal being that multiple and sometimes disparate parties can benefit by participating in research.

REFERENCES

Clutton, E., Bradbury, G., Chennells, D., Dennison, N., Duncan, J., Few, B., Flecknell, P., Golledge, H., McKeegan, D., Murphy, K., Musk, G.C., and Taylor, P. (2017). Pets in clinical trials. *Veterinary Record* 181(8):209–210. PMID:28821702; doi:10.1136/vr.j3913/

Nahama, Alexis (Senior Vice President, Corporate Development (Sorrento Therapeutics) and President, Ark Animal Health (subsidiary)) in discussion with the author (KK), September 2019.

Partners for Healthy Pets. (2018). The opportunity: Pet owners don't always hear what we think we tell them (and how to fix that) [White paper]. www.partnersforhealthypets.org/File.axd?file=PHP_TheOpportunity_WhitePaper_2018.pdf.

14 Ethical Considerations

Steven M. Niemi

CONTENTS

INTRODUCTION

Ethics is defined as "(1) the discipline dealing with what is good and bad and with moral duty and obligation; (2) a set of moral principles; a theory or system of moral values."[*] The objective of this chapter is to describe ethical dimensions concerning the use of pets in research and how those dimensions may be employed. We start with the most important ethical element in these endeavors which is the protection of pets' health and welfare. While other parties involved in the research project (e.g., the scientist, study sponsor, attending veterinarian, the pet's owner[†]) do so with foreknowledge and willingness, the prospective experimental subject possesses neither such mental state. Therefore, it is imperative that precautions be taken to avoid or minimize exposing the pet to more than momentary and mild pain, distress, and other adverse states. A good foundation for humane safeguards and optimal outcomes for pets used in research is provided by the ethical principles and practices established for laboratory animals. Beyond that, the human companion status of a pet raises additional ethical questions that should be considered before a given experiment is initiated on it[‡].

---

[*] Merriam-Webster Dictionary, www.merriam-webster.com/dictionary/ethic#note-1.

[†] "owner" will be used in referring to someone who keeps an animal in the household for companionship and is responsible for the animal's health and welfare. This is not to demean a pet's status as mere inanimate property but to be consistent with other established language (e.g., owner's consent) used by regulatory agencies and professional organizations.

[‡] One may challenge the morality of raising additional ethical elements only for pets and not for laboratory animals since both may share many advanced cognitive and proprioceptive traits even if they are not the same species. This differentiation is posited merely to reflect that a pet is acquired and maintained in expectation of a positive emotional attachment while laboratory animals are not (even though such attachments by laboratory personnel can occur later – see Sharp 2019, 123). This unique contextual status for pets has been acknowledged by at least one animal ethicist (Favre 2018, 194).

FIRST CONSIDERATION: IS THE RESEARCH WORTH DOING?

No matter how benign or trivial a given research protocol is perceived to be or described to others, pets (and their owners) may still experience substantial angst in the course of that research. If the protocol includes procedures that are invasive or expose the pet to emotional or material deprivation, all the more reason that the legitimacy of the proposed research be verified prior to pet recruitment. Questions to address include:

- What is the purpose of the research? Does it intend to identify or characterize a basic biological phenomenon or is it to test a hypothesis constructed specifically to advance human or veterinary medical knowledge?
- Is the research novel or does it replicate a previous or similar study? If the latter, is it intended to confirm an important or puzzling initial finding or is it meant, instead, to demonstrate the superiority of a competing commercial product? Or is the "research" a training exercise, instead, that is needed to gain familiarity and skills with a given technique or technology?
- Does the experimental plan include sound research principles and enough detail so similar results should be obtained if repeated by other investigators (Begley 2014, Lloyd et al. 2016)?

There are no intrinsic "good" or "bad" answers to any of the above questions. Circumstances underlying each protocol and each laboratory or clinic's personnel may guide judgements about their importance or potential value.

To whom should these questions be posed? A first pass review should be performed by the investigator's peers, i.e., other established and reputable scientists conversant in that domain of knowledge. This is to ensure that protocols not worth doing are dismissed before they begin, unless revisions are made, or new pertinent knowledge arises that changes the framework in which the questions are raised. Thus, persons who are likely most familiar with the complexities of the science behind the protocol and its procedures should weigh in sooner rather than later. Reviewers should have no conflicts of interest that could influence their deliberations or taint the results of their review, such as a change in professional standing or personal material gain based on the existence or outcome of the study, or familial or intimate relationships with the researcher. For these reasons and to avoid overly narrow scientific perspectives, much scientific peer review today is undertaken by experts who are neither employed by the institution where the protocol is to be performed nor current collaborators with the investigator proposing the study. Whether intramural or external peer review is appropriate is a decision to be reached for each project, preferably by someone besides the proposed scientist who is familiar with how research, in general, is conducted and holds a position of institutional weight.

SECOND CONSIDERATION: DO NO (UNNECESSARY) HARM

After the scientific merit of the research has been corroborated, the next questions to be addressed involve risk to the animal: (1) what is the likelihood (and degree) of harm to the pet?; (2) are there safeguards, thresholds, or endpoints included in the study design to prevent or reduce that harm?; (3) how may any remaining risks be weighed against actual or potential benefits arising from the research in question? Most established research institutions in the United States have set up ethical review policies and committees to address these and related questions (Page et al. 2016)[*]. Two such intramural bodies commonly used today are a Veterinary Clinical Studies Committee (VCSC) or something similarly named, and an Institutional Animal Care and Use Committee (IACUC). One of these committees may be required or more appropriate instead of the other, depending on regulatory stipulations reviewed in the following section on compliance. The VCSC and the IACUC may co-exist within the same institution, with clear policies dictating which committee is responsible for which kinds of pet research protocols[†]. Or the institution may rely on an IACUC alone for all situations[‡].

Regardless of which committee is engaged, its role, for the purpose of this chapter, is to review and approve research protocols and monitor adherence of those protocols to what was approved. Some questions for committees to address involve general ethics, while other questions are of a local nature regarding the institution's ability to perform the study in the safest possible manner. The first questions to be addressed are provided by the landmark publication, *The Principles of Humane Experimental Technique* (Russell and Burch 1959); three categories of alternatives to using live animals (Replacement, Reduction, Refinement, known collectively as "the Three Rs") should be satisfied to the best of the committee's judgement before an experiment on pets is approved. The questions raised under the Three Rs are: can live animals in the protocol be replaced by either an inanimate system or by a lower, non-sentient order of life?; can the number of animals proposed be reduced to the minimum quantity necessary for scientific validity?; can the protocol be refined to decrease the likely harm to each animal? Note that these principles are independent of deciding the scientific merit of the experiment per se.

Presuming that a protocol passes the Replacement and Reduction tests, then it falls to Refinement to protect the animal from unnecessary harm. If the pet is already ill or injured per the objectives of the study, is the current standard of veterinary care for that condition described in the protocol? [NB: a "standard of care" may not actually be standardized and can vary between states, institutions,

---

[*] While the United States has assigned ethical review responsibilities to local institutional oversight, other countries may provide or require different ethical review bodies and processes (Vasbinder and Locke et seq. 2016).

[†] For example, see www.research.colostate.edu/ricro/crb/ and https://vetmed.tamu.edu/research/crrc/.

[‡] For example, see www.compliance.iastate.edu/committees/iacuc and http://orrp.osu.edu/files/2016/01/IACUC-Oversight-of-Research-or-Teaching-Activities-using-Privately-Owned-Animals.pdf.

and even veterinarians (Block 2018); although the phrase may imply universality, an extensive description in the protocol may still be warranted.] Even if healthy rather than sick pets are desired, there may still be opportunities for Refinement to avoid or lessen the chances for unintended injury or mental distress. This holds especially true if those healthy pets are very old or very young, or if they have conformational traits that pose risks, such as brachycephalic animals prone to dyspnea from high ambient temperature and humidity, or animals with short or arthritic legs expected to climb high steps.

A related issue for the committee to digest is the likely benefit, if any, to the pet itself, particularly if it already is a veterinary patient with fragile health at the time of enrollment. A low likelihood of benefit may be acceptable if the patient's prognosis is otherwise poor and the risk of further harm is minimal. This balancing act can fall under compassionate use criteria because the animal has little to lose and everything to gain at this point. Another situation in which low likelihood of benefit may still be acceptable is when pets, whether healthy or debilitated, are to be used in benign research that is neither invasive nor stressful. Examples include keeping a log of their eating habits, body weights, activity levels, or behavior when provided different versions of safe foods, toys, housing, etc.

If the risk of experimental harm is higher than those scenarios above, then the committee must be thorough in balancing that risk versus the merits of the research for the individual animal and for society in general. One calculus that has become popular for this purpose is the harm–benefit analysis (HBA). Originally designed for laboratory animals, it stipulates that increasing harm should be matched with increasing benefit to justify that research (Bateson 1986). In many cases, it is easier to characterize the harm a pet is likely to experience than predict the benefit of the research study. Regardless if the animal is healthy or not, many adverse effects can be anticipated, such as drug toxicities or post-procedural pain if invasive or lengthy. And it stands to reason that the healthier or more normal the animal, the less risk of harm it should have to experience. However, while HBAs can be useful when the benefits are easy to predict, such as testing vaccine lots for safety or efficacy, they are not helpful when discovery research is involved. In such cases where the experiment aims to venture beyond current knowledge, it is difficult, if not impossible, to predict what benefits will immediately or eventually arise from new findings (Grimm et al. 2017).

This is why the owner's consent to enroll the pet in the study is critical, and all mainstream guidelines include obtaining an owner's informed consent as an ethical prerequisite*. The basic parts of the owner's consent document are well specified, as is the process of reviewing that consent with the owner before signing (Baneux et al. 2014). This includes describing the purpose of the research; the potential benefits and risks of that research to the pet; what, if any, compensation

---

* To be accurate, "consent" should be replaced with "permission" because in human subject research the former is reserved for persons able to reach and convey a decision by themselves, while the latter is used for those who can't (e.g., infants, comatose patients) and ethical convention permits an acceptable surrogate to decide on their behalf. But since "owner's consent" is standard language for pet research, it will be used here, too.

such as discounted or free veterinary care will be included; and what rights and prerogatives the owner retains throughout the study. For an example of an approved owner's consent form for a clinical research project, see University of Pennsylvania (2015). Note that none of this is to be conflated with informed consent sought from owners by practitioners before established yet potentially risky procedures are to be performed on their pets (Flemming and Scott 2004) in the absence of any research.

Even if the owner claims to be conversant in that field of research, it is important that the consent form uses language that avoids technical jargon so it is easy to understand without sacrificing accuracy. The consent form should also not gloss over possible risks, including worst outcomes no matter how remote. Yet there can still be uncertainty about how well the owner comprehends the salient points in the consent form even if consent is given. To confirm the owner understands what has been discussed and before being asked to decide, consider using a tool known as the teach-back method, in which the owner would be asked to repeat to the study representative critical details of the research. This tool was conceived by (human) healthcare professionals to confirm that the patient understands what's in his or her medical discharge plan (US Department of Health & Human Services 2017) and found to be similarly helpful for human clinical trial informed consent purposes (Kripalani et al. 2008).

One could argue that provision of free or discounted veterinary care and experimental treatment in return for consenting to enroll the pet in the study creates a potential conflict of interest for the owner. If that monetary benefit wasn't part of the study package, would the owner still agree to allow the pet to be used in the experiment? A related concern stems from payment for costs by the study sponsor being contingent on the pet completing the entire study and payments made only at the end of the study (Page et al. 2016). How may that influence an owner's decision to consent or continue to the detriment of the pet? Going a little darker, what if the owner couldn't afford veterinary care for a very ill pet and would conclude, in the absence of an offer of a treatment subsidy, that euthanasia is the most humane decision? Is this an unintended kind of ethical coercion? Will the owner feel emotionally obligated to consent in order to cover the pet's veterinary bills so that it won't have to die now (Moses 2018)? And is the animal really better off living longer in poor health?

If the owner is conflicted, who else may serve as the pet's advocate? It may seem that this is an obvious charge assigned to the committee reviewing the protocol and overseeing the study. But some committee members may employ less rather than more critical scrutiny when considering the possible or actual harmful outcomes to the pet. Researcher members may be enamored with the innate elegance of the science; veterinarian and physician members may be excited about the medical advances that could result; administrator members may be enthused about the research dollars that accompany the project, including funding for indirect costs (e.g., administrator salaries); non-exempt employee members may feel uncomfortable challenging those with professional credentials and seniority during protocol deliberations. The only category remaining is the community or non-affiliated member, a person who must have no other relationships or loyalties with that institution and isn't supposed to have prior animal research experience – a background stipulated to avoid any hint of clouded judgement. This is a mandatory IACUC seat under the federal Animal Welfare Act (AWA) and its Regulations enforced by the Department of Agriculture (USDA; US Department of Agriculture 2019a) or the US Public Health Service (PHS) Policy on Humane Care and Use of Laboratory Animals (US Public Health Service 2015), but otherwise not legally required. But its ethical importance as perhaps the only convincingly unbiased voting member should inspire institutions and their animal research review committees to make sure that such a person is included and his or her opinions sought.

What if the owner is willing but the pet is not? Let's consider the situation when pets, healthy or not, are needed only to provide blood or tissue samples. What if the animal expresses signs of fear or hostility severe enough to put itself and personnel at risk of injury when restrained for sample collection? Initial anxiety may be anticipated but what if it doesn't resolve and worsens? One presumes protocol exclusion criteria would include fractious or unmanageable behavior. But what if such behavior isn't obvious at the time of enrollment and appears only later? In either event, the pet is clearly indicating it is not consenting to such treatment even though its owner has. How can mismatches of an owner's consent and a pet being uncooperative be detected and resolved, to provide the animal and its handlers relief and also avoid compromising the quality of the research? In the laboratory animal sector, the IACUC is expected to monitor protocols for compliance after they've been approved. This exercise includes checking on animals most likely to experience harm, in addition to many other components; searching the web for "IACUC post-approval monitoring (PAM)" will yield an abundance of institutional auditing principles and processes from across the country. When pets are involved, the local oversight committee needs to be sensitive to the possibility that pets may not participate in that research (as evidenced by their behavior) to the degree permitted by their owner's consent and expected by the study investigators. Performing post-approval monitoring and maintaining open communication with research staff, institutional veterinarians, veterinary technical and animal husbandry staff, and even the owners can help avoid such problems and remove pets from studies for which they are not cooperating sooner rather than later.

Other components of the Do No Harm dictum for the committee to verify involve institutional competence. Can the institution and its personnel provide an appropriate standard of veterinary care to all pets in the study regardless of which treatment group they may be assigned? Are the research facilities and equipment in good and safe working order, including on-site temporary holding or extended housing accommodations and veterinary support for every animal on the protocol? Are inventories of routine and emergency drugs and supplies in enough quantity, properly stored and handled, and unexpired? Are research and veterinary personnel proficient in requisite skills and knowledge about all aspects of the protocol? If the IACUC is the oversight body, it is required to inspect or evaluate these and other parameters at least every 6 months, under either the AWA or PHS Policy. A sample checklist offered by the National Institutes of Health Office of Laboratory Animal Welfare (OLAW) provides a good starting point (NIH Office of Laboratory Animal Welfare 2018). In addition, potential or actual conflicts of interest (see above) for research personnel and the referring veterinarian (if applicable) should be documented and then avoided or managed to the best extent possible.

THIRD CONSIDERATION: FOLLOW THE RULES

Research involving live animals in the United States is regulated by various federal agencies, as determined by the species involved, who owns the animal, the purpose of the research, and the funding source. Thus, regulatory oversight and determination of compliance may fall under more than one authority or none. State and municipal laws and regulations may apply and possibly complicate the matter further. Therefore, it is recommended that the institution in which the research is to be performed consult with pertinent oversight bodies to avoid confusion and non-compliance. Some of the possibilities in the United States will be reviewed separately below[*].

Let's start with the most straightforward scenario: if the research is funded by PHS or other US government agencies, regardless of whether the animal is individually owned (i.e., a pet) or institutionally owned (e.g., a lab animal or shelter rescue), then OLAW's requirements for IACUC approval and oversight apply in full and irrespective of any ancillary involvement by an institution's VCSC (NIH Office of Laboratory Animal Welfare 2020). OLAW's requirements were introduced in the aforementioned PHS Policy (2015) that provides further links to various directives. Those unfamiliar with these directives are encouraged to contact OLAW for guidance. Note that PHS Policy does not encompass the use of invertebrates or dead vertebrates and their tissues even if the research is federally funded.

If a federal agency is not paying for the research, then other requirements may come into play. The AWA, like the PHS Policy, makes no distinction between privately and institutionally owned animals used in research, but it does cover dead animals if they are a species covered by the AWA[†]. In most cases, the AWA does

---

[*] It may appear odd to rank as an ethical imperative regulatory compliance slightly lower than protecting the pet since one could reasonably expect that by complying with regulations, the pet is protected. But as we shall see, there exist ambiguities or gaps in regulating pet research in the United States that may skirt legal oversight. Hence, the above section on avoiding or minimizing unnecessary harm preceded this one.

[†] The AWA defines "animal" as "any live or dead dog, cat, monkey (nonhuman primate mammal), guinea pig, hamster, rabbit, or such other warm blooded animal, as the Secretary may determine is being used, or is intended for use, for research, testing, experimentation, or exhibition purposes, or as a pet; but such term excludes (1) birds, rats of the genus Rattus, and mice of the genus Mus, bred for use in research, (2) horses not used for research purposes, and (3) other farm animals, such as but not limited to livestock or poultry, used or intended for use as food or fiber, or livestock or poultry used or intended for use for improving animal nutrition, breeding, management, or production efficiency, or for improving the quality of food or fiber. With respect to a dog, the term means all dogs including those used for hunting, security, or breeding purposes" (7 US Code, Section 2132(g), www.aphis.usda.gov/animal_welfare/downloads/bluebook-ac-awa.pdf).

apply to covered pets used in research when those animals are *not* under the clinical care of a veterinarian (commonly designated as a veterinarian–client–patient relationship or VCPR)*, or when the pet is to be subjected to procedures, invasive or not, that fall outside a VCPR (such as evaluation of a new surgical technique or drug). Quoting from a widely used compliance reference vetted by USDA and OLAW,

> The determining factor as to whether or not [the AWA is] applicable is whether the veterinary engagement with the animal is in response to the requirements for research or in the usual care of the patient.... If the treatment plans and monitoring elected by the client-owners are not influenced by the study, then the research use [of the pet] would be incidental and may not fall under the [AWA].
>
> (Huerkamp et al. 2014, 286–287)

Consequently, a USDA veterinarian inspecting veterinary schools, where research on pets is most likely to occur, is instructed that

> For protocols involving regulated animals [covered species] used in regulated teaching [and research] activities, protocol and IACUC oversight requirements [AWA applicability] are the same as for any other research facility. For animals that are not regulated by the AWA (i.e., pets or patients) no protocols or IACUC [and AWA] oversight is required.
>
> **(US Department of Agriculture 2019b)**

The equivocal "may" and "most" are used above rather than the definitive "must" and "all," respectively, because published opinions and guidance sometimes rely on dissecting actual or hypothetical situations to pin down where the AWA applies or to highlight dissimilar interpretations. For example, Kendall et al. (2018) present scenarios involving pets, VCPRs, and research protocols in various combinations, accompanied by opinions from academicians and one regulator as to whether IACUC (and USDA) oversight is required or not. The opinions following one scenario in particular are enlightening in this regard:

> **Proposed study**—A clinician wants to collect blood samples from healthy dogs to serve as control samples for a study evaluating potential biomarkers in dogs with heart disease. The blood samples would be in addition to any blood samples collected for routine veterinary care but would be collected at the same time blood samples were collected for routine diagnostic testing.
>
> **Academicians' interpretation**—The consensus was that the use of animals would require IACUC oversight. There would be no medical need for the additional blood to be collected and doing so would not serve any diagnostic or therapeutic purpose.

---

* Veterinarian–Client–Patient Relationship (VCPR) FAQ (www.avma.org/resources-tools/pet-o wners/petcare/veterinarian-client-patient-relationship-vcpr-faq).

USDA interpretation—Evaluation of USDA guidelines could offer an alternative interpretation. If the owners were present during blood sample collection, the owners provided their consent for collection of additional blood without their being present, or collection of additional blood was not considered an invasive or high-risk procedure with no actual or potential medical benefit[*], then the activity would not be regulated, regardless of whether the samples were collected at the same time as blood samples were collected for routine diagnostic testing or as a separate procedure. Nevertheless, having informed consent is recommended for minimally invasive procedures such as blood sample collection that are not of clear or certain benefit to the animal, as is having the owner present for the procedure, if feasible. This ensures that owners have real-time information on the welfare of their animals and can make informed decisions regarding their welfare.

The American Veterinary Medical Association (AVMA) advises that "When the VCSC determines that the protocol of a clinical research study will influence the management of the animal patient the VCSC shall refer the proposed work for IACUC review" (American Veterinary Medical Association 2015). In other words, if the pet may be denied the current standard of care for its illness or injury or if that care must be altered in any way for scientific necessity, then the institution's VCSC will hand over protocol review and oversight to its IACUC for that research project. In order to ensure seamless coordination between the two committees, the AVMA further recommends that the "VCSC should be composed of veterinarians primarily involved in clinical practice, should work closely with the IACUC, and have at least one member who is a member of the IACUC to serve as a conduit between the two entities."

Despite the above delineations, it still may not always be obvious which type of committee should take the lead and what protocol details are needed for that committee to render a decision. Lack of consistent guidance or precedent makes it imperative that clear and open communication be maintained by the institution's research oversight infrastructure, its scientists, and external regulators. Failure to do so can be frustrating and even contentious (Silverman et seq. 2018).

Finally, if the objectives of the research project include submitting the results to a regulatory review agency for eventual market approval of a new veterinary drug or biologic, then additional requirements must be followed. In the United States, these requirements are promulgated and enforced by the Food and Drug Administration Center for Veterinary Medicine (CVM) for drugs and the USDA Center for Veterinary Biologics (CVB) for products composed of or derived from biological substances (e.g., vaccines, antisera, toxoids) rather than synthetic chemicals. CVM's current Good Clinical Practice document is available as Guidance for Industry #85 (US Food and Drug Administration 2011). CVB's corresponding

---

[*] Reference cited here in the original paper: "Animal Care, USDA APHIS. Animal welfare inspection guide. Section 7–52: special circumstances that may require registration."

directives begin under Title 9 ("Animals and Animal Products") of the Code of Federal Regulations (US Code of Federal Regulations 2019) and Veterinary Services Memorandum No. 800.50 (US Department of Agriculture 2018). There is a myriad of related regulations, recommendations, and subtleties expected with each new product submission and review process that is beyond the scope of this chapter; these are mentioned solely to inform the reader as to their existence and importance, if applicable.

OTHER CONSIDERATIONS (MORE TRANSPARENCY IS BETTER)

Let's consider other pet research situations that may benefit from ethical judgements. First, what if the research project needs tissues from pre-deceased pets? Independent of AWA compliance, is permission required in advance from the pet's owner? Should the owner even be informed? If the owner is known and the death of the pet is recent, then it's reasonable and respectful to ask the owner for permission to obtain the desired samples and be told the purpose of the research. An efficient approach is to have a standard document to this effect available to review with the owner and ask for his or her signature to document that permission was given.

Second, what about sharing research data and outcomes with the owner? If the study is properly blinded so neither the person administering the test materials nor the person collecting the resultant data knows which variation was given to which pet, no one will know the results and their significance until the study is concluded. At that time, it seems reasonable to tell the owner in which arm of the study his or her pet was enrolled and what the overall results mean, as another way of thanking the owner for the use of their pet in the research (Nature 2018). Even if the study design precludes proper blinding so it's obvious to which treatment group the pet belongs, results should not be shared or explained until after all experimental results are analyzed. That's because initially promising or discouraging results may be premature or eventually meaningless, and the owner should not be subjected to possible hope or despair until all the data are collected and examined. This is especially pertinent if the owner is involved in data collection, such as documenting the pet's behavior at home while it's on study; early data and outcome sharing may skew the owner's observations and annul that pet's contribution to the study or the study entirely. But if the research shows convincing efficacy or serious side effects for enough animals and earlier than expected, there should be endpoint thresholds in the study design that permit breaking the blinded treatment codes sooner and sharing the good or bad news with all owners promptly (and terminating inferior or dangerous treatments at the same time). All these stipulations should be covered in the owner's consent or the research protocol, with a copy of the latter document provided to the owner who consents to maintain it as confidential.

Another unanticipated finding is the discovery of a hitherto occult lesion or other clinical abnormality, unrelated to the research, while either evaluating the pet for study inclusion or during its conduct. The owner should be informed immediately of this finding and its implications for the pet's health, regardless of the consequences for the research, and advised to consult with the pet's regular veterinarian. Then, depending on the exclusion criteria, the pet may not be eligible for enrollment or to continue on the study. Or the pet could be withdrawn from consideration or continued participation by the owner, based on the advice of the pet's regular veterinarian. These contingencies should be covered in the owner's consent document. However, things can get muddled if the abnormality is theoretical rather than actual, such as when genotyping the pet indicates possible future risk of (any) disease unrelated to the research. The question of sharing such findings is undergoing heated ethical debate about human patients in clinical trials or population studies (Castellanos et al. 2020) and has been raised for pet genetic testing (Moses et al. 2018), with no consensus established for either case yet. Alternatively, what if the pet develops an illness after the study ends that the owner or someone else concludes was caused by the research itself? That could invite significant liabilities for the investigator, the research institution, and the study sponsor. A waiver of owner's claims to compensation for damages possibly arising from unintended consequences may be wise to include in the consent document to avoid such problems.

Other information that may deserve divulging to the owner pertains to the institution's compliance and accreditation status. If the record is clean, providing those accolades to the owner may relieve concerns about the quality of the research to be performed. On the other hand, should the owner be informed prior to study start about any recent compliance lapses or ongoing investigations, in order to avoid later embarrassment and circulation via social media and certainly if that information may already be available as a public record and not difficult to find? Or does this present an opportunity to explain the facts and reassure the owner that any prior citations have been resolved, and avoid false rumors being widely circulated if discovered by the owner after the fact? Or is there an ethical obligation to disclose any of this?

Third, what if the research yields something of tangible (i.e., profitable) value? For instance, what if the study findings are the basis for a lucrative patent or commercial revenues? Should the pet's owner have a claim to those outcomes since the research relied, in part, on the owner consenting to the pet's participation? Or should the sponsor funding the research or the startup company arising from those findings have exclusive and unfettered economic rights to the data? Separately, what if the results indicate a genetic predisposition to a disease or drug toxicity for that pet but the owner still wants to breed it to sell the offspring for a profit – who is accountable for the confidentiality of those results since they resulted from a research project rather than routine screening? These and other potential questions involving commerce should be anticipated and resolved prior to study initiation, often via appropriate language added to the owner's consent document. Applicable clauses could: (1) waive the owner's claim to any intellectual property resulting from the study, and (2) agree not to propagate offspring from the pet in case an inherited malady is discovered, if that is the stance of the institution.

CONCLUSION

As made evident in earlier chapters, the use of pets in both basic (discovery) and applied (clinical) research offers advantages that complement and may supersede more traditional research relying on laboratory animals. Because of the emotional attachment between pets and their human companions, along with the liberties and obligations accompanying legal ownership, research involving pets comes with other and sometimes unique ethical considerations beyond conventional protections and allowances for laboratory animals. It is incumbent on the pet's owner, the scientist performing the research, and the institution hosting that research to ensure the pet is protected to the maximum degree possible in the pursuit of knowledge. This chapter has raised various ethical questions for all parties to contemplate but not as many answers. The field of pet research ethics will continue to evolve, in step with how our relationship to non-human animal research subjects is perceived (Walker and Fisher 2018) as well as how human clinical trial ethics is being affected by new inputs (Grady et al. 2017). Consequently, more input to this discipline is essential and welcomed.

ACKNOWLEDGEMENTS

The author is grateful for suggestions and critiques kindly provided by Lon Kendall, Lisa Moses, and Lori Palley.

REFERENCES

American Veterinary Medical Association. (2015). Establishment and use of veterinary clinical studies committees. www.avma.org/policies/establishment-and-use-veterinary-clinical-studies-committees.

Baneux PJR, Martin ME, Allen MJ, Hallman TH (2014). Issues related to institutional animal care and use committees and clinical trials using privately owned animals. *Inst Lab Anim Res J* 55(1): 200–209.

Bateson P (1986). When to experiment on animals. *New Scientist* 109(1496): 30–32.

Begley CG (2014). Six red flags for suspect work. *Nature* 497(7450): 433–434.

Block G (2018). A new look at standard of care. *J Amer Vet Med Assoc* 252(11): 1343–1344.

Castellanos A, Phimister EG, Stefánsson K, Clayton EW (2020). Disclosure of genetic risk revealed in a research study. *N Engl J Med* 382(8): 763–765.

Favre DS (2018). *Respecting Animals: A Balanced Approach to Our Relationship with Pets, Food, and Wildlife.* Amherst, NY: Prometheus Books.

Flemming DD, Scott JF (2004). The informed consent doctrine: What veterinarians should tell their clients. *J Amer Vet Med Assoc* 224(9): 1436–1439.

Grady C, Cummings SR, Rowbotham MC, McConnell MV, Ashley EA, Kang G (2017). Informed consent. In The changing face of clinical trials, JM Drazen, DP Harrington, JJV McMurray, JH Ware, J Woodcock, eds. *New Engl J Med* 376(9): 856–867.

Grimm H, Eggel M, Depazes-Zemp A, Biller-Andorno N (2017). The road to hell is paved with good intentions: Why harm–benefit analysis and its emphasis on practical benefit jeopardizes the credibility of research. *Animals* 7(9): 70–75.

Huerkamp MJ, Iten L, Archer DR (2014). Animal acquisition and disposition. In: *IACUC Handbook, 3rd Edition*, JA Silverman, MA Suckow, S Murthy, eds. Boca Raton, FL: CRC Press.

Kendall LV, Petervary N, Bergdall VK, Page RL, Baneux PJR (2018). Institutional Animal Care and Use Committee review of clinical studies. *J Amer Vet Med Assoc* 253(8): 980–984.

Kripalani S, Bengtzen R, Henderson LE, Jacobson TA (2008). Clinical research in low-literacy populations: Using teach-back to assess comprehension of informed consent and privacy information. *IRB Eth Hum Res* 30(2): 13–19.

Lloyd KCK, Niemi SM, Beaver BV, Berridge BRM, Chamberlain PL, Clarke CL, Landi MS, Macleod M, Martinson BC, Silk SB, Anestidou L (2016). ACLAM position statement on reproducibility. *J Amer Assoc Lab Anim Sci* 55(6): 824–825.

Moses L (2018). "Expanding laboratory animal laws to other animal owners: The ethical implications of using pets as research subjects"; a presentation for the workshop, future directions for laboratory animal law in the United States. www.slideshare. net/petrieflom/lisa-moses-expanding-laboratory-animal-laws-to-other-animal-owners; https://vimeo.com/253823511.

Moses L, Niemi S, Karlsson E (2018). Pet genomics medicine runs wild. *Nature* 559(7715): 470–472.

Nature Editorial. (2018). Mutual benefit. Researchers should do much more to involve those who take part in clinical trials. *Nature* 563(7731): 294–295.

NIH Office of Laboratory Animal Welfare. (2018). Semiannual program review and facility inspection checklist. https://olaw.nih.gov/resources/documents/cheklist.htm.

NIH Office of Laboratory Animal Welfare. (2020). Frequently Asked Question A.7. ("Does the IACUC need to approve research studies that use privately owned animals, such as pets?"; https://olaw.nih.gov/guidance/faqs#527) and Frequently Asked Question A.8. ("How can the IACUC determine if activities involving privately owned animals constitute veterinary clinical care or research activities?" https:// olaw.nih.gov/guidance/faqs#528).

Page R, Baneux P, Vail D, Duda L, Olson P, Anestidou L, Dybdal N, Golab G, Shelton W, Salgaller M, Hardy C (2016). Conduct, oversight, and ethical considerations of clinical trials in companion animals with cancer: Report of a workshop on best practice recommendations. *J Vet Intern Med* 30(2): 527–535.

Russell WMS, Burch RL (1959). *The Principles of Humane Experimental Technique.* Charles C. Thomas, Publisher. http://altweb.jhsph.edu/pubs/books/humane_exp/ het-toc.

Sharp LA (2019). *Animal Ethos: The Morality of Human-Animal Encounters in Experimental Lab Science.* Oakland, CA: University of California Press.

Silverman J (2018). Protocols for pets: What authority does an IACUC have?; Braden G and Esmail M. Details necessary for IACUC assessment?; Greer B and Danridge L. Oversight depends on how 'eligibility' is defined; Hallman T, Fusco K, DeAngelis R. IACUC overreach, no bones about it; Brown P. A word from OLAW; Nesline CP and Weston E. Complete details for a complete review. *Lab Anim* 47(5): 113–116.

University of Pennsylvania. (2015). Matthew J. Ryan Veterinary Hospital, University of Pennsylvania, owner informed consent form. www.vet.upenn.edu/docs/default -source/ryan/shelter-canine-mammary-tumor-program/desmopressin-study-inform ed-consent.pdf?sfvrsn=2.

US Code of Federal Regulations. (2019) Title 9 - Animals and animal products, chapter I - Animal and plant health inspection service, department of agriculture, Subchapter E.VIRUSES, SERUMS, TOXINS, AND ANALOGOUS PRODUCTS;

ORGANISMS and VECTORS, Parts 101 to 124, as of January 1, 2019. www.aphis. usda.gov/aphis/ourfocus/animalhealth/veterinary-biologics/biologics-regulations-and-guidance/ct_vb_cfr.

US Department of Agriculture. (2018). Veterinary services memorandum no. 800.50. Basic license requirements and guidelines for submitting materials in support of licensure. www.aphis.usda.gov/animal_health/vet_biologics/publications/memo_800_50.pdf.

US Department of Agriculture. (2019a). Animal welfare act and animal welfare regulations. APHIS 41-35-076. www.aphis.usda.gov/animal_welfare/downloads/bluebook-ac-awa.pdf.

US Department of Agriculture. (2019b). *Animal Welfare Inspection Guide*, Section 7.5 Guidance for Veterinary Schools and Veterinary Technician Programs (VTP) for the Inspector. www.aphis.usda.gov/animal_welfare/downloads/Animal-Care-Inspection-Guide.pdf.

US Department of Health & Human Services. (2017). Teach-back: Intervention. Rockville, MD: Agency for Healthcare Research and Quality. www.ahrq.gov/patient-safety/reports/engage/interventions/teachback.html.

US Food and Drug Administration. (2011). CVM GFI #85 (VICH GL9) good clinical practice. www.fda.gov/media/70333/download.

US Public Health Service. (2015). *Public Health Service Policy on Humane Care and Use of Laboratory Animals*. https://olaw.nih.gov/policies-laws/phs-policy.htm.

Vasbinder MA, Locke P (2016). Introduction: Global laws, regulations, and standards for animals in research. *Inst LAB Anim Res* 57(3): 261–265.

Walker RL, Fisher JA (2018). Companion animal studies: Slipping through a research oversight gap. *Amer J Bioeth* 18(10): 62–63.

Appendix A: Funding for Veterinary Clinical Research

Rebecca A. Krimins

Undoubtedly, one of the most difficult steps in performing a clinical trial is having source(s) for funding. Without appropriate funding it is extremely difficult to perform research. Collecting data and performing research takes time, money, and resources. There is no secret recipe for how to gain funding other than to keep trying. Also, be aware that there may be research funding for a specific topic/subject as well as funding to train investigators on a specific topic/subject. Following is a brief overview of common mechanisms used to gain funding for clinical research (Agencies accessed as of March 2020).

PUBLIC FUNDING, GOVERNMENTAL AGENCIES, AND US STATE FUNDING

Public funding from the government (i.e. National Institutes of Health) is responsible for a large percentage of research funding. In 2008, funding for biomedical research from NIH was equal to approximately $27.9 billion (Dorsey et al. 2010). Public funding sources include the National Science Foundation, United States Department of Agriculture, Department of Defense, the Food and Drug Administration, Defense Threat Reduction Agency, National Academies of Sciences, Engineering, and Medicine, National Cancer Institute, and US National Library of Medicine, amongst numerous additional organizations. The NIH offers a T35 Short-Term Institutional Research Training Grant for students in health professional schools as well as T32 Institutional National Research Service Awards that enable institutions to recruit individuals for predoctoral and postdoctoral research training (a PhD is not required). There are also thousands of awards available at local geographic areas and US state levels. For example, the US Small Business Administration (www.sba.gov/funding-programs/grants) offers grants to small businesses performing research.

PRIVATE BUSINESS AND NOT-FOR-PROFIT FUNDING AGENCIES

Private and not-for-profit funding sources includes charities, foundations, research organizations, and more.

	Accessed March 9th, 2020
Alex's Lemonade Stand	www.alexslemonade.org/
Alfred P. Sloan Foundation	https://sloan.org/

(Continued)

ALS Foundation	www.alsa.org/
American Academy of Veterinary Nutrition	www.aavn.org/about/
American Animal Hospital Association Foundation	www.aaha.org
American Association of Feline Practitioners	https://catvets.com
American Cancer Society	www.cancer.org
American College of Veterinary Dentistry	https://avdc.org
American College of Veterinary Emergency and Critical Care	www.acvecc.org
American College of Veterinary Internal Medicine Foundation	www.acvim.org
American College of Veterinary Ophthalmologists	www.acvo.org
American College of Veterinary Radiology	https://acvr.org
American College of Veterinary Surgeons	www.acvs.org
American Diabetes Association	www.diabetes.org
American Heart Association	www.heart.org
American Holistic Veterinary Medical Foundation	www.ahvmf.org
American Lung Association	www.lung.org
American Kennel Club Canine Health Foundation	www.akcchf.org
American Veterinary Medical Foundation	https://avmf.org
Anicura Research Fund	www.anicuragroup.com
Animal Cancer Foundation	https://acfoundation.org
AO Vet Foundation	https://aovet.aofoundation.org
ASPCA Grants	www.aspca.org/about-us/aspca-grants
The Aspen Institute	www.aspeninstitute.org
Arthritis Foundation	https://arthritis.org
Bill and Melinda Gates Foundation	www.gatesfoundation.org
Brain and Behavior Research Foundation	www.bbrfoundation.org
Burroughs Wellcome Fund	www.bwfund.org
Canines-N-Kids	https://caninesnkids.org
Cavalier Health Foundation	http://cavalierhealthfoundation.org
Comparative Gastroenterology Society	https://vetmed.tamu.edu/cgs/
The Consortium of Universities for Global Health	www.cugh.org
Collie Health Foundation	www.colliehealth.org
The Council on International Veterinary Medical Education	www.aavmc.org/additional-pages/civme.aspx
CSA BioTech	www.csabiotech.com
Cystic Fibrosis Foundation	www.cff.org
The Dana Foundation	www.dana.org
Diabetes Research and Wellness Foundation	www.diabeteswellness.net
Foundation for Veterinary Dentistry	www.veterinarydentistry.org
Frankie's Friends, Inc.	www.frankiesfriends.org
Global Probiotics Council	https://probioticsresearch.com/global-probiotics-council/
Golden Retriever Foundation	www.goldenretrieverfoundation.org

(Continued)

Gray Lady Foundation, Inc.	www.grayladyfoundation.org
Henry Frank Guggenheim Foundation	www.hfg.org
Hirshberg Foundation for Pancreatic Cancer Research	http://pancreatic.org
Human Animal Bond Research Institute	https://habri.org
International Feline Foundation	http://tiffresearch.org
International Sled Dog Veterinary Medical Association	https://isdvma.org
Leap Venture Studio	www.leapventurestudio.com/about/
Maddie's Shelter Medicine Research Grant	www.maddiesfund.org/colleges-of-veterinary-medicine.htm
Markle Foundation	www.markle.org
Melanoma Research Foundation	https://melanoma.org
Merck Animal Health	www.merck-animal-health-usa.com
Michelson Prize & Grants	www.michelsonprizeandgrants.org
Million Dollar Round Table Foundation	www.mdrt.org/about-mdrt/foundation/
Minnesota Ovarian Cancer Alliance	https://mnovarian.org
Morris Animal Foundation	www.morrisanimalfoundation.org
Muscular Dystrophy Association	www.mda.org
Nestle Purina Company	www.purina.com/our-giving-programs
National Association of Animal Breeders	www.naab-css.org
National Institutes of Health	https://grants.nih.gov/grants/oer.htm
National Pancreas Foundation	https://pancreasfoundation.org
Ohio Animal Health Foundation	https://oahf.org
Orthopedic Foundation for Animals	www.ofa.org
The Patterson Foundation	www.thepattersonfoundation.org
The Pet Care Trust	www.petsintheclassroom.org/about/
PETCO Foundation	www.petcofoundation.org/
PetSmart Charities	https://petsmartcharities.org
Pharmaceutical Research and Manufacturers of America Foundation, Inc.	www.asbmr.org/grants/
PKD Foundation	https://pkdcure.org
Poodle Club of America Foundation	https://poodleclubofamericafoundation.org
Portuguese Water Dog Alliance	www.pwdfoundation.org
Radiological Society of North America	www.rsna.org
Robert Wood Johnson Foundation	www.rwjf.org
Sandler Family Supporting Foundation	www.sandlerfoundation.org
The V Foundation for Cancer Research	www.v.org/2018/the-v-foundation-announces-canine-comparative-oncology-grant-program/
Veterinary Cancer Society	http://vetcancersociety.org
Veterinary Comparative Respiratory Society	http://the-vcrs.org
Veterinary Emergency Treatment Fund	https://vet-fund.org

(Continued)

Veterinary Orthopedic Society	www.vosdvm.org
Whitaker Foundation	www.whitaker.org
Winn Feline Foundation	www.winnfelinefoundation.org
Zoetis, Inc.	www.zoetis.commar

Abbreviated list of US funding sources for veterinary biomedical research including public and private businesses, for-profit and not-for-profit organizations. Note
that this list is not all-encompassing. Organizations are created and dissolve, mission changes occur, funding mechanisms change over time; it is important to
check updated resources.

INDUSTRY FUNDING

Industry funding can be a wonderful mechanism by which veterinary clinical
trials are supported. Industry support may come directly from pharmaceutical
companies, biotechnology companies, medical device companies, health IT and
start-up companies. This type of funding may also be accessed through relationships with contract research organizations.

INTERNAL FUNDING FROM COLLEGES AND UNIVERSITIES

Colleges and universities regularly have internal mechanisms for funding. As
research evolves and medicine advances, so do the mechanisms from where funding is sourced. An evaluation of internal research funding mechanisms at the
Louisiana State University School of Veterinary Medicine in 2012, found that
to improve the effectiveness of their internal research funding program investment, there appeared to be a greater return on investment for projects funded with
smaller awards (approximately $10,000) compared to projects funded with larger
awards (approximately $52,000) (Baker and Kearney 2012). Many universities
offer seed grant funding (pilot funding), Hatch funding/awards, and more. Pivot
is a web-based discovery and workflow tool used by many universities that allows
funding organizations to increase their discoverability (https://pivot.proquest.
com/).

CROWDSOURCING TECHNOLOGY

One of the newer sources of funding for biomedical research comes from crowd-
sourcing technology and other social media platforms such as GoFundMe (https://
charity.gofundme.com). Additional sources include experiment.com (https://
experiment.com), Consano (https://consano.org), MedStartr (www.medstartr.
com), and Kickstarter (www.kickstarter.com).

PHILANTHROPY

Philanthropic resources are an important source of funding for veterinary clinical trials. Pet owners (both past, present, and future) can be an ideal source for philanthropic funds to collect pilot data.

REFERENCES

Baker, D. G., and M. T. Kearney. 2012. "Evaluation of an internal research funding program in a school of veterinary medicine." *J Vet Med Educ* 39(1):39–45. doi:10.3138/jvme.0311.039R.

Dorsey, E. R., J. de Roulet, J. P. Thompson, J. I. Reminick, A. Thai, Z. White-Stellato, C. A. Beck, B. P. George, and H. Moses, 3rd. 2010. "Funding of US biomedical research, 2003–2008." *JAMA* 303(2):137–143. doi:10.1001/jama.2009.1987.

Appendix B: Resources for Veterinary Clinical Research

Name	Website
Administrative Applications and the Phased Review Process – Guidance for Industry #132	www.fda.gov/media/70029/download
American Kennel Club Canine Health Foundation	https://akcchf.org
American Veterinary Medical Association Animal Health Studies Database	https://ebusiness.avma.org/aahsd/study_search.aspx
Animal Clinical Investigation, LLC	www.animalci.com
Animal Drugs at FDA	https://animaldrugsatfda.fda.gov/adafda/views/#/search
Animal Drug User Fee Act	www.fda.gov/industry/fda-user-fee-programs/animal-drug-user-fee-act-adufa
Animal Generic Drug User Fee Act	www.fda.gov/industry/fda-user-fee-programs/animal-generic-drug-user-fee-act-agdufa
Animal Health Institute	https://ahi.org
Anivive Clinical Trials Database	www.anitrial.com
APHIS Agreement # 04-9100-0859-MU FDA Serial # 225-05-7000	www.aphis.usda.gov/animal_health/vet_biologics/publications/APHIS_FDA_biologics_MOU.pdf
Association for Clinical and Translational Science	www.actscience.org
Banfield Pet Hospital Dog and Cat Breeds	www.banfield.com/pet-healthcare/additional-resources/breed-information
Banfield Pet Hospital State of Pet Health Report	www.banfield.com/state-of-pet-health
Bioequivalence: Blood Level Bioequivalence Study – Guidance for Industry #224	www.fda.gov/media/89840/download
Bioequivalence Guidance – Guidance for Industry #35	www.fda.gov/media/70115/download
Bionano Genomics	https://bionanogenomics.com
Canine Comparative and Oncology and Genomics Consortium	https://ccogc.net/biospecimen-repository-procedures/
Cell Based Products for Animal Use – Guidance for Industry #218	www.fda.gov/media/88925/download
CVM Policies and Procedures Manual	www.fda.gov/animal-veterinary/guidance-regulations/policies-procedures-manual
Clinical Research Resources	www.nih.gov/research-training/clinical-research-resources

(Continued)

Name	Website
Clinical and Translational Science Award One Health Alliance – Clinical Trials	www.ctsaonehealthalliance.org/resources/resea rch/clinical-trials
Code of Federal Regulations Title 21	www.accessdata.fda.gov/scripts/cdrh/cfdocs/cf cfr/CFRSearch.cfm?CFRPart=516
The Comparative Gastroenterology Society	https://vetmed.tamu.edu/cgs/about/
Comparative Nutrition Society	www.cnsweb.org
Comparative Oncology Program	https://ccr.cancer.gov/comparative-oncology-p rogram
Comparative Oncology Trials Consortium	https://ccr.cancer.gov/comparative-oncology-p rogram/consortium
Conservation Through Public Health	https://ctph.org
Consortium for Canine Comparative Oncology – Duke Cancer Institute & North Carolina State University College of Veterinary Medicine	www.c3oncology.org
Convention on Biological Diversity	www.cbd.int
Cornell University College of Veterinary Medicine Biobank	www.vet.cornell.edu/departments/centers/corne ll-veterinary-biobank/about-biobank
Darwin's Ark	https://darwinsark.org/about-us/
Department of Comparative Medicine – Stanford University	http://med.stanford.edu/compmed.html
Department of Molecular and Comparative Pathobiology – Johns Hopkins University	https://mcp.bs.jhmi.edu/home
Dog Aging Project	https://dogagingproject.org
Dog Genome Project – Broad Institute	www.broadinstitute.org/scientific-community/s cience/projects/mammals-models/dog/dog-g enome-links
Dog (Mixed Breed) Tissue Samples	www.kerafast.com/productgroup/535/dog-mi xed-breed-tissue-samples
DNA Zoo	www.dnazoo.org
EcoHealth Alliance	www.ecohealthalliance.org
Earth Biogenome Project	www.earthbiogenome.org
Electronic Code of Federal Regulations	www.ecfr.gov/cgi-bin/ECFR?page=browse
Eligibility Criteria for Expanded Conditional Approval of New Animal Drugs – Guidance for Industry #261	www.fda.gov/media/130706/download
Embark Veterinary	https://embarkvet.com
Ethos Discovery	www.ethosdiscovery.org/veterinary-clinical-tr ials/
The European Agency for the Evaluation of Medicinal Products	www.ema.europa.eu/en/documents/scientific-gui deline/vich-gl9-good-clinical-practices-step-7_en.pdf
Family Dog Project	https://familydogproject.elte.hu

(Continued)

Name	Website
Federal Drug Administration (FDA)-Approved Drugs	www.accessdata.fda.gov/scripts/cder/daf/index.cfm
Federal Food, Drug, and Cosmetic Act	https://legcounsel.house.gov/Comps/Feder al%20Food,%20Drug,%20And%20 Cosmetic%20Act.pdf
Food and Agricultural Organization of the United Nations	www.fao.org/faostat/en/#home
Genetic Resources Core Facility – Johns Hopkins University	https://grcf.jhmi.edu
GenomeArk – Vertebrate Genomes Project	https://vgp.github.io
Guidance for Industry (Index of FDA-CVM Documents)	www.fda.gov/animal-veterinary/guidance-regula tions/guidance-industry
Guidance for Industry M3(R2) Nonclinical Safety Studies for the Conduct of Human Clinical Trials and Marketing Authorization for Pharmaceuticals	www.fda.gov/media/71542/download
Illumina	www.illumina.com
The Intergovernmental Panel on Climate Change	www.ipcc.ch
International One Health Coalition	https://onehealthplatform.com/ohp/who-we-are/ international-one-health-coalition
International Society for Companion Animal Infectious Diseases	https://iscaid.org
The Journey of an Animal Drug through the Approval Process	www.fda.gov/animal-veterinary/animal-health-l iteracy/idea-marketplace-journey-an imal-drug-through-approval-process
London, Cheryl (Cheryl London, DVM, PhD, DACVIM (Oncology)) TED Talk	www.youtube.com/watch?v=4YooZCkyUsY
Mari Lowe Center for Comparative Oncology Research – PennVet	www.vet.upenn.edu/research/centers-initiatives/ center/mari-lowe-center-for-comparative-onc ology-research
Mouse Genome Informatics	www.informatics.jax.org
NCBI Genomes and Maps	www.ncbi.nlm.nih.gov/guide/genomes-maps/
NIH One Health: Integrating the Veterinarian-Scientist into the Biomedical Research Enterprise	https://orip.nih.gov/comparative-medicine/ini tiatives/one-health-integrating-veterina rian-scientist-biomedical-research
Office of Minor Use and Minor Species Animal Drug Development (Lions and Tigers and Bears! OMUMS!)	www.fda.gov/animal-veterinary/animal-health-l iteracy/lions-and-tigers-and-bears-omums
One Health Commission	www.onehealthcommission.org
One Health Initiative	http://onehealthinitiative.com
Online Mendelian Inheritance in Animals – The University of Sydney	https://omia.org/home/

(Continued)

Name	Website
Online Mendelian Inheritance in Man – Johns Hopkins University	https://omim.org
Oxford Nanopore Technologies	https://nanoporetech.com
Public Responsibility in Medicine and Research (holds the largest annual IACUC conference in the United States)	www.primr.org/conferences/
Rapid Autopsy – Johns Hopkins University	http://pathology.jhu.edu/RapidAutopsy/
Resources for Veterinary Research	www.ncbi.nlm.nih.gov/books/NBK22914/
Society for Comparative Endocrinology	www.veterinaryendocrinology.org
Target Animal Safety for Veterinary Pharmaceutical Products – Guidance for Industry #185	www.fda.gov/media/88925/download
Tissue Collection Bank – University of Missouri Veterinary Health Center	https://vhc.missouri.edu/small-animal-hospital/oncology/tissue-collection-bank/
A Tripartite Guide to Addressing Zoonotic Diseases in Countries	www.fao.org/3/ca2942en/ca2942en.pdf
12 Golden GCP Rules for Veterinary Studies (out of print)	www.amazon.com/Golden-GCP-Rules-Veterinary-Studies/dp/0953117480
US Department of Agriculture National Animal Health Monitoring System – Equine Studies	www.fao.org/faostat/en/#home
US Food and Drug Administration Center for Veterinary Medicine	www.fda.gov/animal-veterinary
Vermillion, Krista	www.linkedin.com/in/krista-vermillion-01ba2428/
Veterinary Clinical Research Office – Virginia-Maryland College of Veterinary Medicine	www.vetmed.vt.edu/clinical-trials/
Veterinary Clinical Trials Network – Johns Hopkins University	www.hopkinsvctn.org
Veterinary Innovation Program	www.fda.gov/animal-veterinary/animals-intentional-genomic-alterations/vip-veterinary-innovation-program
Wildlife Conservation Society	https://oneworldonehealth.wcs.org
Wisdom Panel	www.wisdompanel.com/en-us
World Organization for Animal Health	www.oie.int/for-the-media/onehealth
World Small Animal Veterinary Association – One Health Committee	https://wsava.org/committees/one-health-committee/
World Wildlife Fund	https://wwf.panda.org/knowledge_hub/all_publications/living_planet_report_2018/

A copy of this list can be found online at www.routledge.com/9780367173104. If you have a resource that you would like added to this list, please send an email to Dr. Krimins (rkrimin1@jhmi.edu) with the resource information and it will be added during an update.

Index